COLOR ATLAS & SYNOPSIS OF
CLINICAL OPHTHALMOLOGY

Wills Eye Institute

Uveitis

EDITOR

Sunir J. Garg, MD

Associate Professor of Ophthalmology
MidAtlantic Retina
The Retina Service of Wills Eye Institute
Jefferson Medical College of Thomas Jefferson University
Philadelphia, Pennsylvania

SECTION EDITORS

Bahram Bodaghi, MD, PhD
Robert Nussenblatt, MD, MPH
S. R. Rathinam, MNAMS, PhD
H. Nida Sen, MD, MHSc

SERIES EDITOR

Christopher J. Rapuano, MD

Director and Attending Surgeon, Cornea Service
Co-Director, Refractive Surgery Department
Wills Eye Institute
Professor of Ophthalmology
Jefferson Medical College of Thomas Jefferson University
Philadelphia, Pennsylvania

COLOR ATLAS & SYNOPSIS OF CLINICAL OPHTHALMOLOGY

Wills Eye Institute

Uveitis

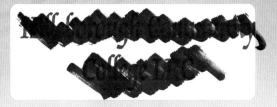

Wolters Kluwer | Lippincott Williams & Wilkins
Health

Philadelphia · Baltimore · New York · London
Buenos Aires · Hong Kong · Sydney · Tokyo

Senior Executive Editor: Jonathan W. Pine, Jr.
Senior Product Managers: Emilie Moyer and Grace Caputo
Senior Manufacturing Coordinator: Benjamin Rivera
Marketing Manager: Lisa Lawrence
Creative Director: Doug Smock
Production Services: Aptara, Inc.

Two Commerce Square
2001 Market Street
Philadelphia, PA 19103 USA
LWW.com

Printed in China

Library of Congress Cataloging-in-Publication Data
Uveitis / editor, Sunir J. Garg ; section editors, Bahram Bodaghi . . . [et al.].
   p. ; cm. – (Color atlas and synopsis of clinical ophthalmology–Wills Eye Institute)
  Includes bibliographical references and index.
  ISBN 978-1-4511-0146-1 (alk. paper)
  1. Uveitis–Handbooks, manuals, etc.   I. Garg, Sunir J.   II. Series: Color atlas and synopsis of clinical ophthalmology series.
  [DNLM: 1. Uveitis–Handbooks. WW 39]
  RE351.U87 2011
  617.7'2–dc23

             2011025132

Care has been taken to confirm the accuracy of the information presented and to describe generally accepted practices. However, the authors, editors, and publisher are not responsible for errors or omissions or for any consequences from application of the information in this book and make no warranty, expressed or implied, with respect to the currency, completeness, or accuracy of the contents of the publication. Application of the information in a particular situation remains the professional responsibility of the practitioner.

The authors, editors, and publisher have exerted every effort to ensure that drug selection and dosage set forth in this text are in accordance with current recommendations and practice at the time of publication. However, in view of ongoing research, changes in government regulations, and the constant flow of information relating to drug therapy and drug reactions, the reader is urged to check the package insert for each drug for any change in indications and dosage and for added warnings and precautions. This is particularly important when the recommended agent is a new or infrequently employed drug.

Some drugs and medical devices presented in the publication have Food and Drug Administration (FDA) clearance for limited use in restricted research settings. It is the responsibility of the health care provider to ascertain the FDA status of each drug or device planned for use in their clinical practice.

To purchase additional copies of this book, call our customer service department at (800) 638-3030 or fax orders to (301) 223-2320. International customers should call (301) 223-2300.

Visit Lippincott Williams & Wilkins on the Internet: at LWW.com. Lippincott Williams & Wilkins customer service representatives are available from 8:30 am to 6 pm, EST.

10 9 8 7 6 5 4 3 2 1

RRS1107

To my Mom, Dad, Ravin, and Chottu Mama—thank you for your love and support; and to my Stella, for brightening my day.

Editors

SERIES EDITOR

Christopher J. Rapuano, MD
Director and Attending Surgeon, Cornea Service
Co-Director, Refractive Surgery Department
Wills Eye Institute
Professor of Ophthalmology
Jefferson Medical College of Thomas Jefferson
  University
Philadelphia, Pennsylvania

EDITOR

Sunir J. Garg, MD
Associate Professor of Ophthalmology
MidAtlantic Retina
The Retina Service of Wills Eye Institute
Jefferson Medical College of Thomas Jefferson
  University
Philadelphia, Pennsylvania

SECTION EDITORS

Bahram Bodaghi, MD, PhD
Professor of Ophthalmology
University of Pierre and Marie Curie
Hôpital de la Pitié-Salpêtrière
Paris, France

Robert Nussenblatt, MD, MPH
Head, Laboratory of Immunology
National Eye Institute
National Institutes of Health
Bethesda, Maryland

S. R. Rathinam, MNAMS, PhD
Professor of Ophthalmology
Head of Uveitis Service
Aravind Eye Hospital and Post Graduate Institute
  of Ophthalmology
Madurai, Tamil Nadu, India

H. Nida Sen, MD, MHSc
Director, Uveitis and Ocular Immunology
  Fellowship Program
National Eye Institute
National Institutes of Health
Bethesda, Maryland

Contributors

Bhupesh Bagga, DOMS, FRCS
Consultant
Cornea and Anterior Segment Services
L.V. Prasad Eye Institute
Hyderabad, India

Manohar Babu Balasundaram, MS
Uvea Clinic
Aravind Eye Hospital
Coimbatore, India

Andrea D. Birnbaum, MD, PhD
Clinical Assistant Professor
Department of Ophthalmology
Feinberg School of Medicine
Northwestern University
Attending Physician
Jesse Brown VA Medical Center
Chicago, Illinois

Jyotirmay Biswas, MS, FAMS
Director, Department of Uvea and Ocular
    Pathology
Sankara Nethralaya
Chennai, India

Bahram Bodaghi, MD, PhD
Professor of Ophthalmology
University of Pierre and Marie Curie
Hôpital de la Pitié-Salpêtrière
Paris, France

Roy D. Brod, MD
Clinical Associate Professor
Department of Ophthalmology
Pennsylvania State University School of Medicine
Hershey, Pennsylvania
Attending Surgeon
Division of Ophthalmology
Lancaster General Hospital
Lancaster, Pennsylvania

Leon D. Charkoudian, MD
Fellow
Department of Ophthalmology
Emory Eye Center
Associate in Ophthalmology
Emory University Hospital
Atlanta, Georgia

Emmett T. Cunningham, Jr., MD, PhD, MPH
Adjunct Clinical Professor
Department of Ophthalmology
Stanford University School of Medicine
Stanford, California
Director, The Uveitis Service
Department of Ophthalmology
California Pacific Medical Center
San Francisco, California

Matthew A. Cunningham, MD
Resident
Department of Ophthalmology
Cullen Eye Institute
Baylor College of Medicine
Houston, Texas

Sam S. Dahr, MD
Retina Center of Oklahoma
Oklahoma City, Oklahoma

Janet L. Davis, MD
Professor
Department of Ophthalmology
Bascom Palmer Eye Institute
University of Miami Miller School of Medicine
Miami, Florida

Carlos Alexandre de Amorim Garcia, MD, PhD
Chairman
Department of Ophthalmology
Federal University of Rio Grande do Norte
Natal, Brazil

Rishi R. Doshi, MD
Resident Physician
Department of Ophthalmology
California Pacific Medical Center
San Francisco, California

Allison Dublin, MD
Resident
Department of Ophthalmology
George Washington University
Washington, DC

Lisa J. Faia, MD
Clinical Fellow
Vitreoretinal Surgery
Associated Retinal Consultants, P. C.
Royal Oak, Michigan

Harry W. Flynn, Jr., MD
Professor of Ophthalmology
Bascom Palmer Eye Institute
University of Miami Miller School of Medicine
Miami, Florida

Sunir J. Garg, MD
Associate Professor of Ophthalmology
Mid Atlantic Retina
The Retina Service of Wills Eye Institute
Jefferson Medical College of Thomas Jefferson
    University
Philadelphia, Pennsylvania

Debra A. Goldstein, MD, FRCS(C)
Professor of Ophthalmology
Director, Uveitis Service
University of Illinois Eye and Ear Infirmary
Chicago, Illinois

Chloe Gottlieb, MD, FRCSC, Dip ABO
Assistant Professor of Ophthalmology
University of Ottawa Eye Institute
Ottawa, Ontario, Canada

Julie Gueudry, MD
Department of Ophthalmology
Charles Nicolle Hospital
Paris, France

Amod Gupta, MD
Professor
Department of Ophthalmology
Advanced Eye Centre
Post Graduate Institute of Medical Education and
    Research
Chandigarh, India

Vishali Gupta, MD
Associate Professor
Department of Ophthalmology, Advanced Eye
    Centre
Post Graduate Institute of Medical Education and
    Research
Chandigarh, India

William Hodge, MD, PhD
Professor and Chair
Department of Ophthalmology
University of Western Ontario
Ophthalmologist in Chief
Department of Ophthalmology
St Joseph's Health Care Ivey Eye Institute
London, Ontario, Canada

Jason Hsu, MD
The Retina Service of Wills Eye Institute
Clinical Instructor
Thomas Jefferson University
Philadelphia, Pennsylvania

Ann O. Igbre, MD, MPH
Resident, Department of Ophthalmology
Temple University Hospital
Philadelphia, Pennsylvania

Rajeev Jain, MBBS, MS
Clinical Lecturer
Discipline of Ophthalmology and Visual Sciences
University of Adelaide
Adelaide, South Australia
Head of the Vitreoretina Services
Sharp Sight Centre
Delhi, India

Karina Julian, MD
Instructor
Department of Ophthalmology
Universidad Austral
Buenos Aires, Argentina
Assistant
Department of Ophthalmology
Hôpital de la Pitié-Salpêtrière
Paris, France

Moncef Khairallah, MD
Professor of Ophthalmology
Faculty of Medicine
University of Monastir
Chief, Department of Opthalmology
Fattouma Bourguiba University Hospital
Monastir, Tunisia

Jaclyn L. Kovach, MD
Assistant Professor of Clinical Ophthalmology
Bascom Palmer Eye Institute, Naples
University of Miami Miller School of Medicine
Miami, Florida

Nupura Krishnadev, MD, FRCSC
Clinical Fellow
Department of Epidemiology and Clinical
  Research
National Eye Institute
National Institutes of Health
Bethesda, Maryland

Shree Kurup, MD
Assistant Professor
Vitreoretinal Diseases and Surgery
Uveitis and Ocular Immunology
Wake Forest University Eye Center
Winston-Salem, North Carolina

Theresa Larson, MD
Clinical Fellow
Ocular Immunology, Uveitis, and Medical Retina
National Eye Institute
National Institutes of Health
Bethesda, Maryland

Phuc LeHoang, MD, PhD
Professor of Ophthalmology
University of Pierre and Marie Curie
Chairman, Department of Ophthalmology
Hôpital de la Pitié-Salpêtrière
Paris, France

Julie Lew, MD
Clinical Ophthalmologist
Holzer Clinic
Athens, Ohio

Parthopratim Dutta Majumder, MS
Associate Consultant
Department of Uvea and Ocular Pathology
Sankara Nethralaya
Chennai, India

Annal D. Meleth, MD, MS
Medical Retina Fellow
National Institutes of Health
Bethesda, Maryland

Somasheila I. Murthy, MS
Consultant
Cornea and Anterior Segment Service
Ocular Immunology and Uveitis Service
L.V. Prasad Eye Institute, Kallam Anji Reddy Campus
Hyderabad, India

Robert Nussenblatt, MD, MPH
Head, Laboratory of Immunology
National Eye Institute
National Institutes of Health
Bethesda, Maryland

Jason F. Okulicz, MD
Assistant Professor of Medicine
Department of Medicine
Uniformed Services University of the Health
  Sciences
Bethesda, Maryland
Staff Physician
Infectious Disease Service
Brooke Army Medical Center
Fort Sam Houston, Texas

John F. Payne, MD
Fellow in Vitreoretinal Surgery
Department of Ophthalmology
Emory University
Atlanta, Georgia

Uwe Pleyer, MD, FEBO
Professor of Ophthalmology
Department of Ophthalmology
Humboldt University
Charité
Berlin, Germany

S. Lalitha Prajna, MD
Department of Ocular Microbiology
Aravind Eye Hospital
Madurai, India

Patrick Prendergast
Medical Student
Schulich School of Medicine and Dentistry
University of Western Ontario
London, Ontario, Canada

Kim Ramasamy, DNB
Professor of Ophthalmology
Retina and Vitreous Service
Aravind Eye Hospital and Postgraduate Institute of
  Ophthalmology
Chief, Retina and Vitreous Service
Aravind Eye Hospital
Madurai, India

P. Kumar Rao, MD
Associate Professor
Department of Ophthalmology
Washington University in St. Louis
St. Louis, Missouri

S. R. Rathinam, MNAMS, PhD
Professor of Ophthalmology
Head of Uveitis Service
Aravind Eye Hospital and Post Graduate Institute
    of Ophthalmology
Madurai, Tamil Nadu, India

Swapnali Sabhapandit, MS
Clinical Associate
Cornea and Anterior Segment Service
L.V. Prasad Eye Institute, Kallam Anji Reddy
    Campus
Hyderabad, India

Virender S. Sangwan, MS
Head, Cornea and Anterior Segment Service
Ocular Immunology and Uveitis Services
Associate Director
L.V. Prasad Eye Institute, Kallam Anji Reddy
    Campus
Hyderabad, India

Nehali V. Saraiya, MD
Fellow
Department of Ophthalmology
University of Illinois Eye and Ear Infirmary
Chicago, Illinois

Anita Schadlu, MD
Department of Ophthalmology
Scottsdale Healthcare
Scottsdale, Arizona

Stephen G. Schwartz, MD, MBA
Associate Professor of Clinical Ophthalmology
Medical Director
Bascom Palmer Eye Institute at Naples
University of Miami Miller School of Medicine
Miami, Florida

**Dinesh Selva, MBBS (Hons), FRACS,
FRANZCO**
Professor
Discipline of Ophthalmology and Visual Sciences
University of Adelaide
Chairman, Department of Ophthalmology
Royal Adelaide Hospital
Adelaide, South Australia

H. Nida Sen, MD, MHSc
Director, Uveitis and Ocular Immunology
Fellowship Program
National Eye Institute
National Institutes of Health
Bethesda, Maryland

Carol L. Shields, MD
Professor of Ophthalmology
Thomas Jefferson University
Co-Director, Ocular Oncology Service
Wills Eye Institute
Philadelphia, Pennsylvania

Wendy M. Smith, MD
Clinical Fellow
Uveitis and Ocular Immunology
National Eye Institute
National Institutes of Health
Bethesda, Maryland

Sunil K. Srivastava, MD
Staff Physician
Cole Eye Institute
Cleveland Clinic Foundation
Cleveland, Ohio

Johnny Tang, MD
Assistant Professor of Ophthalmology
Department of Ophthalmology and Visual
    Sciences
Case Western Reserve University
University Hospitals Eye Institute
University Hospitals Case Medical Center
Cleveland, Ohio

Céline Terrada, MD, PhD
Fellow
Department of Ophthalmology
Paris-Est Creteil University
Clinic Eye University of Creteil
Creteil, France

Valérie Touitou, MD, PhD
Fellow
Department of in Ophthalmology
University of Pierre and Marie Curie
Hôpital de la Pitié-Salpêtrière
Paris, France

Roxana Ursea, MD
Assistant Professor of Ophthalmology
Director, Cornea and Refractive Surgery Division
Department of Ophthalmology
University of Arizona
Tucson, Arizona

Virginia M. Utz, MD
Chief Resident
University Hospitals Eye Institute
University Hospitals Case Medical Center
Cleveland, Ohio

P. Vijayalakshmi, MS, DO
Professor of Ophthalmology
Chief
Paediatric Ophthalmology and Adult Strabismus
    Department
Aravind Eye Hospital
Madurai, Tamil Nadu, India

Henry Wiley, MD
Division of Epidemiology and Clinical
    Applications
National Eye Institute
National Institutes of Health
Bethesda, Maryland

Robert W. Wong, MD
Retina Research Center, PLLC
Austin, Texas

Keith Wroblewski, MD
Chief, Ophthalmology Service
Walter Reed Army Medical Center
Washington, DC

Steven Yeh, MD
Assistant Professor of Ophthalmology
Uveitis, Vitreoretinal Diseases and Surgery
Emory Eye Center
Emory University School of Medicine
Atlanta, Georgia

Joseph R. Zelefsky, MD
Assistant Professor
Department of Ophthalmology and Visual
    Sciences
Albert Einstein College of Medicine
Director, Glaucoma Service
Department of Ophthalmology
Bronx Lebanon Hospital Center
Bronx, New York

About the Series

The beauty of the atlas/synopsis concept is the powerful combination of illustrative photographs and a summary approach to the text. Ophthalmology is a very visual discipline that lends itself nicely to clinical photographs. While the seven ophthalmic subspecialties in this series—Cornea, Retina, Glaucoma, Oculoplastics, Neuroophthalmology, Pediatrics, and Uveitis—employ varying levels of visual recognition, a relatively standard format for the text is used for all volumes.

The goal of the series is to provide an up-to-date clinical overview of the major areas of ophthalmology for students, residents, and practitioners in all the healthcare professions. The abundance of large, excellent quality photographs and concise, outline-form text will help achieve that objective.

Christopher J. Rapuano, MD
Series Editor

Preface

Even though most of the work we do at the Retina Service of Wills Eye Institute is for traditional vitreoretinal diseases, the cases that often generate the most discussion are the uveitis cases. They are engaging for a number of reasons: They are interesting to look at, the differential diagnosis often covers a wide range of disparate diseases, and they typically have a number of extraocular manifestations that serve as reminders that we are physicians who are eye specialists. However, the same things that make these diseases interesting can also make uveitis cases frustrating and challenging.

This book is intended to provide comprehensive ophthalmologists, ophthalmology residents, and retina and cornea fellows with a single-volume, easily accessible resource covering all the major aspects of ocular inflammatory disease. It will also be useful for subspecialists who are looking for an up-to-date, concise review of the field.

The first two chapters provide a basic overview of the immune response and the anatomic classification of uveitis, an understanding of which will help to narrow down a differential diagnosis. The next several chapters cover both common and the not-so-common but nonetheless important diseases that are likely to be encountered. These topics are subdivided primarily based on their main anatomic localization. The final chapter is a general overview of the treatment approach to these patients.

This volume has a few unique attributes that will hopefully make it a go-to text for the busy clinician. While all the chapters provide a comprehensive, current discussion of a particular disease and treatment, they do so concisely. We have included a large number of high-quality images assembled from the libraries of international experts in the field. These photographs include not only the ocular manifestations but also systemic manifestations of the diseases whenever possible. Finally, the editors and authors are experts that practice around the world, lending this atlas a truly global perspective.

Sunir J. Garg, MD
Editor

Acknowledgments

I would like to thank Chris Rapuano, MD, for the opportunity to create this new volume for what is an already excellent series, and the associate editors, authors, and Grace Caputo, our developmental editor, who all contributed their time and expertise to this text. David Fischer, MD, and Russ Van Gelder, MD, PhD, got me interested in ocular inflammatory disease, have been wonderful teachers, and are now trusted colleagues. Lloyd Jacobs, MD, Michael Roth, MD, and Terry Bergstrom, MD, encouraged me to go to Wills Eye Institute for my retina training, and I am fortunate to have been invited to remain on the staff of such an incredible place. Our photographers, Julia Monsonego, Tom Walker, and Elaine Liebenbaum, are consummate professionals and are responsible for a number of images in this text. Finally, I would like to thank my patients, residents, fellows, colleagues, and teachers for giving me the opportunity to work with them.

Contents

Editors   vi

Contributors   vii

About the Series   xii

Preface   xiii

Acknowledgments   xiv

CHAPTER 1   **Immune Response Overview**   **1**

    Sunir J. Garg

    Basic Concepts   1

    Building Blocks of the Immune Response   2

    Plasma-Derived Enzyme Systems: The Complement System   5

    Hypersensitivity Reactions   5

    Immunity and the Eye   6

CHAPTER 2   **Anatomic Classification of Uveitis**   **7**

    Wendy M. Smith, Lisa J. Faia, Sunir J. Garg, and H. Nida Sen

    Classification   7

    SUN Terminology for Activity of Uveitis   11

CHAPTER 3   **Episcleritis, Scleritis, and Keratitis**   **13**

    Theresa Larson, H. Nida Sen, S. R. Rathinam, Patrick Prendergast,
    William Hodge, Joseph R. Zelefsky, Emmett T. Cunningham, Jr., and Roxana Ursea

    Episcleritis   13

    Scleritis   15

        Anterior Scleritis   15

        Posterior Scleritis   19

    Phylectenulosis   21

    Herpetic Keratouveitis   24

        Herpes Simplex Virus   24

        Varicella Zoster Virus   26

    Mooren's Ulcer   28

    Peripheral Ulcerative Keratitis   31

CHAPTER 4   **Anterior Uveitis**   **35**

    Julie Gueudry, Bahram Bodaghi, Phuc LeHoang, Karina Julian, and Sunir J. Garg

    Human Leucocyte Antigen B27–Associated Uveitis   35

        Seronegative Spondyloarthropathies   36

    Posner-Schlossman Syndrome   41

    Fuchs' Uveitis Syndrome (Fuchs' Heterochromic Iridocyclitis)   43

    Juvenile Idiopathic Arthritis–Associated Uveitis (Juvenile Rheumatoid/
        Chronic Arthritis)   46

    Tubulointerstitial Nephritis and Uveitis Syndrome   51

CHAPTER 5 **Cataract- and Lens-Induced Uveitis   53**

Somasheila I. Murthy, Swapnali Sabhapandit, and Anita Schadlu

Phacoantigenic/Phacoanaphylactic/Phacolytic Uveitis   53

Cataract Surgery-Related Uveitis   56

CHAPTER 6 **Intermediate Uveitis   59**

Andrea D. Birnbaum and Debra A. Goldstein

CHAPTER 7 **Posterior Uveitis and Collagen Vascular Diseases   65**

H. Nida Sen, Robert Nussenblatt, Rishi R. Doshi, S. R. Rathinam, Emmett T. Cunningham, Jr., Nupura Krishnadev, Bhupesh Bagga, Virender S. Sangwan, Robert W. Wong, Virginia M. Utz, Johnny Tang, Jyotirmay Biswas, Parthopratim Dutta Majumder, Keith Wroblewski, Leon D. Charkoudian, Sunil K. Srivastava, Julie Lew, and Shree Kurup

Sarcoidosis-Associated Uveitis   65

Sympathetic Ophthalmia   72

Vogt-Koyanagi-Harada Syndrome   76

Ocular Complications of Rheumatoid Arthritis   81

Behçet's Disease   85

Systemic Lupus Erythematosus   91

Antiphospholipid Syndrome   95

Eales' Disease   101

Granulomatosis with Polyangiitis (Wegener's Granulomatosis)   104

Kawasaki's Disease   108

Relapsing Polychondritis   110

Scleroderma   114

Dermatomyositis and Polymyositis   119

Polyarteritis Nodosa   122

CHAPTER 8 **White Dot Syndromes   124**

Céline Terrada, Bahram Bodaghi, P. Kumar Rao, Matthew A. Cunningham, Steven Yeh, Annal D. Meleth, Jaclyn L. Kovach, Janet L. Davis, and Jason Hsu

Acute Posterior Multifocal Placoid Pigment Epitheliopathy   124

Serpiginous Chorioretinopathy   128

Multiple Evanescent White Dot Syndrome   132

Multifocal Choroiditis/Subretinal Fibrosis Syndrome   135

Punctuate Inner Choroidopathy   141

Ocular Histoplasmosis Syndrome   145

Birdshot Chorioretinopathy (Vitiliginous Chorioretinitis)   149

Acute Zonal Occult Outer Retinopathy   153

Acute Macular Neuroretinopathy   155

Unilateral Acute Idiopathic Maculopathy   157

Acute Retinal Pigment Epitheliitis   159

CHAPTER 9 **Infectious Posterior Uveitis   163**

Karina Julian, Bahram Bodaghi, Phuc LeHoang, P. Vijayalakshmi, Sunir J. Garg, Moncef Khairallah, S. Lalitha Prajna, S. R. Rathinam, Julie Gueudry, Vishali Gupta, Amod Gupta, Chloe Gottlieb, Robert Nussenblatt, H. Nida Sen, Uwe Pleyer, Valérie Touitou, Carlos Alexandre de Amorim Garcia, Jason F. Okulicz, Rajeev Jain, Dinesh Selva, and Kim Ramasamy

Viral Infection 163
Herpetic 163
  Acute Retinal Necrosis Syndrome 163
  Progressive Outer Retinal Necrosis 169
Congenital Rubella Syndrome 172
West Nile Virus 176
Chikungunya 179

Spirochetes 181
Syphilis 181
Lyme Disease 188
Leptospirosis 191

Mycobacteria 194
Intraocular Tuberculosis 194
Hansen's Uveitis (Leprosy) 200

Parasites, Bacteria, Fungi, and Nematodes 204
Ocular Toxoplasmosis 204
Ocular Toxocariasis 208
Cat-Scratch Disease 212
Whipple's Disease 217
Diffuse Unilateral Subacute Neuroretinitis 220
Onchocerciasis 224
Loiasis 229
Ocular Cysticercosis 232
Rhinosporidosis 235

CHAPTER 10 **Endophthalmitis 238**
  Stephen G. Schwartz, Harry W. Flynn, Jr., Roy D. Brod, Manohar Babu Balasundaram,
  S. R. Rathinam, Bahram Bodaghi, and Phuc LeHoang
  Postoperative Endophthalmitis 238
    Acute-Onset Postoperative Endophthalmitis 238
    Delayed-Onset (Chronic) Postoperative Endophthalmitis 241
    Filtering Bleb-Associated Endophthalmitis 243
  Endogenous Endophthalmitis 245
  Endogenous Fungal Endophthalmitis 249

CHAPTER 11 **AIDS-Related Eye Disease 253**
  Annal D. Meleth and Allison Dublin
  HIV Retinopathy 253
  Cytomegalovirus Retinitis 255
  Immune Recovery Uveitis 260
  Acute Retinal Necrosis 261
  Progressive Outer Retinal Necrosis 263
  Fungal Retinitis 265
  Pneumocystis carinii (jirovecii) Choroiditis 267
  Kaposi's Sarcoma 268

CHAPTER 12 **Drug-Induced Uveitis** **270**

Nehali V. Saraiya and Debra A. Goldstein

Rifabutin 270
Cidofovir 272
Bisphosphonates 273
Sulfonamides 274
Metipranolol 276
Brimonidine 277
Prostaglandin Analogues 278

CHAPTER 13 **Masquerade Syndromes** **279**

H. Nida Sen, Bahram Bodaghi, Carol L. Shields, Henry Wiley, Ann O. Igbre, Sunir J. Garg, John F. Payne, and Sunil K. Srivastava

Primary Intraocular Lymphoma 279
Retinoblastoma Simulating Uveitis 285
Metastatic Cancer 288
Retinitis Pigmentosa 290
Ocular Ischemic Syndrome 293
Cancer-Associated Retinopathy Syndrome 297

CHAPTER 14 **Treatment of Uveitis** **300**

Sam S. Dahr, Theresa Larson, and H. Nida Sen

Local Therapy **300**
Topical Therapy 300
    Prednisolone and Difluprednate 300
    Cycloplegics and Mydriatics 301
Periocular Therapy 301
    Triamcinolone 301
Intravitreal Therapy 302
    Triamcinolone 302
    Ranibizumab and Bevacizumab 302
    Fluocinolone Implant (Retisert) 303
    Dexamethasone Implant (Ozurdex) 304
    Methotrexate 304
    Rituximab (Rituxan) 305
    Ganciclovir 305
    Foscarnet 306
    Clindamycin 306
Systemic Therapy **307**
Steroids 307
Immunosuppressive Agents 307
Antimetabolites 309
T-Cell Inhibitors 309
Alkylating Agents 309
Biologics 309

Index 310

Immune Response Overview

Sunir J. Garg

BASIC CONCEPTS

- The immune response is a complex system that protects the body from harm. Ideally, the immune response recognizes pathologic material and then eliminates it with minimal collateral damage. Autoimmune diseases occur when these responses malfunction.

- The eye has no lymphatic drainage, so it protects itself in other ways.

  - The first way is physical protect on from the skin, eyelids, eyelashes, blink reflex, tears, and tear pH.

  - If the physical defenses do not work, soluble inhibitors, such as immunoglobulin A (IgA) and lysozymes, can block the effects of an antigen.

  - If that does not work, the body can attempt to kill or neutralize the antigen through both innate and adaptive immunity.

  - If the body still cannot get rid of a particular pathogen, it can tolerate it through anterior chamber–associated immune deviation (ACAID).

Innate Immunity

- Innate immunity is an inborn immune response.

- Innate immunity targets a variety of common infections, foreign toxins, and damaged host "self" material.

- This type of reaction does not improve with subsequent exposures and has a limited repertoire.

Adaptive Immunity

- In contrast, adaptive immunity is antigen specific. When challenged by a novel organism or virus, the naïve immune system recognizes the material as foreign, processes the material, and then responds with an antigen-specific immune reaction.

- Upon exposure to new antigens, the naïve adaptive immune system typically responds slowly, requiring several days to mount an appropriate response.

- In contrast, subsequent (secondary) exposures lead to a more potent and rapid response to the same antigen; an antigen (a protein, carbohydrate, lipid, etc.) triggers a response specific to that antigen by using an antibody or T-cell receptor specific to that antigen.

BUILDING BLOCKS OF THE IMMUNE RESPONSE

- A variety of mechanisms work together to generate an immune response: leukocytes, antibodies, T-cell receptors, major histocompatibility complex (MHC) molecules, complement, cytokines, various enzyme systems, vasoactive amines, and lipid mediators.
- Hypersensitivity reactions also play a role.

Leukocytes

- A common stem cell gives rise to the following cells: neutrophils, monocytes/macrophages, eosinophils, lymphocytes (B cells and T cells), mast cells, basophils, megakaryocytes (which give rise to platelets), and red blood cells.

Phagocytes (Fig. 1-1)

Polymorphonuclear Neutrophils

- Polymorphonuclear neutrophils (PMNs, or "polys") are cells that travel in the bloodstream. When recruited toward inflamed tissues, they adhere to the blood vessel wall and exit via diapedesis through gaps between cells that make up the vessel wall.

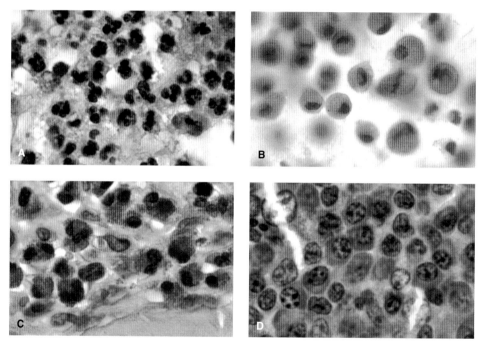

FIGURE 1-1. **A.** Polymorphonuclear leukocytes "neutrophils" are the most common phagocytes and can rapidly leave the bloodstream to engulf bacteria and damaged tissue. They have a multilobed nucleus. **B.** Macrophages play a critical role in eradicating microbes and damaged and/or dysplastic cells, in antigen presentation, and in inflammatory regulation. They are called histiocytes when they enter tissue. In this example, the cytoplasm is filled with lens material in a patient with phacolytic glaucoma. **C.** Eosinophils play an important role in fighting parasites and bacteria; they also play a role in the allergic response and in asthma. These cells characteristically have multiple, red cytoplasmic granules that surround a large nucleus. **D.** Plasma cells are white blood cells that are antigen specific. They can rapidly produce a large quantity of antibodies. (Note the characteristic "cart wheel" appearance.) Plasma cell dysregulation can lead to diseases such as multiple myeloma and Waldenström's macroglobulinemia. (Courtesy of Ralph Eagle, MD.)

- Once in the inflamed site, they engulf (phagocytize) and destroy the targeted antigens.
- These cells have a brief lifespan.

Mononuclear Phagocytes

- These are a second group of cells that phagocytize abnormal material. Examples include monocytes in the blood and Kupffer cells in the liver. These cells live much longer than PMNs. Blood-borne monocytes migrate into tissues and become tissue macrophages (histiocytes).
- Macrophages serve three main functions:
  - They play a scavenging role.
  - They present antigens to T cells (in conjunction with their MHC molecules).
  - They serve an important inflammatory effector role.

Eosinophils

- Eosinophils constitute 2% to 5% of blood leukocytes.
- They are seen in skin infiltrates (late phase reaction), atopic reactions, asthma, and around parasites.
- Certain immune stimuli cause these cells to degranulate and fuse their granules to the plasma membrane.
- In theory, large pathogens, such as parasitic worms, are too large to be engulfed. Eosinophils surround them and release their granules into the extracellular space in order to destroy the parasite.

Auxiliary Cells

Basophils and Mast Cells

- These cells constitute less than 0.2% of leukocytes in the bloodstream.
- The IgE receptor is activated by IgE (which is in turn activated by allergens). This leads to cell degranulation (with release of histamine, heparin, leukotrienes, and eosinophil chemotactic factor of anaphylaxis).

Platelets

- When endothelial cells are injured, platelets are attracted to the area and then release serotonin and thrombin. This activates complement, which increases vessel permeability, and attracts leukocytes to the site of injury.

Lymphocytes

B Cells (Bursa)

- Antigen specificity of the B cell is based on molecular recognition by antibodies.
- Upon exposure to an antigen, most B cells become plasma cells (antibody-forming cells), whereas a small group become memory cells (once they are exposed to an antigen, they remember it).
- Upon repeat exposure to an antigen, the B cells that have antibodies targeted against the antigen respond and make more antibodies.

Antibodies (aka Immunoglobulins)

- Antibodies are molecules produced in response to antigen exposure, and they can bind with a high degree of affinity to the antigen that stimulated its production.
- Antigens have highly variable antigen-binding sites that can attach to sites on antigens (epitopes). The antigen-binding site is located within the Fab (fragment-antigen binding) portion of the molecule.
- A different region of the antibody molecule called Fc (Fragment crystallizable) then activates the host immune response.
- The root structure of any immunoglobulin is made of four polypeptide chains (two identical heavy and two identical light chains).
  - The heavy chain determines the class and isotype of the Ig (i.e., IgG vs. IgA).
  - Each light chain interacts with a heavy chain forming the Fab portion of the antibody. The two heavy chains are then cross-linked and form the Fc portion of the molecule.

- There are several mechanisms that lead to the rich assortment of antibody specificities that may be seen. These range from gene recombination to somatic mutation.

  ▪ The repertoire is not genetically preprogrammed, but rather the result of amazing molecular genetics.

- A brief discussion of each of the major Ig classes follows:

  ▪ IgG Class

    ▸ These constitute the majority (70% to 75%) of serum immunoglobulins.

    ▸ They play an important role in secondary immune responses, and their presence signifies previous antigen exposure.

    ▸ IgG can cross into the placenta and also passes freely into extravascular spaces.

    ▸ IgG also activates complement.

  ▪ IgM Class

    ▸ These make up between 5% and 10% of serum immunoglobulins.

    ▸ They are important in primary immune responses (signifies recent/current infection).

    ▸ IgM remains (mostly) in the intravascular space because of its large size.

    ▸ IgM can activate complement.

  ▪ IgA Class

    ▸ IgA constitutes approximately 15% to 20% of serum immunoglobulins.

    ▸ IgA dimers are actively transported across mucosal membranes and are found in the various mucosal surfaces (i.e., the conjunctiva and the respiratory, intestinal, and genitourinary tracts).

  ▪ IgE Class

    ▸ IgE makes up less than 1% of serum immunoglobulins.

    ▸ IgE binds to eosinophils, basophils, and mast cells, resulting in release of histamine and other pro-inflammatory mediators. It plays a role in helminthic infections and allergic reactions.

T Cells (Thymus) and T-Cell Receptors

- T-cell receptors (TCRs) are the basis for T-cell antigen specificity.

- Positive and negative selection eliminates 95% of potential TCRs during thymic "education."

- Antigen recognition requires that the antigen be presented by an antigen-presenting cell (APC; usually a macrophage or a dendritic cell). Antigenic peptide fragments are presented in conjunction with an MHC molecule on the surface of the APC. A T cell with CD3 protein and either a CD4 or a CD8 protein also needs to be present on the cell for the TCR complex to work properly.

- The ability of a T cell to recognize and respond to a specific antigen is critical to an effective immune system. The TCR is the basis for T-cell antigen specificity.

- Unlike antibodies, which recognize antigens in their native state, the TCR recognizes antigen fragments presented by APCs in concert with human leukocyte antigen (HLA) proteins (major histocompatibility complex [MHC]) on cell surfaces.

- TCRs share some basic molecular building blocks with antibodies, yet they play a different role. Diversification of the TCR results from gene recombination that is similar to that of antibodies.

Large Granular Lymphocytes (not B, not T)

- Another subset of lymphocytes that comprises ≈15% of circulating lymphocytes. These cells are adept at killing virally infected cells and tumor cells.

- Natural killer (NK) cell activity is not antibody dependent. Instead, cells that do not display a "friendly" MHC are killed by NK cells (this is a form of negative identification).

Major Histocompatibility Complex

- The MHC holds an antigenic peptide fragment in a binding groove and present these fragments to TCRs. CD4 and CD8 proteins on the T-cell surface function as co-receptors (with TCRs) for the MHC molecule.

- The MHC, like TCRs and antibodies, are members of the immunoglobulin superfamily with many of the same basic domain structural units as antibodies. In humans, the human leukocyte antigen (HLA) proteins are located within the MHC on chromosome 6.

- Each individual has six pairs of HLA haplotypes (six from each parent: there are two HLA-As, two HLA-Bs, etc.).

- MHC haplotype affects a number of different aspects of the immune system, including disease susceptibility to specific infections and autoimmune diseases, the ability to produce antibodies, and organ transplant rejection.

Cytokines and Cytokine Receptors

- Cytokines are a group of more than 200 small signaling proteins that are traditionally named based upon their functions. They allow communication between cells. The main types of cytokines are:

  - Interleukins, which control intracellular communications

  - Interferons, which play a role in limiting viral infections

  - Tumor necrosis factor, which regulates tumor apoptosis, as well as macrophage and PMN activation

  - Growth factors, which can mediate cell proliferation and maturation

  - Colony stimulating factors, which drive cell division, and

  - Chemokines, which affect chemotaxis.

PLASMA-DERIVED ENZYME SYSTEMS: THE COMPLEMENT SYSTEM

- Complement (aka the complement system) plays a very important role in inflammation and immunity. There are more than 20 complement proteins, and together they constitute 10% of serum proteins.

- There are two major pathways for complement activation: the classical and the alternative (innate) pathways.

- Complement helps control inflammation, the action of phagocytes, and the membrane attack complex.

- Complement performs three basic functions:

  - Cell lysis by the membrane attack complex

  - Recruitment of PMNs via chemotaxis and induction of inflammation via anaphylotoxins

  - Coating of antigen/pathogen by C3b to enhance phagocytosis; this process is called opsonization.

HYPERSENSITIVITY REACTIONS

- These are excessive immune reactions.

- A useful mnemonic to remember the different reactions is ACIDS (Type 1 is Anaphylactic, Type 2 is Cytotoxic, Type 3 is Immune complex, Type 4 is Delayed-type hypersensitivity, Type 5 is Stimulatory).

- Types 1, 2, 3, and 5 are all antibody mediated.

- Type 4 is unique because it is T-cell mediated.

Hypersensitivity Type 1: Anaphylactic

- This is the production of IgE in response to antigen exposure (i.e., molds, pollens). Antigen cross-links IgE on the surface of mast cells and basophils, which release histamine, leukotrienes, and cytokines.

■ Systemic examples: Anaphylaxis, hay fever, allergic asthma, and atopic dermatitis

■ Ocular examples: Seasonal allergic conjunctivitis, atopic and vernal keratoconjunctivitis, and giant papillary conjunctivitis

Hypersensitivity Type 2: Cytotoxic

● This is typified by antibodies directed at cell membranes. Together with complement activation, it can lead to cell lysis.

■ Systemic examples: Myasthenia gravis, Goodpasture's syndrome

■ Ocular examples: Ocular cicatricial pemphigoid, herpes dermatitis, pemphigus vulgaris

Hypersensitivity Type 3: Immune Complex Deposition

● These are antibody–antigen complex deposition-related diseases.

■ Systemic examples: Serum sickness, lupus, Stevens-Johnson syndrome, rheumatoid arthritis, polyarteritis nodosa, Behçet disease

■ Ocular examples: Effects of the preceding systemic diseases on the eye

Hypersensitivity Type 4: Delayed Type Hypersensitivity

● This is unique because these are T-cell–mediated inflammatory reactions that take ≥12 hours to develop.

■ Systemic examples: Tuberculosis (TB) and the purified protein derivative (PPD) test, sarcoidosis, Wegener's granulomatosis, sympathetic ophthalmia

■ Ocular examples: The PPD test and the preceding systemic diseases

Hypersensitivity Type 5: Stimulatory

● Antibodies directed against receptors activate the receptors. For instance, in Graves' disease, an antibody against the thyroid stimulating hormone (TSH) receptor is believed to activate the receptor driving hyperthyroidism. Myasthenia gravis provides another example of an antibody that has an effect on a receptor. In this case, anti-acetylcholine antibodies lead to internalization of the acetylcholine (ACH) receptor and a depletion of the number of active receptors.

■ Ocular examples: Myasthenia gravis, Graves' disease

IMMUNITY AND THE EYE

Intraocular Immune Privilege

● The eye—along with the brain, the pregnant uterus, the adrenal cortex, hair follicles, testes, and ovaries—resists immune rejection.

● There are several passive reasons for this, including the blood–eye barrier, minimal lymphatic drainage, and little MHC expression in the eye. A number of cell-surface proteins also inhibit the immune system in the eye.

● Several proteins secreted in the eye also confer tolerance: Transforming growth factor beta (TGF-β), α-melanocyte stimulating hormone, and vasointestinal peptide.

Anterior Chamber–Associated Immune Deviation

● Antigens that are delivered into the anterior chamber can lead to an immune response that is different than if the antigen were delivered elsewhere (e.g., the skin).

● If the body cannot get rid of an antigen, it can learn to tolerate it without causing an inflammatory response.

REFERENCES

Delves P, Martin S, Burton D, et al. *Roitt's Essential Immunology (Essentials),* 11th ed. Hoboken, NJ: Wiley-Blackwell; 2006.

Nussenblatt RN, Whitcup SM. *Uveitis: Fundamentals and Clinical Practice,* 4th ed. Philadelphia: Mosby Elsevier; 2010.

Anatomic Classification of Uveitis

Wendy M. Smith, Lisa J. Faia,
Sunir J. Garg, and H. Nida Sen

The uvea—made up of the iris, ciliary body, and choroid—is a pigmented, vascular structure of the eye. These anatomic components can be used to divide the uveal tract into anterior (iris and ciliary body), intermediate (ciliary body and pars plana), and posterior (choroid) locations. Inflammation of the uveal tract, or uveitis, may also involve the retina and the retinal vasculature.

CLASSIFICATION

In 2004, the First International Workshop on Standardization of Uveitis Nomenclature (SUN) endorsed an anatomic classification of uveitis based on the International Uveitis Study Group (IUSG) criteria.

Prior to these working groups, there were several grading systems in use. Standardization of classification criteria, inflammation grading schema, and outcomes allows comparisons of clinical research from different centers. Use of these criteria confers several advantages, including better definition of the clinical course of disease and more efficient evaluation of new therapies.

The SUN Classification contains several important features.

- The type of uveitis is determined by the predominant site(s) of uveal inflammation.

  - The anatomic localizations are anterior, intermediate, posterior, and panuveitis (**Table 2-1**).

  - Identifying the predominant site of inflammation also helps to narrow the differential diagnosis (**Table 2-2**). Significant inflammation of the anterior chamber and vitreous is not panuveitis. (These should be classified as anterior and intermediate uveitis, respectively.)

- Anatomic classification is not influenced by the presence of structural complications.

  - For example, the presence of macular edema or optic disk edema alone is not enough to classify an eye as "posterior uveitis." Macular edema due to anterior chamber inflammation would be correctly categorized as anterior uveitis.

  - Vitritis plus peripheral vascular sheathing or macular edema is defined

TABLE 2-1. SUN Working Group Anatomic Classification of Uveitis

Type	Primary Site of Inflammation	Includes
Anterior uveitis	Anterior chamber	Iritis, iridocyclitis, anterior cyclitis
Intermediate uveitis	Vitreous	Pars planitis, posterior cyclitis, hyalitis
Posterior uveitis	Retina or choroid	Focal, multifocal, or diffuse choroiditis; chorioretinitis, retinochoroiditis, retinitis, neuroretinitis
Panuveitis	Involves all compartments of the eye without one predominating	

Adapted from Jabs DA, Nussenblatt RB, Rosenbaum JT. Standardization of Uveitis Nomenclature (SUN) Working Group. Standardization of uveitis nomenclature for reporting clinical data. Results of the First International Workshop. *Am J Ophthalmol.* 2005;140(3):509–516.

TABLE 2-2. Differential Diagnosis of the Major Causes of Uveitis

ANTERIOR UVEITIS*

Granulomatous

Sarcoidosis
Syphilis
Tuberculosis
Herpes simplex
Leptospirosis
Brucellosis
Phacoanaphylactic
Idiopathic

Nongranulomatous

Human leukocyte antigen-B27–associated (including ankylosing spondylitis, Reiter's syndrome, inflammatory bowel disease, psoriatic arthritis)
Juvenile rheumatoid arthritis
Fuchs' heterochromic iridocyclitis
Posner-Schlossman (glaucomatocyclitic crisis)
Masquerade syndromes
Uveitis-glaucoma-hyphema syndrome
Trauma
Kawasaki's disease
Drug-induced (rifabutin, cidofovir)

INTERMEDIATE UVEITIS

Sarcoid, syphilis
Inflammatory bowel disease
Multiple sclerosis
Pars planitis (idiopathic)
Lymphoma, Lyme
Other (tuberculosis, Behçet's, Vogt-Koyanagi-Harada, Whipple's disease, toxoplasmosis, endophthalmitis)

(continued)

*This category is usually divided up into granulomatous (mutton fat KP) and nongranulomatous uveitis. All of the granulomatous ones can look nongranulomatous, but the nongranulomatous ones do not look granulomatous.
Pearl: Sarcoid, syphilis, tuberculosis, Lyme, and lymphoma can look like anything.

TABLE 2-2. Differential Diagnosis of the Major Causes of Uveitis (*Continued*)

POSTERIOR UVEITIS

Focal Retinitis

Toxoplasmosis
Onchocerciasis
Cysticercosis
Masquerade syndromes

Multifocal Retinitis

Syphilis
Herpes simplex virus (acute retinal necrosis)
Cytomegalovirus
Sarcoidosis
Masquerade syndromes
Candidiasis
Progressive outer retinal necrosis
Eales' disease
Diffuse unilateral subacute neuroretinitis

PANUVEITIS

Sympathetic ophthalmia
Vogt-Koyanagi-Harada
Behçet's disease
Endophthalmitis
Sarcoidosis
Phacoanaphylaxis
Lyme disease
Masquerade syndromes
Toxoplasmosis
Syphilis
Tuberculosis

CHOROIDITIS

Focal Choroiditis

Tuberculosis
Toxocariasis
Nocardia
Candidiasis
Masquerade syndromes

Multifocal Choroiditis

Histoplasmosis
Pneumocystis choroiditis
Serpiginous choroiditis
Birdshot
Lymphoma
Acute multifocal placoid pigment epitheliopathy
Multifocal choroiditis/punctate inner choroiditis
Masquerade syndromes
Cryptococcus
Mycobacterium

---

as intermediate uveitis, as this is the pre-dominant site of inflammation.

- Pars planitis is a specific, idiopathic disease entity defined by the presence of snowball or snowbank formation in the absence of an associated infection or systemic disease; otherwise, the correct term is intermediate uveitis.

The SUN working group criteria currently has a few limitations:

- It does not provide criteria for diagnosis of specific uveitic entities.

- It does not address the classification of neuroretinitis.

- It is still undergoing validation.

The SUN working group also standardized the descriptors of uveitis in order to facilitate clinical descriptions of diseases both for clinical care as well as for research purposes.

- Onset

  ▪ Sudden

  ▪ Insidious

- Duration
  - Limited (≤3 months)
  - Persistent (>3 months)
- Course of disease
  - Acute (sudden onset and limited duration)
  - Chronic (persistent uveitis with relapse <3 months after discontinuing therapy)
  - Recurrent (repeat episodes of uveitis separated by at least 3 months without treatment)
- Grading
  - Anterior chamber cell and flare (**Tables 2-3 and 2-4**)
    - ▸ Presence of hypopyon should be noted separately
  - Vitreous haze
    - ▸ The SUN working group adopted the National Eye Institute System (**Fig. 2-1** and **Table 2-5**).
    - ▸ A more recent grading system using calibrated Bangerter diffusion filters and color photographs for assessing vitreous haze is a promising technique that requires further validation (Davis et al.).

TABLE 2-3. SUN Working Group Grading Scheme for Anterior Chamber Cells

Grade	Cells in High-Powered Field*
0	<1
0.5+	1–5
1+	6–15
2+	16–25
3+	26–50
4+	>50

*Field size: 1 mm × 1 mm slit beam.
Adapted from Jabs DA, Nussenblatt RB, Rosenbaum JT. Standardization of Uveitis Nomenclature (SUN) Working Group. Standardization of uveitis nomenclature for reporting clinical data. Results of the First International Workshop. *Am J Ophthalmol.* 2005;140(3):509–516.

TABLE 2-4. The SUN Working Group Grading Scheme for Anterior Chamber Flare

Grade	Description
0	None
1+	Faint
2+	Moderate (iris and lens details clear)
3+	Marked (iris and lens details hazy)
4+	Intense (fibrin or plastic aqueous)

Adapted from Jabs DA, Nussenblatt RB, Rosenbaum JT. Standardization of Uveitis Nomenclature (SUN) Working Group. Standardization of uveitis nomenclature for reporting clinical data. Results of the First International Workshop. *Am J Ophthalmol.* 2005;140(3):509–16.

  - There is no SUN Working Group consensus on vitreous cell. Although not adopted by the SUN group, **Table 2-6** shows the National Eye Institute Grading Scheme with Hruby lens.
- Unilateral or bilateral
- Appearance (granulomatous or nongranulomatous keratic precipitates). Although this is useful during clinical care, this has not yet been standardized.

TABLE 2-5. The National Eye Institute Grading Scheme for Vitreous Haze

Grade	Description
0	Clear
0.5+ (trace in the NEI scheme)	Trace
1+	Few opacities, mild blurring
2+	Significant blurring but still visible
3+	Optic nerve visible, no vessels seen
4+	Dense opacity obscures the optic nerve head

*Based on the view of the posterior retina and optic disc using indirect ophthalmoscopy and 20D lens.
Adapted from Nussenblatt RB, Palestine AG, Chan CC, Roberge F. Standardization of vitreal inflammatory activity in intermediate and posterior uveitis. *Ophthalmology.* 1985;92(4):467–471.

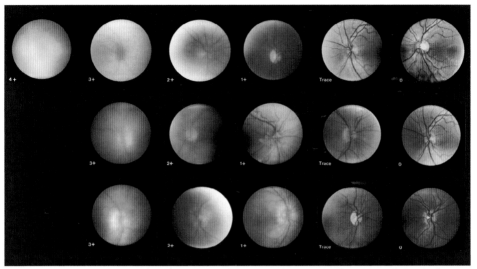

FIGURE 2-1. Vitreous haze grading. (From Nussenblatt RB, Palestine AG, Chan CC, et al. Standardization of vitreal inflammatory activity in intermediate and posterior uveitis. *Ophthalmology.* 1985;92(4): 467–471.)

TABLE 2-6. The National Eye Institute Grading Scheme for Vitreous Cells with Hruby Lens

Grade	Cells in Retroilluminated Field	Description
0	0–1	Clear
Trace	2–20	Few opacities
1+	21–50	Scattered opacities
2+	51–100	Moderate opacities
3+	101–250	Many opacities
4+	>251	Dense opacities

Not endorsed by SUN.
Adapted from Nussenblatt RB, Whitcup SM. *Uveitis: Fundamentals and Clinical Practice.* 4th ed. Location: Elsevier; 2010.

SUN TERMINOLOGY FOR ACTIVITY OF UVEITIS

Although the ultimate goal of uveitis treatment is to suppress inflammation completely, it is also important to assess short-term changes in inflammation, especially when evaluating the efficacy of treatment.

- Inactive uveitis is defined as:
  - Zero to rare anterior chamber cells (less than one cell per high-power field)
  - There was no consensus for definition of inactive vitritis on the basic of vitreous cells.
- Worsening activity
  - Two-step increase in inflammation (anterior chamber cell or vitreous haze) or increase from grade 3+ to 4+

- Improved activity

  - Two-step decrease in inflammation (anterior chamber cell or vitreous haze) or decrease to grade 0

- Remission

  - Inactive disease for 3 months or more after discontinuing all treatments for eye disease

- Definition of successful corticosteroid sparing outcomes

  - For adults, long-term steroid use should be limited to 10 mg per day or less.

REFERENCES

Davis JL, Madow B, Cornett J, et al. Scale for photographic grading of vitreous haze in uveitis. *Am J Ophthalmol.* 2010;150:637–641.

Jabs DA, Nussenblatt RB, Rosenbaum JT. Standardization of Uveitis Nomenclature (SUN) Working Group. Standardization of uveitis nomenclature for reporting clinical data. Results of the First International Workshop. *Am J Ophthalmol.* 2005;140(3):509–516.

Nussenblatt RB, Palestine AG, Chan CC, et al. Standardization of vitreal inflammatory activity in intermediate and posterior uveitis. *Ophthalmology.* 1985;92(4):467–471.

Nussenblatt RB, Whitcup SM. *Uveitis: Fundamentals and Clinical Practice,* 4th ed. Philadelphia: Elsevier; 2010.

Episcleritis, Scleritis, and Keratitis

EPISCLERITIS

Theresa Larson and H. Nida Sen

Episcleritis is a self-limited, generally benign inflammation of the episclera.

Etiology and Epidemiology

- Episcleritis occurs most frequently in young to middle-aged women (20 to 40 years old).
- It is frequently unilateral (70%).
- The etiology is unknown in most cases, but it is believed to be immune mediated, and it is occasionally associated with systemic disease.

Symptoms

- Redness, minimal eye pain
- Foreign-body sensation
- Minimal to no changes in vision

Signs

- Bright red or salmon-pink color in natural light (Fig. 3-1)

- The superficial episcleral vessels are injected, and the redness can be sectoral (70%), diffuse, or, rarely, nodular.
- The vessels are easily mobile with a cotton-tipped applicator and blanch with topical administration of 10% phenylephrine.
- Small peripheral corneal opacities are present in 10% of cases.

Differential Diagnosis

- Scleritis
  - In contrast to scleritis, episcleritis has minimal pain, less common systemic disease association, and essentially no complications.
- Pinguecula
- Phlyctenule
- Subconjunctival hemorrhage
- Conjunctival neoplasia
- Anterior uveitis

Diagnostic Evaluation

- Although systemic disease is not commonly associated with episcleritis, a thorough review of systems and targeted systemic

This contribution to the work was done as part of the authors' official duties as NIH employees and is a work of the United States Government.

workup is indicated. Systemic workup can be considered in recurrent cases. Up to 30% of patients are found to have an underlying disease association.

Treatment

- Episodes are self-limited and rarely require treatment beyond artificial tears, topical NSAIDs, and topical corticosteroids. If the episcleritis does not resolve promptly with therapy, consider another diagnosis.

Prognosis

- The prognosis is usually very good.
- Episodes may recur but rarely are there lasting sequelae.

REFERENCES

Foster CS, and Sainz de la Maza M. Clinical consideration of episcleritis and scleritis. In *The Sclera*. New York: Springer-Verlag; 1994:107.

Jabs DA, Mudun A, Dunn JP, et al. Episcleritis and scleritis: clinical features and treatment results. *Ophthalmology.* 2000;130:469–476.

Sainz de la Maza M, Jabbur NS, Foster CS. Severity of scleritis and episcleritis. *Ophthalmology.* 1994;101:389–396.

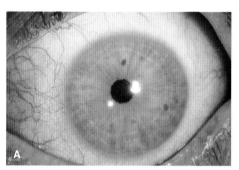 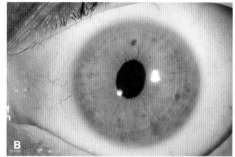

FIGURE 3-1. **Episcleritis. A.** This patient has episcleritis with a salmon pink hue. **B.** The same eye with blanching of the episclera after administration of 10% phenylephrine.

SCLERITIS

Theresa Larson and H. Nida Sen

Scleritis is characterized by inflammation and edema of scleral and episcleral tissue. It is classified as anterior or posterior, and further subclassified as diffuse, nodular, and necrotizing (**Table 3-1**).

ANTERIOR SCLERITIS

Etiology and Epidemiology

● Anterior scleritis is the most common form, making up 80% to 85% of all scleritis cases. Diffuse and nodular scleritis occur with equal frequency.

● Scleritis occurs most frequently in middle-aged women (40 to 60 years old)

● 25% to 50% of patients have a history of systemic disease, most commonly rheumatoid arthritis (**Table 3-2**).

● Necrotizing scleritis is the most severe and destructive form of scleritis and is most often associated with sight-threatening sequelae.

   ▪ Necrotizing scleritis is divided into "with inflammation" and "without inflammation" (scleromalacia perforans).

TABLE 3-1. Scleritis Clinical Subtypes and Their Prevalence

Anterior scleritis	80%–85%
Diffuse	40%–45%
Nodular	40%
Necrotizing scleritis	10%–15%
With inflammation	10%
Without inflammation	1%–5%
(scleromalacia perforans)	
Posterior scleritis	1%–5%

Adapted from Nussenblatt RB, Whitcup SM. *Uveitis: Fundamentals and Clinical Practice,* 4th ed. Philadelphia: Elsevier; 2010.

This contribution to the work was done as part of the authors' official duties as NIH employees and is a work of the United States Government.

Symptoms

● Patients present with a red, painful eye. They may have a boring eye pain.

● Vision loss is rare.

● Patients with scleromalacia perforans typically have no pain.

Signs

● The sclera has a violaceous hue in natural light with inflamed vessels that are immobile with a cotton-tipped applicator (**Fig. 3-2**). It is easier to appreciate scleritis by looking at the eye without the slit lamp.

● Areas of repeated attacks may demonstrate scleral thinning with a bluish hue.

● Eyes with diffuse scleritis have generalized edema, while eyes with sectoral or nodular scleritis have localized erythema (**Fig. 3-3**).

● Necrotizing scleritis has a white avascular area surrounded by injection and edema (**Fig. 3-4**).

● Topical (10%) phenylephrine will not blanch the vessels in scleritis.

Differential Diagnosis

● Episcleritis

● Subconjunctival hemorrhage

● Conjunctival mucosa–associated lymphoid tissue lymphoma

● Sentinel vessels

● Anterior uveitis or panuveitis

● Acute angle-closure glaucoma

● Keratitis

● Endophthalmitis

● Carotid or dural sinus fistula

Diagnostic Evaluation

● Testing is guided by history and review of systems.

   ▪ Rheumatoid factor, anti-citrullinated cyclic protein (CCP), classical

TABLE 3-2. Systemic Disease Associations

Noninfectious	Infectious	Other
Connective tissue disease	Herpes zoster ophthalmicus	Gout
Rheumatoid arthritis	Herpes simplex keratitis	Rosacea
Juvenile rheumatoid arthritis	Acanthamoeba keratitis	Foreign body reaction
Reiter's syndrome	Syphilis	Drugs (bisphosphonates)
Systemic lupus erythematosus	Lyme disease	
Relapsing polychondritis	Bartonellosis	
Polymyositis	Tuberculosis	
Inflammatory bowel disease		
Spondyloarthropathy		
Vasculitides		
Wegner's granulomatosis		
Polyarteritis nodosa		
Allergic angiitis of Churg-Strauss		
Cogan syndrome		
Takayasu disease		
Adamantiades—Behçet's disease		
Sarcoidosis		

antineutrophil cytoplasmic antibody (c-ANCA), protoplasmic-staining antineutrophil cytoplasmic antibodies (p-ANCA), myeloperoxidase, antinuclear antibody (ANA), and anti-dsDNA may be considered if an underlying rheumatologic disease is suspected.

▪ Rule out infectious causes with the appropriate tests, including: fluorescent treponemal antibody absorption (FTA-Abs), rapid plasma reagin (RPR) or Venereal Disease Research Laboratory (VDRL), purified protein derivative (PPD) and/or QuantiFERON, trauma, and foreign body.

● Orbital CT should be considered in atypical cases.

Treatment

● Oral NSAIDs for milder (nonnecrotizing) scleritis cases

● Nodular scleritis often can respond to an injection of triamcinolone over the nodule. Periocular triamcinolone can also be used selectively for cases of diffuse scleritis.

● Oral prednisone

● Immunosuppressive therapy is indicated for recurrent or severe cases (particularly for necrotizing scleritis).

● ANCA positive patients may have a more severe course of disease and thus require more aggressive therapy.

● In patients with necrotizing scleritis associated with a systemic disorder such as rheumatoid arthritis (Fig. 3-5) or Wegener's granulomatosis, aggressive systemic therapy is necessary because it is associated with a high mortality rate without systemic treatment.

Prognosis

● The prognosis varies based on the site of inflammation, associated complications, underlying conditions, and response to therapy. Diffuse anterior scleritis has the best prognosis, whereas necrotizing scleritis has the worst prognosis with the highest rates of visual loss and complications.

REFERENCES

Albini TA, Zamir E, Read RW, et al. Evaluation of subconjunctival triamcinolone for nonnecrotizing anterior scleritis. *Ophthalmology.* 2005;112(10): 1814–1820.

Foster CS, Sainz de la Maza M. Clinical consideration of episcleritis and scleritis. In *The Sclera.* New York: Springer-Verlag; 1994:107.

Foster CS, Forstot SL, Wilson LA. Mortality rate in rheumatoid arthritis patients developing necrotizing scleritis or peripheral ulcerative keratitis: effects of immunosuppression. *Ophthalmology.* 1984;91: 1253–1263.

Jabs DA, Mudun A, Dunn JP, et al. Episcleritis and scleritis: clinical features and treatment results. *Ophthalmology.* 2000;130:469–476.

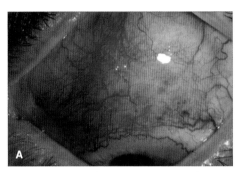
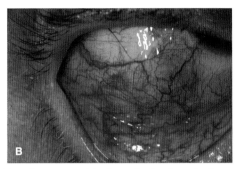

FIGURE 3-2. **A.** Diffuse anterior scleritis is characterized by inflammation of the deep scleral and episcleral vessels, which have a dark red/violaceous hue. **B.** Diffuse anterior scleritis with inferotemporal thinning. Note the scleral injection and adjacent scleral thinning evidenced by the blue color of the underlying choroid.

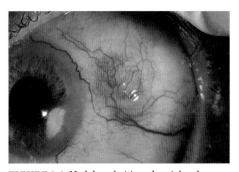

FIGURE 3-3. Nodular scleritis and peripheral ulcerative keratitis. The immobile nodule is surrounded by scleral injection. There is a focal, peripheral corneal opacity resulting from past episodes of peripheral ulcerative keratitis.

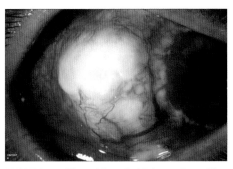

FIGURE 3-4. Necrotizing scleritis in a patient with Wegener's granulomatosis with one suture remaining from a past scleral biopsy. Note the white, avascular patch of sclera with surrounding scleritis.

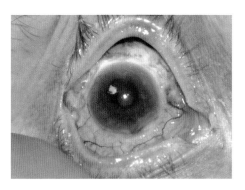

FIGURE 3-5. This elderly woman had poorly treated rheumatoid arthritis that caused painless scleral thinning through which the underlying blue choroid is visible (necrotizing scleritis without inflammation, or scleromalacia perforans). (Courtesy of Sunir J. Garg, MD.)

POSTERIOR SCLERITIS

It is an inflammatory disease of the sclera that begins posterior to the spiral of Tillaux/ora serrata and involves the posterior aspect of the eye.

Etiology and Epidemiology

- Posterior scleritis is more common in women. It has the lowest incidence of the various subtypes of scleritis; however, it is often underrecognized because of its many manifestations.

Symptoms

- Patients often present with an "achy, deep" pain, decreased vision, and redness.

Signs

- Unlike anterior scleritis, the vision is often affected.
- Pain
- Elevated intraocular pressure, associated anterior scleritis, a swollen optic disc, choroidal folds, serous retinal detachment, and/or a subretinal mass or lesion (Fig. 3-6)
- T-sign on B-scan ultrasound (Fig. 3-7)

Differential Diagnosis

- Choroidal tumors
- Uveal effusion syndrome
- Rhegmatogenous retinal detachment
- Vogt-Koyanagi-Harada syndrome
- Central serous chorioretinopathy
- Optic neuritis
- Masquerade syndromes (lymphoma, metastatic carcinoma, choroidal melanoma)

Diagnostic Evaluation

- Laboratory evaluation for an underlying systemic disease is warranted based on the results of a thorough history and review of systems.

- Rule out treatable infectious causes such as syphilis and tuberculosis (RPR, VDRL, FTA-Abs, PPD, Quantiferon)
- B-scan: This is critical to establish the diagnosis. It demonstrates scleral wall thickness >2 mm in either a diffuse or nodular fashion. Classically, a T-sign that represents a sonographically empty space due to edema surrounding Tenon's capsule and the optic nerve is seen.
- Fluorescein angiography can be used to rule out other causes such as Vogt-Koyanagi-Harada syndrome and sarcoidosis.

Treatment

- Most patients respond to oral NSAIDs; however, those with more severe chronic disease will require more aggressive systemic therapy with corticosteroids and/or immunosuppressive therapy.

Prognosis

- The prognosis depends on the timeliness of treatment and severity of disease. Patients older than 50 years, patients with an associated systemic disease, and patients requiring more aggressive treatment have a greater risk of vision loss.

REFERENCES

Benson WE. Posterior scleritis (review). *Surv Ophthalmol.* 1988;32(5):297–316.

Foster CS, Sainz de la Maza M. Clinical consideration of episcleritis and scleritis. In *The Sclera.* New York: Springer-Verlag; 1994:107.

Foster CS, Forstot SL, Wilson LA. Mortality rate in rheumatoid arthritis patients developing necrotizing scleritis or peripheral ulcerative keratitis: effects of immunosuppression. *Ophthalmology.* 1984;91:1253–1263.

Jabs DA, Mudun A, Dunn JP, et al. Episcleritis and scleritis: clinical features and treatment results. *Ophthalmology.* 2000;130:469–476.

McCluskey PJ, Watson PG, Lightman S, et al. Posterior scleritis: clinical features, systemic associations, and outcome in a large series of patients. *Ophthalmology.* 1999;106:2380–2386.

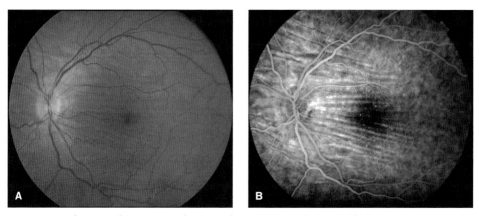

FIGURE 3-6. This patient has posterior scleritis. **A.** There are horizontal choroidal folds consistent with a mass (in this cases scleral inflammation) behind the globe. **B.** The fluorescein angiogram shows the choroidal striations. (Courtesy of William Benson, MD.)

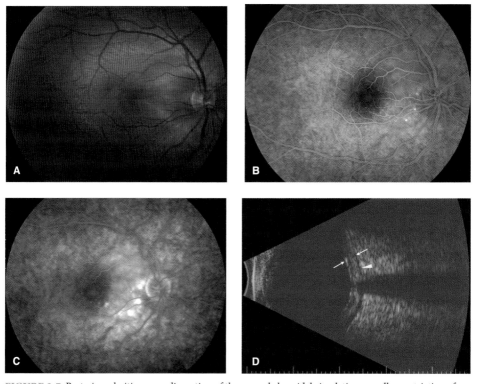

FIGURE 3-7. Posterior scleritis causes disruption of the normal choroidal circulation as well as restriction of scleral outflow through the vortex veins. This causes subsequent dysfunction of the retinal pigment epithelium. **A.** This can result in a serious retinal detachment. Fluorescein angiography can demonstrate pinpoint choroidal leakage (**B**) with pooling of dye in the late frames (**C**). **D.** B-scan ultrasonography demonstrates thickening of the sclera and choroid (*arrows*). Edema of Tenon's capsule behind the globe, and along the optic nerve, creates the T-sign. (Courtesy of William Benson, MD, and Eliza Hoskins, MD.)

PHYLECTENULOSIS

S. R. Rathinam

Phlyctenular keratoconjunctivitis is a non-specific, delayed hypersensitivity (type IV) reaction of the cornea and/or conjunctiva toward a variety of antigens.

Etiology and Epidemiology

- Phlyctenulosis is seen in the first two decades of life.
- It is more common in persons with poor personal hygiene and in those of lower socio-economic status.
- It is often associated with chronic mei-bomitis and chalazia.
- Less commonly, it has been associated with pulmonary and extra pulmonary tuber-culosis, staphylococcal infection, worm infes-tation, and focal sepsis.

Symptoms

- Lacrimation, photophobia, decreased vision, and blepharospasm

Signs

- Phlyctenulosis is a focal inflammatory disease characterized by an elevated, trans-lucent nodule or vesicle with an ulcerated summit surrounded by a zone of hyperemia (**Figs. 3-8 and 3-9**).
- Often, conjunctival phlyctens are transient and asymptomatic.
- However, larger phlyctens can result in frank pustular conjunctivitis.
- If the corneal phlycten migrates from its lim-bal origin to the central cornea, it is called *fas-cicular keratitis*, which causes severe vision loss.

Differential Diagnosis

- Pingueculum
- Episcleritis
- Foreign-body granuloma
- Scleral abscess

Diagnostic Evaluation

- Examination of the lid margin for blepha-ritis, meibomitis, and chalazia.
- In countries such as India, consider:
  - Systemic workup for pulmonary/extrapulmonary tuberculosis
  - Screening for palpable lymph node to biopsy
  - Pulmonary radiological studies to rule out tuberculosis
  - Stool examination for worm infestation

Treatment

- The primary treatment is good lid hygiene to eliminate staphylococcal lid infection; this includes warm moist compresses, lid scrubs with baby shampoo, and topical erythromy-cin eye ointment.
- If another systemic cause is found, treat-ment of the underlying disease is essential:
  - If due to a parasite, albendazole 400 mg/day can be used.
  - In cases of tuberculosis, multidrug anti-tubercular treatment (rifampicin 10 mg/kg/day, isoniazid 5 mg/kg/day q.d. for 6 to 9 months, ethambutol 15 mg/kg/day, and pyrazinamide 25 to 30 mg/kg/day q.d. for first 2 months should be considered).
- Prednisolone acetate 1% or dexametha-sone 0.1% every two hours for 1 week fol-lowed by a slow taper hastens resolution.
- In severe cases, or those that require lon-ger-term steroid use, topical cyclosporine A 2% has been found to be effective.

Prognosis

- Conjunctival phlyctens heal without scar-ring and carry a good prognosis.

- Corneal phlyctens may cause stromal scarring, which can cause vision loss (Fig. 3-10).

- Recurrences are more common in patients with tuberculosis (Fig. 3-11).

REFERENCE

Doan S, Gabison E, Gatinel D, et al. Topical cyclosporine A in severe steroid-dependent childhood phlyctenular keratoconjunctivitis. *Am J Ophthalmol.* 2006;141: 62–66.

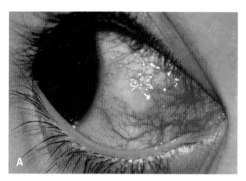

FIGURE 3-8. This is a typical, moderate to severe phlyctenule with an elevated, translucent nodule with an ulcerated summit surrounded by a ring of hyperemia.

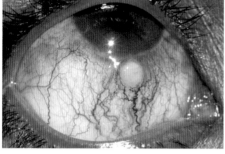

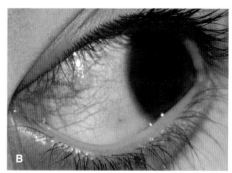

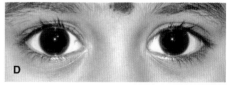

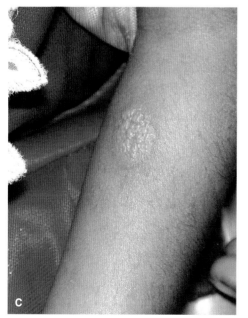

FIGURE 3-9. This child had bilateral phlyctenules. There is a small, elevated vesicle with surrounding hyperemia on the right (**A**) and left (**B**) eyes. **C.** Given the lack of eyelid disease, a search for a systemic cause was undertaken. The child had a positive Mantoux reaction. **D.** After receiving systemic antitubercular treatments and topical steroids, there was resolution of symptoms.

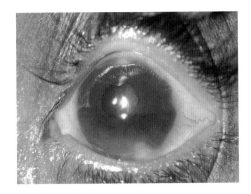

FIGURE 3-10. Multiple healed limbal phlyctenules with residual corneal scarring.

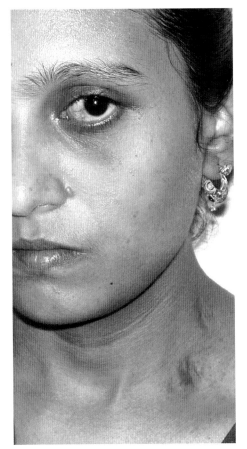

FIGURE 3-11. This woman has an active phlyctenule in her left eye and a healed cervical tubercular sinus, which has left a scar above the left clavicle. Treatment of her underlying tuberculosis with concomitant topical steroids caused resolution of her eye disease.

HERPETIC KERATOUVEITIS

Patrick Prendergast and William Hodge

Inflammation of the cornea and uveal tract arising from infection with varicella zoster virus (VZV) or herpes simplex virus (HSV) infection is a common cause of anterior uveitis.

HERPES SIMPLEX VIRUS

Etiology and Epidemiology

- Nearly all people are infected with HSV 1 and 2 during their lifetime. The initial infection is usually asymptomatic. The virus can then become a latent infection, often residing in the trigeminal nerve ganglion. It can then reactivate at any time along one of the trigeminal nerves, including those that go to the eye.

- Herpes simplex keratouveitis most commonly results from reactivation of latent infection, and is the most common cause of infectious uveitis. It presents at all ages and occurs in both sexes with equal frequency.

- HSV is the leading cause of corneal blindness in developed countries. In the United States, there are 20,000 new ocular cases per year, and 28,000 reactivations per year. One in 10,000 infants are born with neonatal HSV annually.

- Risk factors for viral reactivation include primary or secondary immunosuppression, and less commonly illness or stress, menstruation, local injury and UV light exposure.

- The ocular inflammation may be due to the viral infection itself or from the inflammatory response to the infection.

Symptoms

- Patients may develop redness, itching, burning, tearing, and/or discharge.

- Photophobia, moderate to severe pain, and blurry vision are common.

- Blisters may occur on or near the eyelid.

Signs

- The hallmark of the infection is epithelial dendritic keratitis, which is most notable with fluorescein staining (**Fig. 3-12**).

- Conjunctival injection, decreased corneal sensation, corneal scarring, and decreased visual acuity are common.

- A thickened, edematous cornea (disciform keratitis), fibrinous flare with heavy anterior chamber cell and medium-sized granulomatous keratic precipitates present on the endothelium; synechiae and increased intraocular pressure arising from trabeculitis may also be seen (**Figs. 3-13 and 3-14**).

Differential Diagnosis

- Bacterial, viral, fungal, or allergic conjunctivitis, acute angle-closure glaucoma, iritis or scleritis, corneal abrasion, recurrent corneal erosion, or toxic conjunctivitis

Diagnostic Evaluation

- Slit-lamp examination classically reveals branching dendrites with terminal end bulbs that tend to show fluorescein staining in the ulcer base and rose bengal staining at the border.

- A corneal swab for HSV DNA can be tested with polymerase chain reaction (PCR) can be used or antibody titers from an aqueous sample can be obtained to assess exposure.

Treatment

- HSV epithelial keratitis usually resolves without treatment. Topical antiviral medication such as trifluorothymidine 1% drops q.i.d. or topical gancyclovir 0.15% five times daily can reduce the duration of the episode.

- Patients with HSV stromal keratitis or uveitis (without epithelial disease) can be treated with cycloplegia with scopolamine 0.25% or cyclopentolate 1% drops t.i.d. Prednisolone acetate 1% drops q.i.d. should be used with a slow taper. Systemic steroids should be considered in severe uveitis. Trifluorothymidine 1% drops q.i.d. should be used for prophylaxis while on topical steroids. Oral acyclovir can reduce the risk of recurrence.

- Trophic epithelial defects can be prevented with preservative-free lubricant drops and ointments.

- Tarsorrhaphy can facilitate healing and prevent recurrent surface breakdown.

- A bandage lens and tissue adhesive can be used to promote epithethial healing and prevent corneal melts.

Prognosis

- Most VZV and HSV infections respond to antiviral treatment, steroids, or both.

Complications depend on the severity of the eye disease as well as patient characteristics.

- Potential complications of HSV infection includes corneal neovascularization and scarring, cataract formation, neurotrophic ulcers, bacterial or fungal infection, secondary glaucoma, postherpetic neuralgia, or vision loss arising from optic neuritis or chorioretinitis.

- Corneal transplantation may be necessary in some individuals.

REFERENCE

Wilhelmus KR, Gee L, Hauck WW, et al. Herpetic Eye Disease Study. A controlled trial of topical corticosteroids for herpes simplex stromal keratitis. *Ophthalmology.* 1994;101(12):1883–1895.

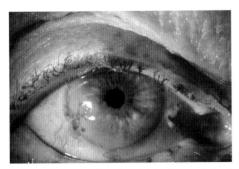

FIGURE 3-12. Dendritic keratitis is characteristic of HSV epithelial keratitis. Dendritic keratitis has active virus replicating in the epithelium; therefore, it is typically treated with topical antiviral agents, while corticosteroids are avoided.

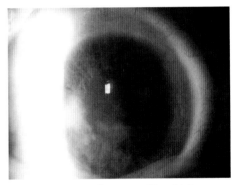

FIGURE 3-13. Disciform stromal keratitis is an immune-mediated condition resulting from chronic HSV infection. Disciform keratitis is the most common cause of blinding infectious keratitis in the United States. Topical corticosteroids are the mainstay of treatment and antiviral medications are used to avoid breakthrough of active infection, not to treat the disciform keratitis.

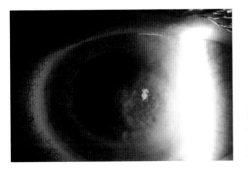

FIGURE 3-14. Disciform keratitis and anterior uveitis from HSV. The inflammatory disciform corneal lesions often occur along with a low-grade uveitis that produces small keratic precipitates as seen inferiorly in this photo.

VARICELLA ZOSTER VIRUS

Etiology and Epidemiology

- Herpes zoster ophthalmicus is caused by reactivation of latent varicella zoster virus. VZV also causes chicken pox and shingles.

- Over 90% of adults have been exposed to VZV.

- Exposure to affected individuals, increasing age, and immunosuppression are important risk factors for VZV reactivation.

- Iridocyclitis occurs in approximately 40% to 60% cases of herpes zoster ophthalmicus.

- The lifetime risk of reactivation is 10% to 20%.

Symptoms

- Onset of the disease may be preceded by a flu-like illness with malaise, nausea, and mild fever, along with progressive pain, skin hyperesthesia, and tingling.

- Within a few hours or days after onset of symptoms, a diffuse erythematous or maculopapular rash presenting over a single dermatome appears. It progresses to vesicles and pustules, which rupture and form crusts within 3 to 5 days.

- The uveitis usually starts 1 to 2 weeks after onset of the rash. Patients can develop foreign-body sensations, eye pain, decreased vision, and/or photophobia.

Signs

- Decreased visual acuity, increased intraocular pressure, and miosis

- Hutchinson's sign is a unilateral vesicular rash along the nasociliary branch of trigeminal nerve distribution

- Anterior chamber cells and flare, granular infiltrates in the anterior corneal stroma, pseudodendrites, keratitis, ciliary injection, and corneal edema may occur (Figs. 3-15 and 3-16).

- Sector iris stromal atrophy is a specific sign of herpetic keratouveitis.

- Mucous plaque keratopathy can occur late in the disease course.

- Patients may also develop rash and vesicles on the eyelids along with conjunctivitis, retinal necrosis, and optic nerve involvement.

- Compared to HSV, slit-lamp examination may reveal dendrites that are slightly elevated, broader, and have less regular branching; there are fewer terminal end bulbs, and there is less central rose bengal staining. Fluorescein pools along the edge.

Differential Diagnosis

- Bacterial, viral, fungal, or allergic conjunctivitis, acute angle-closure glaucoma, iritis or scleritis, corneal abrasion, recurrent corneal erosion, or toxic conjunctivitis

Diagnostic Evaluation

- The diagnosis is made clinically, and no laboratory tests are routinely ordered, although PCR can be helpful in certain cases.

Treatment

- Systemic antivirals: Immunocompetent patients (>50 years of age) with keratouveitis should be treated with:

  - Acyclovir 800 mg PO five times per day for 10 to 14 days or

  - Valacyclovir 1 g t.i.d. PO for 7 to 10 days or

  - Famciclovir 500 mg PO q8h for 7 to 10 days

  - Patients with recurrent disease may benefit from long-term therapy.

- Antivirals are typically used for primary disease within the first week of onset.

- Topical steroids: Prednisolone acetate 1% q.i.d. on a gradually tapering regimen should be administered concomitantly with antiviral agents. Strong evidence exists for improved quality of life with a combination of an anti-viral medication and topical steroid; however, not all patients are candidates.

- Cycloplegic agents such as scopolamine 0.25% t.i.d. should be used.

- Increased intraocular pressure should be aggressively managed with aqueous suppressants including timolol 0.5% b.i.d., brimonidine 0.2% t.i.d., and dorzolamide 2% t.i.d.

Prognosis

- Most VZV infections respond to antiviral treatment and/or steroids.

- Complications depend on severity of the eye disease as well as patient characteristics. Potential complications of VZV infection include dry eye, corneal neovascularization and scarring, cataract formation, corneal ulcer formation, bacterial or fungal infection, secondary glaucoma, postherpetic neuralgia or vision loss arising from optic neuritis or chorioretinitis.

- Immunocompetent patients may benefit from the herpes virus vaccination, as it can reduce the incidence of herpes zoster.

REFERENCES

Cobo LM, Foulks GN, Liesegang T, et al. Oral acyclovir in the treatment of acute herpes zoster ophthalmicus. *Ophthalmology.* 1986;93(6):763–770.

Gnann JW, Whitley RJ. Herpes zoster. *N Engl J Med.* 2002;347(5):340–346.

Tseng HF, Smith N, Harpaz R, et al. Herpes zoster vaccine in older adults and the risk of subsequent herpes zoster disease. *JAMA.* 2011 12;305(2):160–166.

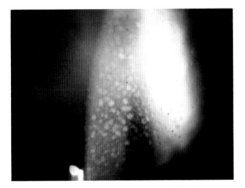

FIGURE 3-15. Granulomatous uveitis from herpes zoster. Both herpes zoster and herpes simplex can cause a granulomatous uveitis. Both can also create nongranulomatous uveitis and produce spine-like keratic precipitates called stellate keratic precipitates (not shown). Isolated uveitis from HSV or HZV in the absence of cornea disease is rare but can occur.

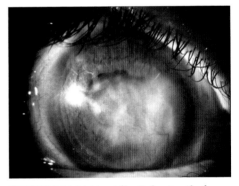

FIGURE 3-16. Lipid and fibrotic keratopathy from severe herpes zoster ophthalmicus. These are late-stage complications of herpes zoster ophthalmicus that occur after multiple episodes of inflammation and typically take years to develop.

MOOREN'S ULCER

Joseph R. Zelefsky and
Emmett T. Cunningham, Jr. ▪

Mooren's ulcer is a rare, progressive, inflammatory keratopathy characterized by severe pain, conjunctival and episcleral injection, and peripheral corneal ulceration without loss of adjacent sclera.

Epidemiology and Etiology

● Mooren's ulcer is most commonly seen in the developing world, particularly in Western Africa and India.

● Men are affected more often than women.

● It can develop in both young and old patients. To a large extent, age at presentation varies by region. It can affect one or both eyes.

● Risk factors include prior corneal trauma or surgery, previous corneal infection, and concurrent intestinal hookworm infestation.

● Patients with the HLA-DR17 haplotype have an increased risk of developing Mooren's ulcer, and both cell-mediated and humoral immune-mediated mechanisms antibodies have been suggested.

Symptoms

● Severe pain

● Photophobia

● Tearing

● Decreased vision

Signs

● Conjunctival and episcleral injection in the absence of scleral injection.

● Ulceration may follow three specific patterns (Fig. 3-17):

▪ **Partial peripheral:** Peripheral ulceration of most, but not all, of the cornea, characterized by deep vessels extending into the ulcer bed from the limbus, and an

overhanging and frequently opacified "leading edge" (Fig. 3-18)

▪ **Complete peripheral:** Extensive peripheral ulceration leaving a central island of corneal tissue

▪ **Total corneal ulceration:** Complete loss of all stromal tissue, which leaves a residual fibrovascular membrane overlying an intact Descemet's membrane.

● Bilateral involvement occurs in up to 50% of patients.

● Corneal perforation occurs in up to 15% of cases and tends to occur most frequently in patients with the complete peripheral pattern of ulceration.

Differential Diagnosis

● Peripheral ulcerative keratopathy (secondary to rheumatoid arthritis, Wegener's granulomatosis, polyarteritis nodosa, systemic lupus erythematosus, and relapsing polychondritis)

● Ocular rosacea

● Infectious keratitis

● Terrien's marginal degeneration

Diagnostic Evaluation

● Review of systems and laboratory tests to rule out underlying rheumatologic diseases (e.g., rheumatoid factor, ANCA, ANA, HSV) and for hookworm infestation are useful. There are no tests specific for Mooren's ulcer.

● Although earlier work suggested an association with hepatitis C, more recent work found no such association.

Treatment

● Aggressive immunosuppressive therapy is the mainstay of treatment.

● Initially, patients may be treated with topical corticosteroids, acetylcysteine, or topical cyclosporine.

● Most patients require systemic therapy including corticosteroids and one or more noncorticosteroid immunosuppressive agents.

- In recalcitrant cases, surgical interventions such as limbal conjunctival excision have been employed with varying degrees of success, and corneal or scleral patch grafts may be necessary in cases with corneal perforation. (Fig. 3-19).

Prognosis

- The prognosis is generally variable and likely depends on how quickly and aggressively therapy is initiated.

- A recent large cohort study reported that less than 15% of patients maintained 20/40 vision or better.

REFERENCES

Chow C, Foster CS. Mooren's ulcer. *Int Ophthalmol Clin.* 1996;36:1–13.

Srinivasan M, Zegans ME, Zelefsky JR, et al. Clinical characteristics of Mooren's ulcer in South India. *Br J Ophthalmol.* 2007;91:570–575.

Tandon R, Chawla B, Verma K, et al. Outcome of treatment of Mooren ulcer with topical cyclosporine a 2%. *Cornea.* 2008;27(8):859–861.

Watson PG. Management of Mooren's ulcer. *Eye.* 1997; 11:349–356.

Zegans ME, Srinivasan M, McHugh T, et al. Mooren ulcer in South India: serology and clinical risk factors. *Am J Ophthalmol.* 1999;128(2):205–210.

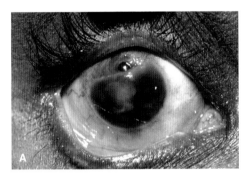
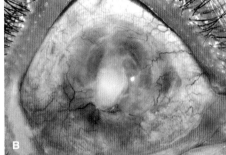
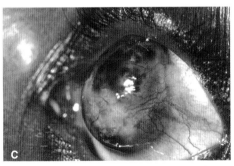

FIGURE 3-17. The clinical spectrum of Mooren's ulcer. **A.** Partial peripheral Mooren's ulcer showing conjunctival and episcleral injection, with ulceration up to, but sparing, the sclera, with deep vessels in the ulcer bed, and an overhanging and opacified central ulcer margin. There is a small descemetocele within the ulcer. **B.** A total peripheral Mooren's ulcer with a central island of edematous, opacified cornea. **C.** Complete Mooren's ulcer with loss of all stromal tissue, replaced here with a fibrovascular membrane overlying an intact Descemet's membrane. (Reproduced with permission from Srinivasan M, Zegans ME, Zelefsky JR, et al. Clinical characteristics of Mooren's ulcer in South India. *Br J Ophthalmol.* 2007; 91:570–575, with permission from BMJ Publishing Group Ltd.)

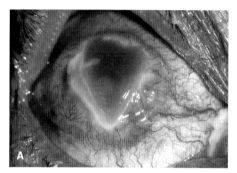
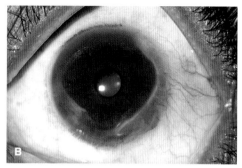

FIGURE 3-18. A. Active Mooren's ulcer showing extensive peripheral ulceration, vascularization of the ulcerated bed, and overhang of the active leading edge. **B.** Inactive Mooren's ulcer in a different patient has residual corneal thinning with persistent vascularization of the ulcer bed and opacification of the leading edge.

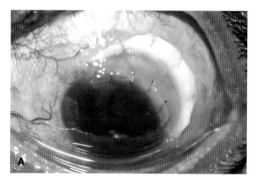
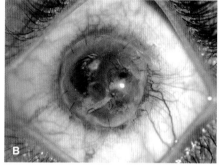

FIGURE 3-19. A. A tectonic patch graft was used to treat peripheral perforation in a patient with Mooren's ulcer. **B.** A total tectonic graft used to treat central perforation in a patient with complete Mooren's ulcer.

PERIPHERAL ULCERATIVE KERATITIS

Roxana Ursea

Peripheral ulcerative keratitis (PUK) is an ocular inflammatory condition with potentially devastating consequences. It is often associated with a coexisting systemic collagen vascular disease, but it may also be due to an infectious etiology.

Pathophysiology

● The periphery of the cornea has unique anatomic and physiologic characteristics that predispose it to involvement in autoimmune and inflammatory conditions.

  ▪ The limbus and peripheral cornea are adjacent to the highly vascular conjunctiva and derive part of their nutrient supply from the capillary arcades. The conjunctiva is rich in immunocompetent cells, including macrophages, lymphocytes, and plasma cells, and these cells have easy access to the peripheral cornea.

  ▪ The peripheral cornea also has a high concentration of Langerhans cells, which are involved in antigen presentation and secretion of inflammatory mediators. This leads to recruitment of inflammatory cells and mediators with subsequent release of proteases and collagenases that result in peripheral corneal stromal degradation, necrosis, and ulceration.

  ▪ The release of these keratolytic enzymes is dysregulated; the matrix metalloprotease-2, (member of a family of enzymes involved in the degradation of extracellular matrix) is overexpressed.

  ▪ The conjunctival lymphatic drainage begins at the limbus.

  ▪ The limbal vessels terminate at the peripheral cornea, which affects the diffusion of high-molecular-weight molecules. This facilitates the deposition of immune complexes, IgM, and C1, which further contributes to the immunologic activity and inflammatory response.

Etiology

● Systemic diseases (noninfectious): Collagen vascular diseases are responsible for approximately 50% of noninfectious cases of PUK.

  ▪ Rheumatoid arthritis is the most commonly associated condition.

  ▪ Other commonly associated diseases are Wegener's granulomatosis, relapsing polychondritis, polyarteritis nodosa, microscopic polyangiitis, Churg-Strauss syndrome, and systemic lupus erythematosus

  ▪ Rarely: Crohn's disease and temporal arteritis are associated with PUK.

● Secondary to infection: Organisms that can cause PUK include *Staphylococcus* and *Streptococcus* species (the most common pathogens), *Pseudomonas, Acanthamoeba, Neisseria* species, gram-negative bacilli, tuberculosis, syphilis, and human immunodeficiency virus (HIV).

  ▪ Mooren's ulcer is a subtype of PUK that is idiopathic and, by definition, occurs without scleral involvement and in the absence of any systemic findings. Mooren's ulcer is a diagnosis of exclusion made only after the presence of collagen vascular disease or infectious causes have been ruled out.

Symptoms

● Ocular pain and redness (typical presentation)

● Tearing, photophobia, and decreased visual acuity (due to corneal opacity or astigmatism)

Signs

- A crescent-shaped corneal ulcer found within 2 mm of the limbus is the typical lesion

- There is often an epithelial defect overlying the ulcer with thinning of the underlying stroma.

- There can be a stromal infiltrate followed by progressive corneal thinning (also known as "corneal melt") (Fig. 3-20).

- Descemetocele formation leading to perforation rarely occurs.

- One third of patients have associated scleritis.

Diagnostic Evaluation

- A thorough history and examination is the most important part of the workup.

- Cultures of the ulcer should be considered.

- Evaluation for underlying systemic diseases, including testing for serum antibodies should be considered.

- Occasionally a corneal biopsy is needed to establish the diagnosis.

Differential Diagnosis

- Conditions that lead to peripheral corneal thinning or scarring include Terrien's marginal ulceration, corneal degeneration, pellucid marginal degeneration, phlyctenulosis, trachomatous pannus, marginal keratitis, rosacea keratitis, and vernal keratoconjunctivitis.

- Local insults that lead to peripheral corneal pathology include poor-fitting contact lenses, corneal exposure, trichiasis, keratoconjunctivitis sicca, and meibomian gland dysfunction.

Treatment

- The goal of treatment is to halt progressive corneal ulceration, preserve globe integrity, encourage healing of the epithelial defect, and address the underlying cause.

- If PUK is secondary to an infectious etiology, patients should be treated with medications appropriate for the offending agent.

- If PUK is associated with systemic disease, patients should be treated with systemic immunosuppressive therapy.

- The choice of cytotoxic agent depends on the underlying disease.

  - If vision loss is imminent, pulsed, short-term IV methylprednisolone should be administered.

  - If patients have underlying rheumatoid arthritis, systemic corticosteroids plus and agent such as methotrexate can be effective.

  - Wegener's granulomatosis and polyarteritis nodosa should be treated with systemic corticosteroids and another medication such as mycophenolate mofetil. Azathioprine, cyclosporine A, and chlorambucil have also been used with variable efficacy depending on the underlying collagen vascular disease.

  - Consider reserving agents with higher toxicity, such as cyclophosphamide, for cases with therapeutic failure, drug intolerance, or rapidly progressive disease.

- If no underlying systemic disease is found, consider topical drops or surgery. Drops include:

  - Inhibitors of collagenase synthesis (i.e., 1% medroxyprogesterone drops)

  - Competitive inhibitors of collagenase (i.e., topical 20% N-acetylcysteine and systemic tetracycline)

  - Lubricating agents should promote epithelial healing.

- Surgical management is primarily used in cases of impending perforation in order to preserve globe integrity.

  - Conjunctival resection decreases conjunctival production of proteases and collagenases and reduces local access of immune cells and inflammatory mediators to the peripheral cornea.

▣ Ulcer debridement and application of cyanoacrylate adhesive may be beneficial.

▣ Tissue adhesive can be used to prevent further stromal loss by excluding acute inflammatory cells from the cornea. It has been successfully used in cases of impending perforation.

▣ Continuous-wear bandage soft contact lens may help prevent perforation.

▣ Lamellar or penetrating keratoplasty generally carry a poor prognosis. Graft failure due to a recurrent melt occurs in 80% of eyes by 6 months after penetrating keratoplasty.

▣ Superior forniceal advancement of a conjunctival pedicle in conjunction with systemic immunosuppressive therapy has been used with some success in recent case reports.

● PUK *refractory* to conventional therapies should be treated with a tumor necrosis factor-alpha inhibitor such as infliximab or adalimumab or rituximab, which is an anti-CD20 antibody.

Prognosis

● The finding of PUK in the setting of systemic disease is extremely significant, as it can serve as a marker for the presence of a potentially lethal systemic vasculitis. The progression is rapid and visual loss can occur over a matter of days. The most feared ocular complication is corneal perforation (corneal melt), which can result in abrupt and permanent loss of vision.

● Topical glucocorticoids are contraindicated. They may further aggravate the disease process and produce accelerated corneal melting through inhibition of collagen synthesis.

● Local treatment of PUK alone without simultaneous systemic treatment will almost invariably fail. Cytotoxic agents not only improve the systemic disease but have also been shown to improve graft survival in patients with rheumatoid arthritis.

REFERENCES

Galor A, Thorne JE. Scleritis and peripheral ulcerative keratitis. *Rheum Dis Clin N Am.* 2007;33:835–854.

Ladas JG, Mondino BJ. Systemic disorders associated with peripheral corneal ulceration. *Curr Opin Ophthalmol.* 2000;11:468–471.

Messmer EM, Foster CS. Vasculitic peripheral ulcerative keratitis. *Surv Ophthalmol.* 1999;43(5):379–396.

Sainz de la Maza M, Foster CS, Jabbur NS, et al. Ocular characteristics and disease associations in scleritis-associated peripheral keratopathy. *Arch Ophthalmol.* 2002;120(1):15–19.

Tauber J, Sainz de la Maza M, Hoang-Xuan T, et al. An analysis of therapeutic decision making regarding immunosuppressive chemotherapy for peripheral ulcerative keratitis. *Cornea.* 1990;9(1):66–73.

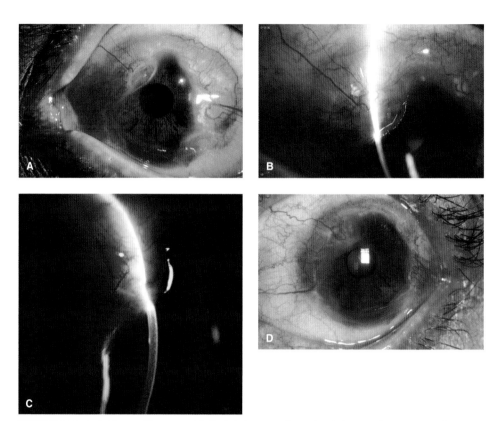

FIGURE 3-20. A. A 39-year-old woman with Crohn's disease and peripheral ulcerative keratitis. Note the circumferential pannus with injected conjunctival vessels and active PUK with a "bullous-like" lesion in the peripheral cornea. **B and C.** Residual thinning in the area of inflammation after the resolution of active inflammation. **D.** The same patient has 360 degrees of pannus after multiple episodes of PUK.

CHAPTER

4

Anterior Uveitis

HUMAN LEUCOCYTE ANTIGEN B27–ASSOCIATED UVEITIS

Julie Gueudry and Bahram Bodaghi

Anterior uveitis constitutes up to 75% of all cases of uveitis and human leucocyte antigen (HLA)-B27–associated uveitis is the most commonly diagnosed cause of acute anterior uveitis. This haplotype is frequently associated with systemic diseases such as ankylosing spondylitis, inflammatory bowel disease, reactive arthritis, psoriatic arthritis, and undifferentiated spondyloarthropathies. This group of diseases is also referred to as seronegative spondyloarthropathies ("seronegative" meaning negative rheumatoid factor, and "spondylo" meaning spine).

Etiology and Epidemiology

- Genetic, geographic, and environmental factors are involved.
- The prevalence of HLA-B27 is 5% to 8% in Western populations. HLA-B27 is less frequent in nonwhite populations.

- The lifetime cumulative incidence of acute anterior uveitis is 0.2% in the general population, but increases to 1% in the HLA-B27–positive population.
- Depending upon the population studied, the HLA-B27 haplotype accounts for 40% to 70% of cases of acute anterior uveitis.
- More than half of the patients with an HLA-B27–associated acute anterior uveitis present with an associated systemic disease.
- HLA-B27–associated uveitis has been thought to be more common in males than in females, but recent work has called this into question.
- It more commonly occurs in younger people.
- The risk of developing spondyloarthritis or uveitis in a B27-positive patient is 25%.
- In patients with spondyloarthropathy, the prevalence of uveitis is as high as 32.7%.

Symptoms

- Sudden onset of redness, pain, photophobia, and blurred vision.
- Associated systemic complaints may include low back pain, arthritis, psoriasis, oral ulcers, chronic diarrhea, and urethritis.

Signs

- Most commonly, patients have acute and/or recurrent episodes of uveitis, usually lasting several days to weeks. However, it may be chronic in 25% of cases.

- Rarely are both eyes simultaneously inflamed.

- Fine keratic precipitates (KPs) and endothelial dusting occur, but the uveitis is always nongranulomatous.

- Severe anterior chamber reaction with fibrin can occur, and a hypopyon is common and is associated with disease severity (Figs. 4-1 and 4-2).

- A fibrin net may form across the pupillary margin.

- Posterior synechiae are frequently present.

- Posterior segment involvement is underrecognized, even though vitritis, vasculitis, papillitis, and macular edema may occur, especially in chronic, undertreated cases.

SERONEGATIVE SPONDYLOARTHROPATHIES
(Figs. 4-3 to 4-7)

- Ankylosing spondylitis is a chronic arthritis that mainly affects the spine and sacroiliac joints.

  - The major symptoms are lower back pain and stiffness.

  - 90% of patients are HLA-B27–positive.

  - Uveitis may be the first manifestation of the disease and may occur prior to onset of joint pain.

  - Nonsteroidal anti-inflammatory medications and physical therapy are the mainstays of treatment. Methotrexate and anti-TNF agents have also been successfully used.

- Reactive arthritis syndrome (Reiter's syndrome)

  - The classic triad is papillary conjunctivitis, urethritis, and polyarthritis ("can't see,

can't pee, can't climb a tree"). However, these symptoms may be mild or absent.

  - Anterior uveitis is usually less common (10% of cases).

  - Most of the patients are young male adults.

  - The HLA-B27 positivity rate is 60%.

  - Bacteria such as *Chlamydia, Salmonella, Yersinia,* and *Shigella* have been associated with the disease, and may trigger the disease in a susceptible patient, however their role remains controversial.

  - Keratoderma blennorrhagicum (scaling skin), circinate balanitis (rash around the penis), aphthous stomatitis, plantar fasciitis, and uncommonly iritis are additional diagnostic criteria.

- Inflammatory bowel disease (IBD)

  - Ulcerative colitis and Crohn's disease are the main diagnostic entities.

  - The risk of developing uveitis is up to five times higher in patients with ulcerative colitis than those with Crohn's disease.

  - Patients with IBD who develop uveitis may develop sacroiliitis and are HLA-B27 positive in 60% of cases.

  - Patients may also have erythema nodosum and pyoderma gangrenosum.

  - Behçet's disease and Whipple's disease are the main differential diagnoses to consider.

- Psoriatic arthritis

  - One-fifth of patients with psoriatic arthritis may develop sacroiliitis.

  - Patients present with cutaneous, joint, and ungual involvement.

    - The typical skin lesions are elevated, well-circumscribed plaques.

    - Patients may have central arthritis affecting the spine, or distal arthritis affecting the fingers. In advanced cases, patients may have "sausage digit deformity."

▶ Nail changes include nail pitting, ridging, and discoloration can occur.

- ▪ The rate of uveitis in patients with psoriatic arthritis is 25%.

- ▪ Uveitis in this subgroup of patients has some specific characteristics such as bilaterality, chronicity, and severity.

- ▪ Posterior segment involvement (CME, retinal vasculitis, and papillitis) is not uncommon.

- Undifferentiated spondyloarthropathies

- ▪ There is an HLA-B27 positivity rate of 25%, and uveitis occurs somewhat less frequently in this group.

Differential Diagnosis

- Idiopathic anterior uveitis
- Sarcoidosis
- Other nongranulomatous uveitis

- ▪ Behçet's disease–associated uveitis

- ▪ Infectious uveitis (herpetic uveitis, syphilis, Lyme disease, Whipple's disease, or infectious endophthalmitis)

- ▪ Drug-induced uveitis: rifabutin, biphosphonates, prostaglandin analogues, and cidofovir

- ▪ Tubulointerstitial nephritis and uveitis (TINU)

- ▪ Lens-induced uveitis

- ▪ Masquerade syndromes (retinoblastoma and metastatic tumors)

Diagnostic Evaluation

- HLA-B27 typing
- ESR, C-reactive protein
- Work-up to rule out items on the differential diagnosis, including serum angiotensin-converting enzyme (ACE), chest radiograph, Lyme titer, VDRL/RPR/FTA-Abs, tuberculin skin test

- If indicated:

- ▫ MRI of the sacroiliac joint and lumbar spine

- ▫ Swab for chlamydia, *Shigella*, *Yersinia*, and other gram-negative bacteria.

- ▫ Specialized consultations: rheumatology, gastrointestinal, dermatology, and infectious disease

Treatment

- Cycloplegic and mydriatic drops will relieve pain and break posterior synechiae.

- Topical corticosteroids are the mainstay of treatment for ocular disease and usually need to be administered every hour for the first 48 hours, then slowly tapered.

- If the uveitis is severe, subconjunctival injections of dexamethasone can be considered daily for 3 consecutive days. Sub-Tenon's triamcinolone injection can also be used.

- If there is no improvement on topical/periocular steroids, systemic corticosteroids and/or systemic immunosuppressive agents may be proposed.

- Systemic NSAIDs may decrease the recurrence rate as well as exposure to corticosteroids.

- Anti-TNF-α treatment may be useful in treatment-resistant and/or sight-threatening cases.

- Prophylactic treatment using sulfasalazine remains controversial.

Prognosis

- Generally favorable with aggressive therapy

- Uveitis often recurs and may become chronic. Presence of chronic inflammation is the main prognostic factor.

- Posterior iris synechiae, band keratopathy, posterior subcapsular cataract, ocular hypertension, hypotony, cystoid macular edema, and epiretinal membrane formation are the major complications.

REFERENCES

Braun J, Baraliakos X, Listing J, et al. Decreased incidence of anterior uveitis in patients with ankylosing spondylitis treated with the anti-tumor necrosis factor agents infliximab and etanercept. *Arthritis Rheum.* 2005; 52(8):2447–2451.

Chang JH, McCluskey PJ, Wakefield D. Acute anterior uveitis and HLA-B27. *Surv Ophthalmol.* 2005;50:364–388.

Durrani K, Foster CS. Psoriatic uveitis: a distinct clinical entity? *Am J Ophthalmol.* 2005;139:106–111.

Loh AR, Acharya NR. Incidence rates and risk factors for ocular complications and vision loss in HLA-B27-associated uveitis. *Am J Ophthalmol.* 2010;150: 534–542.

Zamecki KJ, Jabs DA. HLA typing in uveitis: use and misuse. *Am J Ophthalmol.* 2010;149(2):189–193.

Zeboulon N, Dougados M, Gossec L. Prevalence and characteristics of uveitis in the spondyloarthropathies: a systematic literature review. *Ann Rheum Dis.* 2008;67: 955–959.

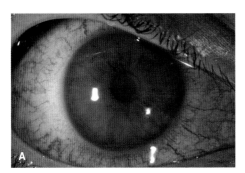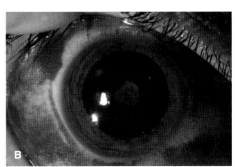

FIGURE 4-1. A. Slit-lamp photograph shows severe acute anterior uveitis with fibrin in the anterior chamber and 360 degrees of posterior synechiae in a patient with reactive arthritis. **B.** Remission occurred with maximal topical corticosteroids, cycloplegic and subconjunctival injection of dexamethasone each day for 3 days.

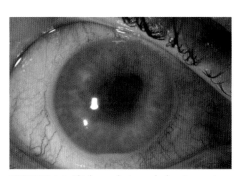

FIGURE 4-2. Slit-lamp photograph showing acute anterior uveitis with fibrin in the anterior chamber and a hypopyon in a patient who is HLA-B27 positive with ankylosing spondylitis.

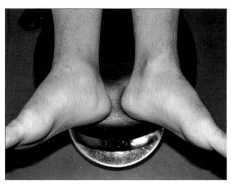

FIGURE 4-3. Right ankle arthritis in a patient with ankylosing spondylitis.

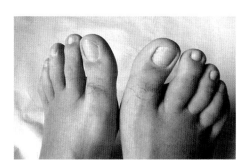

FIGURE 4-4. Sausage toes of the right foot in a case of seronegative spondyloarthritis. (Courtesy of P. Quartier.)

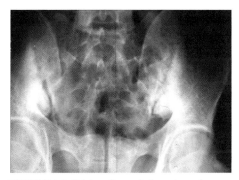

FIGURE 4-5. Pelvis radiograph shows irregular margins and sclerosis of the sacroiliac joints. (Courtesy of P. Quartier.)

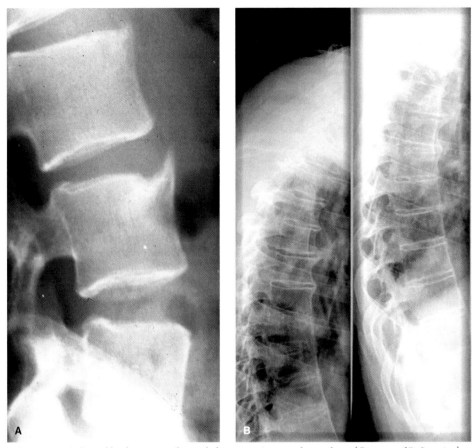

FIGURE 4-6. **A.** Lateral lumbar spine radiograph demonstrating a syndesmophyte. (Courtesy of P. Quartier.) **B.** This person has vertical syndesmophytes on multiple vertebrae causing a "bamboo spine." (Courtesy of V. Vuillemin.)

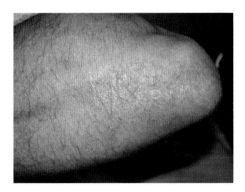

FIGURE 4-7. Plaque psoriasis on the elbow of a patient with HLA-B27–associated uveitis and psoriatic arthritis.

POSNER-SCHLOSSMAN SYNDROME

Bahram Bodaghi

The Posner-Schlossman syndrome (PSS), also known as recurrent glaucomatocyclitic crisis syndrome, is an unusual clinical entity that occurs in young to middle-aged adults. Initially considered an immune-mediated condition, it may be due to a viral infection.

Epidemiology

- It predominantly occurs in young to middle-aged patients but it may also be diagnosed in the elderly.
- There seems to be a clear male preponderance.
- The disease remains rare but must be considered in all cases of unilateral uveitis associated with high intraocular pressure (IOP).

Etiology

- Since its initial description in 1948, there has been much speculation regarding its pathogenesis. Despite lack of evidence, developmental abnormalities of the angle, allergic factors, primary vascular abnormalities, sympathetic nervous system defects, and inflammatory mechanisms have all been proposed as possible mechanisms for this disorder.
- Recent data based on specific intraocular antibody production and molecular biology suggest cytomegalovirus infection as the inciting agent in PSS.

Symptoms

- Patients present with moderate blurred vision, often due to mild corneal edema secondary to an acute rise in IOP.
- It is almost always unilateral with recurrent attacks in the same eye.
- Patients may experience very mild pain or discomfort.

Signs

- Mild decrease in vision
- Dilated conjunctival vessels
- White keratic precipitates of different sizes predominantly located at the central cornea (Fig. 4-8)
- Minimal aqueous flare without cells
- Posterior synechiae are not present.
- The IOP is markedly elevated, ranging from 40 to 60 mm Hg.
- The angle is open, although anterior synechiae may be present.
- There is usually no iris heterochromia.
- Vitritis is absent and there is no posterior segment involvement.
- Between the attacks, the examination is unremarkable (with the exception of glaucomatous optic atrophy).

Differential Diagnosis

- CMV-induced anterior uveitis
- Herpetic anterior uveitis
- Atypical cases of Fuchs' iridocyclitis
- Nonspecific hypertensive iridocyclitis
- Sarcoidosis
- Tuberculosis
- Multiple sclerosis

Diagnostic Evaluation

- An anterior chamber tap may be performed for viral PCR and analysis of specific antibody production, confirming the presence of CMV.
- Visual field testing and/or retinal nerve fiber layer analysis can be used to identify glaucomatous visual field abnormalities that may occur in severe or recurrent forms of the disease.
- Ancillary tests to exclude other causes of unilateral uveitis and secondary glaucoma should be performed as clinically indicated.

Treatment

- Treatment to lower the IOP is usually required during attacks in order to protect the optic disc.

- Before the identification of PSS as a viral disorder, many authors found the use of short-term topical corticosteroids useful.

- In CMV-associated PSS, specific antiviral therapy with topical or systemic drugs may be initiated.

- The duration of antiviral therapy depends on the clinical presentation and the severity of visual field alteration. In severe cases with high clinical suspicion, a 2- to 3-month regimen may be considered.

- Cycloplegic agents are not required.

- Filtering surgery is usually not recommended but may be successfully used to treat glaucoma that progresses despite maximum medical therapy.

Prognosis

- Generally speaking, recurrences decrease with increasing age, so the visual prognosis is usually good.

- However, in the absence of specific ocular antihypertensive medications or surgery, permanent visual loss may occur in approximately 25% of cases due to chronic ocular hypertension.

REFERENCES

Bloch-Michel E, Dussaix E, Cerqueti P, et al. Possible role of cytomegalovirus in the etiology of Posner-Schlossman syndrome. *Int Ophthalmol.* 1987;11:95–96.

Chee SP, Bacsal K, Jap A, et al. Clinical features of cytomegalovirus anterior uveitis in immunocompetent patients. *Am J Ophthalmol.* 2008;145(5):834–840.

Posner A, Schlossman A. Treatment of glaucoma associated with iridocyclitis. *JAMA.* 1949; 139:82–86.

Teoh SB, Thean L, Koay E. Cytomegalovirus in aetiology of Posner-Schlossman syndrome: evidence from quantitative polymerase chain reaction. *Eye (Lond).* 2005; 19(12):1338–1340.

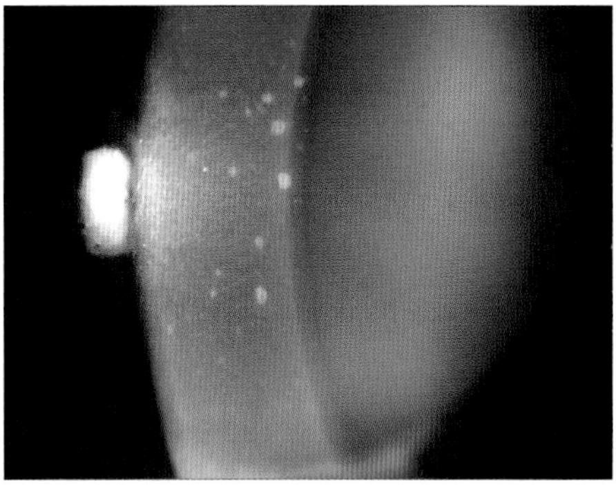

FIGURE 4-8. Typical white keratic precipitates that are most concentrated in the central cornea in a case of CMV-induced Posner-Schlossman syndrome.

FUCHS' UVEITIS SYNDROME (FUCHS' HETEROCHROMIC IRIDOCYCLITIS)

Bahram Bodaghi and Phuc LeHoang

In 1906, Ernst Fuchs described the clinical characteristics of a series of 38 patients with a previously undescribed condition that now bears his name. Usually considered a benign disease, the diagnosis of Fuchs' uveitis syndrome (FUS) may be challenging, leading to the misuse of corticosteroids, which can result in further complications. Recent studies have highlighted the role of a viral agent in the pathogenesis of FUS, expanding the spectrum of viral-induced anterior uveitis.

Epidemiology

- The prevalence of the disease varies from 1.2% to 5% of patients with uveitis.

- The disease affects men and women equally and has no racial predilection, even though it may be more difficult to recognize in individuals with brown eyes.

- FUS generally occurs in young adults.

Etiology and Pathogenesis

- Different theories have been proposed to explain the pathogenesis of this disease.

- Studies on HLA associations and other genetic factors have been contradictory.

- Due to the common clinical features observed in patients with congenital Horner's syndrome, a congenital paralysis of the sympathetic system was considered, but convincing evidence is lacking.

- Based on different immunologic findings it was thought to be an immune-mediated disorder triggered by some inciting event.

- The infectious theory has always been preferred. As chorioretinal scars are observed in 33% to 56% of patients with FUS, it was initially thought to be related to a *Toxoplasma* infection.

- However, compelling evidence suggesting infection with *Rubella* virus in patients with FUS has been recently reported.

Symptoms

- Patients usually have minimal symptoms, and the disease is usually discovered during a routine eye examination.

- Floaters are the main complaint of patients with FUS.

- Visual loss occurs late in the disease course and is usually due to cataract progression.

- The patient may note heterochromia (Fig. 4-9).

Signs

- FUS is a chronic, anterior, granulomatous uveitis with vitreous involvement.

- FUS is mainly unilateral (90% of cases) with a long, insidious course.

- Careful bilateral slit-lamp examination is important. Importantly, ciliary injection and posterior synechiae are never present and should be viewed as exclusion criteria.

- Keratic precipitates (KP) are present in most cases and are typically small, white, and stellate, and are scattered over the entire corneal endothelium (Fig. 4-10). They are never confluent. In most other diseases, KPs are more prominent on the inferior cornea. The other condition that can cause diffuse KPs is herpetic iridocyclitis.

- Heterochromia is a major sign but may be absent in brown-eyed patients. Daylight (or natural light) examination before dilation facilitates the diagnosis.

- Sectoral iris atrophy is not observed in FUS.

- Iris nodules may be observed at the level of the papillary margin (Koeppe nodules) or the iris surface (Busacca nodules).

- Due to iris atrophy, the iris blood vessels are more visible and narrower than in normal eyes.

- Peripheral synechiae and abnormal angle vessels are seen in about 20% to 30% of cases.

- A hyphema may occur with a minor trauma or spontaneously (Amsler's sign).

- Anterior chamber flare and cells are minor.

- Initially, the cataracts are usually posterior subcapsular, but may progress and become hypermature, requiring urgent surgery.

- Secondary glaucoma may occur in two-thirds of cases. This is often due to misuse of topical corticosteroids.

- Vitritis with large cellular aggregates and debris is a typical finding (Fig. 4-11).

- Fundus examination is usually normal even though optic disc hyperfluorescence may be observed on fluorescein angiography. Macular edema is absent in phakic eyes. Small, focal chorioretinal scars may be observed in the periphery.

Differential Diagnosis

- Viral anterior uveitis

- Intermediate uveitis

- Primary intraocular lymphoma

Diagnostic Evaluation

- Often it is a clinical diagnosis. However, ancillary laboratory tests, including PCR, to exclude other etiologies of anterior uveitis can be considered.

- Anterior chamber paracentesis may induce a mild hyphema (Amsler's sign).

- Visual field testing should be performed in cases of suspected glaucoma.

Treatment

- Topical and systemic corticosteroids or immunosuppressants should be avoided.

- Data on the efficacy of topical NSAIDs are controversial.

- Cataract surgery can be performed with an excellent visual outcome, however patients may develop a hyphema. Care should be taken to avoid manipulations of the iris and angle.

- Topical and systemic glaucoma medications are necessary in up to 60% of cases.

- Filtering surgery with adjunctive wound modulators may be considered in resistant cases.

- Vitrectomy is rarely needed to clear vitreous debris and aggregates.

Prognosis

- The prognosis of FUS is usually excellent in the absence of secondary glaucoma.

REFERENCES

Birnbaum AD, Tessler HH, Schultz KL, et al. Epidemiologic relationship between Fuchs heterochromic iridocyclitis and the United States rubella vaccination program. *Am J Ophthalmol.* 2007;144(3):424–428.

Fuchs E. Über Komplicationen der Heterochromic. *Z. Augenheilkd.* 1906;15:191–212.

Liesegang TJ. Clinical features and prognosis in Fuchs' uveitis syndrome. *Arch Ophthalmol.* 1982;100:1622–1626.

Liesegang TJ. Fuchs uveitis syndrome. In: Pepose JS, Holland GN, Wilhelmus KR. *Ocular Infection and Immunity.* St. Louis: Mosby; 1996:495–506.

Quentin CD, Reiber H. Fuchs heterochromic cyclitis: rubella virus antibodies and genome in aqueous humor. *Am J Ophthalmol.* 2004;138(1):46–54.

Van Gelder RN. Idiopathic no more: clues to the pathogenesis of Fuchs heterochromic iridocyclitis and glaucomatocyclitic crisis. *Am J Ophthalmol.* 2008;145:769–771.

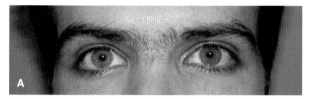 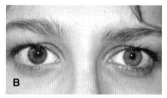

FIGURE 4-9. **A.** Heterochromia in a young male patient with Fuchs' uveitis syndrome of the right eye. **B.** Heterochromia in a young woman with FUS of the left eye.

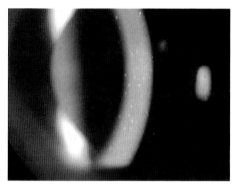 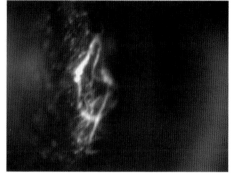

FIGURE 4-10. This patient has the white, small, diffusely distributed stellate keratic precipitates typical of FUS.

FIGURE 4-11. Occasionally, patients with FUS may have vitreous cells and debris.

JUVENILE IDIOPATHIC ARTHRITIS–ASSOCIATED UVEITIS (JUVENILE RHEUMATOID/CHRONIC ARTHRITIS)

Karina Julian and Bahram Bodaghi

Juvenile idiopathic arthritis (JIA) is the main cause of both uveitis and arthritis in children. It is a bilateral, nongranulomatous, chronic anterior uveitis. As it is usually asymptomatic, the diagnosis may be delayed and major visual complications may have already occurred at the time of presentation. Children with JIA must have regular eye exams in order to identify the onset of intraocular inflammation and to initiate effective treatment.

Epidemiology and Etiology

● JIA is defined as arthritis of unknown etiology occurring in children under the age of 16 years and lasting for at least 6 weeks. Seven subgroups of the disease have been defined. Among them, oligoarthritis (pauciarticular arthritis) is the most commonly associated with uveitis. Oligoarthritis is defined as arthritis affecting 1 to 4 joints within the first 6 months of disease onset, and uveitis may occur in a substantial minority of these patients. The level of activity of the arthritis does not necessarily reflect the level of uveitis.

● Young girls (<4 years old) with oligoarthritis and antinuclear antibodies (ANA+) are at highest risk of developing chronic, asymptomatic, nongranulomatous anterior uveitis, which is the only important extra-articular manifestation of JIA (**Tables 4-1 and 4-2**).

● Pathogenic mechanisms in JIA and JIA-uveitis are not well understood. Ethnic differences, family history, and association with particular human leukocyte antigen (HLA) alleles underscore the possibility of a genetic predisposition to the development of JIA and JIA-uveitis.

● Uveitis most commonly occurs within the first 4 years after joint involvement. Occasionally, the eye and joints may be affected simultaneously or, rarely, the eye disease may precede arthritis.

● Other subgroups of JIA include polyarthritis (RF negative), which affects 5 or more joints. Uveitis occurs in approximately 10% of children in this group. Patients with systemic arthritis (one or more inflamed joints along with rash, lymphadenopathy, hepatomegaly/splenomegaly) rarely develop uveitis.

Symptoms

● Patients are usually asymptomatic until sight-threatening complications develop.

Signs

● Anterior nongranulomatous uveitis of varying intensity (granulomatous uveitis is

TABLE 4-1. Risk Factors for Developing Uveitis in Children with JIA

- Oligoarticular form of JIA
- Young girls
- ANA positivity
- Young age at disease onset

TABLE 4-2. Schedule for Uveitis Screening in Children with JIA

	Onset <7 Years Old	Onset ≥7 Years Old
ANA positive (regardless of pauci- or poly-articular	q3mo	q6mo
ANA negative	q6mo	q6mo
Systemic disease or enthesitis-related arthritis	Annually	Annually

possible, even though rare) in an externally quiet eye (i.e., no prominent ciliary injection)

- Anterior chamber cellular reaction is usually present.

- Keratic precipitates usually do not occur, but endothelial dusting may be present.

- Most patients have a lot of flare, which enhances the development of posterior synechiae and other complications (Fig. 4-12).

- No posterior segment inflammation occurs, but there can be some cells in the anterior vitreous as a result of spill-over from the anterior chamber.

- Maculopathy is present in almost 80% of patients at some point during the disease course. Optical coherence tomography (OCT) shows four different patterns of macular involvement in JIA patients (Fig. 4-13):

  ▪ Perifoveolar thickening

  ▪ Macular edema (diffuse or cystoid)

  ▪ Foveal detachment

  ▪ Atrophic macular changes

- In cases with longstanding inflammation, a cataract may be present at the time of diagnosis or it may develop during the course of the disease.

- Calcific band keratopathy can also occur and suggests chronic inflammation (Fig. 4-14).

- The intraocular pressure may be low (due to ciliary body dysfunction), normal, or high (due to inflammatory mediators or anterior segment anatomic changes associated with chronic inflammation).

- Bilateral involvement is the rule and occurs in 85% of cases. However, after 1 year of unilateral disease, the risk of bilateralization is low.

- Amblyopia may be present.

Differential Diagnosis

- Idiopathic anterior uveitis
- HLA-B27–associated anterior uveitis
- Sarcoidosis

Diagnostic Evaluation

- To confirm the diagnosis, patients should have:

  ▪ The classical clinical picture

  ▪ Nonspecific, low titer ANA positivity

  ▪ HLA-B27 negativity

- Patients with oligoarthritis are almost always rheumatoid factor (RF) negative, but patients with polyarthritis may be RF positive (but they rarely develop uveitis).

- To determine inflammatory status and follow disease progression and response to treatment, the following tests can be considered:

  ▪ Laser flare photometry (LFP), a more reliable technique to measure protein levels in aqueous humor than clinical grading of flare. High measurements correlate positively with development of complications such as posterior synechiae, cataract, and macular edema.

  ▪ Macular scanning with OCT at the time of diagnosis and at regular intervals.

    ▸ Whenever signs of maculopathy are present, anti-inflammatory and immunosuppressive treatment should be intensified.

Treatment (Figs. 4-15 and 4-16)

- Medical

  ▪ Topical corticosteroids can be used with the goal of using the least amount of drops possible to achieve a quiet eye. If drops are needed more than four times a day, systemic treatment should be considered.

  ▪ Methotrexate, a disease-modifying antirheumatic drug (DMARD), is a very effective second-line agent for uveitis control and it should be considered for patients with uveitis regardless of their joint inflammatory status. It can be administered orally or via subcutaneous injections. Side effects included gastrointestinal distress, hepatotoxicity, and bone marrow suppression.

■ Systemic steroids may be an important therapeutic tool for short-term control, but due to its effects on bone growth and development, it is not a long-term solution.

■ Periocular steroid injections can be used in cases of hypotony maculopathy or chronic cystoid macular edema. However, they should be used with caution due to a high incidence of cataract formation in children.

■ Biologic agents or anti-TNF-α therapy

▶ Etanercept: Even though very useful for the control of arthritis, it does not control uveitis well and new onset of uveitis has been reported in children being treated with etanercept. It should be avoided for the treatment of JIA-uveitis.

▶ Infliximab: Often achieves excellent control of the uveitis. There is a concern regarding side effects, including a possible increase in tumor occurrence. It is administrated only by inpatient intravenous infusion.

▶ Adalimumab, a humanized monoclonal anti-TNF-α antibody, is given by a subcutaneous injection. It seems to be highly effective in controlling intraocular inflammation with acceptable mild side effects

▶ Even though anti-TNF drugs may be highly effective for the treatment of uveitis, long-term follow-up is lacking. Patients must be monitored for systemic side effects.

■ Systemic cyclosporine, mycophenolate mofetil, and azathioprine have all been used with variable success.

● Surgical

■ Cataract surgery is performed if the cataracts are visually significant. However, perioperative medical control of the uveitis, ideally for at least 3 months.

Delay in surgery needs to be balanced by the risk of developing amblyopia as well as the risk of increased, intractable inflammation if good preoperative inflammatory control is not achieved. is imperative. Intraocular lens implantation remains controversial and must be avoided in young children or in the absence of long-term immunosuppression.

■ Glaucoma: Control of glaucoma can be challenging in these patients. Trabeculectomy or glaucoma drainage devices often have disappointing long-term results. The best treatment of secondary glaucoma remains controlling the underlying disease in order to avoid onset of intractable glaucoma.

■ Band keratopathy is a common complication. Disodium EDTA chelation is effective.

■ Cystoid macular edema is treated by controlling the underlying disease process. Topical NSAIDS and topical steroids can be used for short periods of time.

Prognosis

● Severity of JIA-associated uveitis varies from a self-limiting disease to one causing bilateral blindness (**Table 4-3**).

● Despite advances in immunosuppressive therapy, visual impairment still occurs, with vision loss to 20/200 or less in 15% of cases and legal blindness in 10% of cases.

TABLE 4-3. Risk Factors Predicting Severity in Children with JIA-Associated Uveitis

- Disease severity at onset
- Short interval between joint and ocular involvement
- Female gender
- Persistent flare in phakic eyes, even in the absence of anterior chamber cellular activity

- Early diagnosis of JIA, early patient referral for slit-lamp examination and universal childhood vision screening is the best strategy for reducing disabilities related to JIA uveitis.

REFERENCES

Davis JL, Dacanay LM, Holland GN, et al. Laser flare photometry and complications of chronic uveitis in children. *Am J Ophthalmol*. 2003;135:763–771.

Ducos de Lahitte G, Terrada C, Tran TH, et al. Maculopathy in uveitis of juvenile idiopathic arthritis: An optical coherence tomography study. *Br J Ophthalmol*. 2008;92:64–69.

Foeldvari I, Nielsen S, Kummerle-Deschner J, et al. Tumor necrosis factor-alpha blocker in treatment of juvenile idiopathic arthritis-associated uveitis refractory to second-line agents: Results of a multinational survey. *J Rheumatol*. 2007;34:1146–1150.

Julian K, Terrada C, Quartier P, et al. Uveitis related to juvenile idiopathic arthritis: Familial cases and possible genetic implication in the pathogenesis. *Ocul Immunol Inflamm*. 2010;18:172–177.

Kump LI, Castaneda RA, Androudi SN, et al. Visual outcomes in children with juvenile idiopathic arthritis-associated uveitis. *Ophthalmology*. 2006;113:1874–1877.

Lam LA, Lowder CY, Baerveldt G, et al. Surgical management of cataracts in children with juvenile rheumatoid arthritis-associated uveitis. *Am J Ophthalmol*. 2003;135:772–778.

Petty RE, Southwood TR, Manners P, et al. International league of associations for rheumatology classification of juvenile idiopathic arthritis: Second revision, Edmonton, 2001. *J Rheumatol*. 2004;31:390–392.

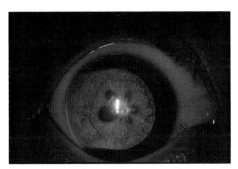

FIGURE 4-12. There are posterior synechiae and a posterior subcapsular cataract in a case with severe anterior uveitis.

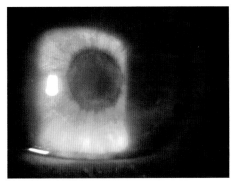

FIGURE 4-14. This child has formation of band keratopathy as well as more extensive posterior synechiae.

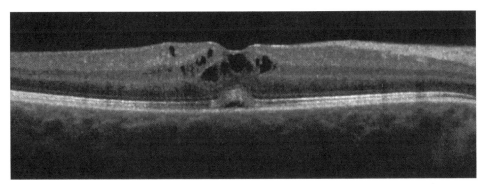

FIGURE 4-13. OCT shows a subfoveal subretinal detachment and cystoid macular edema in a case of severe, chronic JIA uveitis.

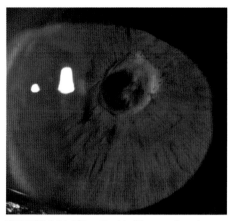

FIGURE 4-15. This patient had been on long-term immunosuppression with good inflammatory control. Although there are large keratic precipitates on the surface of the intraocular lens, the vision remains 20/25.

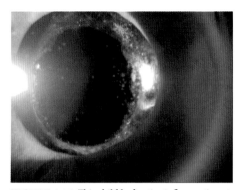

FIGURE 4-16. This child had active inflammation at the time of cataract surgery. There is an early band keratopathy forming. Extensive posterior synechiae and keratic precipitates are present on the intraocular lens.

TUBULOINTERSTITIAL NEPHRITIS AND UVEITIS SYNDROME

Sunir J. Garg

Tubulointerstitial nephritis and uveitis syndrome (TINU) is an acute, idiopathic, bilateral anterior uveitis that occurs along with fever, fatigue, and malaise. It occurs more often in children.

Etiology and Epidemiology

- TINU constitutes up to 2% of all uveitis cases. However, it accounts for up to one-third of cases of acute, bilateral anterior uveitis in patients under age 20.
- In Japan, TINU is the second most frequent diagnosis of childhood uveitis (behind sarcoidosis).
- There is a slight male predominance.
- Generally, the uveitis occurs up to 1 year prior to onset of renal symptoms.

Symptoms

- Patients usually present with sudden onset of bilateral blurry vision, pain, redness, and photophobia.
- These patients often have symptoms of renal insufficiency, including fatigue, fever, malaise, loss of appetite, and weight loss.
- Patients with nephritis may also have mid-back/abdominal pain.

Signs

- Typical of bilateral acute anterior uveitis.
- Most patients have 1 + 1 to 2+ anterior chamber cells.
- Usually the presenting vision is good, and the majority of patients have vision of 20/40 or better, and the vision is rarely worse than 20/100.
- Patients less commonly have optic disk edema, cystoid macular edema, cataract, and posterior synechiae at the time of presentation.
- Older patients have more renal damage at presentation.

Differential Diagnosis

- Systemic lupus erythematosus (SLE): Patients with SLE usually have retinal vasculitis or scleritis.
- Drug-induced nephritis: Usually has an accompanying rash, along with fever and kidney failure.
- Sarcoidosis: Usually has more posterior segment involvement, may be granulomatous, and usually occurs in older people.
- Rheumatoid arthritis: Can cause renal insufficiency, but causes scleritis and dry eye.
- Wegener's granulomatosis: Causes scleritis, keratitis, and orbital inflammation, along with sinus and pulmonary involvement.
- Sjögren's syndrome: Causes tubulointerstitial nephritis. It also causes dry eye but no uveitis.
- Behçet's disease: These patients have an obliterative vasculitis.

Diagnostic Evaluation

- Blood urea nitrogen (BUN) and creatinine levels, CBC for anemia, ESR (sedimentation rate) and C-reactive protein are often elevated, but these are nonspecific.
- Urinalysis looking for proteinuria, hematuria, and pyuria. β_2-microglobulin levels should be specifically ordered. They are elevated in up to 60% of patients with TINU.
- Renal biopsy may be needed to confirm the diagnosis.
- HLA-DRB1*01, HLA-DQA1*01, and HLA-DBQ1*01 are strongly associated with TINU (but are generally not needed).

Treatment

- Most patients with uveitis and normal renal function respond well to topical steroids alone, and treatment beyond 1 year is usually not needed. Patients with more significant ocular and/or renal disease may benefit from judicious use of oral steroids, and some patients may need systemic immunosuppression with mycophenolate mofetil or another steroid-sparing agent.

- Often the renal dysfunction resolves spontaneously. Rarely is the renal function severe enough to require dialysis.

Prognosis

- The majority of patients (70%) will maintain 20/25 vision with normal renal function.

- Fewer than 10% of patients have vision less than 20/40 and/or significant renal impairment.

REFERENCES

Goda C, Kotake S, Ichiishi A, et al. Clinical features in tubulointerstitial nephritis and uveitis (TINU) syndrome. *Am J Ophthalmol.* 2005;140:637–641.

Levinson RD, Park MS, Rikkers SM, et al. Strong associations between specific HLA-DQ and HLA-DR alleles and the tubulointerstitial nephritis and uveitis syndrome. *Invest Ophthalmol Vis Sci.* 2003;44:653–657.

Mackensen F, Billing H. Tubulointerstitial nephritis and uveitis syndrome. *Curr Opin Ophthalmol.* 2009;20(6): 525–531.

Mackensen F, Smith JR, Rosenbaum JT. Enhanced recognition, treatment, and prognosis of tubulointerstitial nephritis and uveitis syndrome. *Ophthalmology.* 2007; 114:995–999.

Mandeville JT, Levinson RD, Holland GN. The tubulointerstitial nephritis and uveitis syndrome. *Surv Ophthalmol.* 2001;46:195–208.

Cataract- and Lens-Induced Uveitis

PHACOANTIGENIC/ PHACOANAPHYLACTIC/ PHACOLYTIC UVEITIS

Somasheila I. Murthy and Swapnali Sabhapandit

Phacoantigenic/phacoanaphylactic uveitis is the result of an immunologic response from disruption of the lens capsule with subsequent release of lens proteins. The clinical diagnosis of phacoanaphylaxis, particularly in an eye with an intraocular lens implant, can be difficult, and on routine examination the condition may be indistinguishable from infectious endophthalmitis. Phacoantigenic uveitis is usually unilateral. The inflammation is predominantly anterior, with zonal granulomatous inflammation centered around the lens material. Traditionally, phacolytic uveitis refers to nongranulomatous inflammation resulting from lens proteins leaking through an intact lens capsule in an eye with a hypermature cataract. All of these entities may represent varying manifestations of a similar disease process and can all be considered lens-induced uveitis.

Etiology and Epidemiology

● It can occur after cataract surgery or trauma, and occasionally occurs spontaneously if there is a hypermature cataract with a leaking capsule.

● The immune system creates inflammation against previously sequestered lens proteins.

Symptoms

● Pain, redness, photophobia, and decreased vision

Signs (Figs. 5-1 to 5-5)

● Circumciliary injection (ciliary flush)

● Corneal edema

● "Mutton fat" keratic precipitates

● Marked flare, abundant cells, lens matter in anterior chamber and/or a hypopyon

● Posterior or peripheral anterior synechiae

● A pupillary membrane

● Irregular lens capsule, opaque lens, intense vitritis

● Glaucoma due to trabeculitis, lens debris in angles or synechiae

- Hypotony due to cyclitic membranes, ciliary shutdown, or choroidal effusion
- Phthisis bulbi

Differential Diagnosis

- Phacolytic glaucoma
- Sympathetic ophthalmia (a bilateral disease)
- Low-grade endophthalmitis (e.g., *Propionibacterium acnes*)
- Bacterial/fungal endophthalmitis

Diagnostic Evaluation

- A high degree of clinical suspicion is important.
- An anterior chamber tap with histopathology may help differentiate lens-induced inflammation from infectious endophthalmitis.
- Histopathology may reveal zonal granulomatous inflammation.

Treatment

- Definitive treatment involves removal of the inciting agent (i.e., the lens or residual lens matter).

- Control of inflammation and glaucoma with corticosteroids and ocular antihypertensive medications is important in order to prevent long-term morbidity.

Prognosis

- There is often a good outcome with prompt and aggressive management.
- If the lens is not promptly removed, complications such as glaucoma, hypotony, macular edema, or macular scarring can lead to visually significant morbidity.

REFERENCES

Kalogeropoulos CD, Malamou-Mitsi VD, Asproudis I, et al. The contribution of aqueous humor cytology in the differential diagnosis of anterior uvea inflammations. *Ocul Immunol Inflamm.* 2004;12(3):215–225.

Thach AB, Marak GE Jr, McLean IW, et al. Phacoanaphylactic endophthalmitis: a clinicopathologic review. *Int Ophthalmol.* 1991;15(4):271–279.

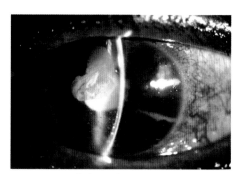

FIGURE 5-1. Slit-lamp photograph of a case of trauma-related phacoantigenic uveitis. Note the granulomatous keratic precipitates and ruptured anterior lens capsule with cortical material in the anterior chamber.

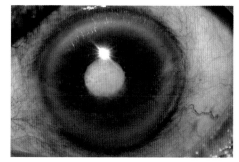

FIGURE 5-2. A 45-year-old woman presented with a 1-month history of pain, redness, and vision loss. She developed these symptoms shortly after blunt trauma to the eye. The fellow eye was normal. Slit-lamp photograph shows moderate anterior chamber inflammation, an intumescent cataract, and posterior synechia. (Courtesy of S. R. Rathinam, MD.)

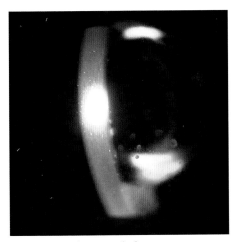

FIGURE 5-3. This patient had cataract surgery with intraocular lens implantation; however, a significant amount of lens material remained in the eye. The patient developed anterior uveitis with granulomatous keratic precipitates. (Courtesy of S. R. Rathinam, MD.)

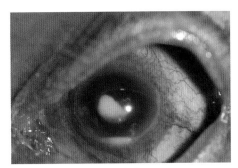

FIGURE 5-4. This person had a Morgagnian cataract, in which the liquefied cortical material caused inflammation due to lens material leaking through an intact capsule into the anterior chamber. The nucleus is inferiorly displaced within the capsular bag. Due to the longstanding nature of this process, this patient has signs of chronic, rather than acute, inflammation. (Courtesy of S. R. Rathinam, MD.)

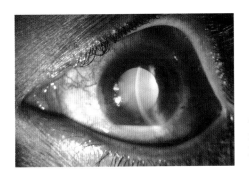

FIGURE 5-5. This patient has a hypermature cataract. There is diffuse injection, corneal edema (due to increased intraocular pressure and diffuse keratic precipitates), a 1-mm hypopyon, and a white cataract. (Courtesy of J. Biswas, MD.)

CATARACT SURGERY-RELATED UVEITIS

Anita Schadlu

Uveitis following cataract or other intraocular surgery is due to retained lens material after cataract surgery, a traumatically ruptured lens capsule, or iris/ciliary body chafing from a malpositioned lens implant.

Etiology and Epidemiology

Lens-induced uveitis may be caused by any of the following:

- Retained lens material in the anterior segment or vitreous cavity following cataract surgery

- Malpositioned intraocular lens (IOL) implant

- Placement of a single-piece IOL in the ciliary sulcus (Fig. 5-6)

Symptoms

- Decreased vision

- Pain, photophobia, redness, floaters

Signs

- Elevated intraocular pressure, often from clogging of the trabecular meshwork with lens protein.

- Conjunctival injection

- Keratic precipitates (KP; can have nongranulomatous or granulomatous KP with a "mutton-fat" appearance)

- Anterior chamber cell and flare (the uveitis may be acute or chronic, and mild to severe)

- Hyphema in severe cases of IOL-induced uveitis, which is termed the *uveitis-glaucoma-hyphema (UGH) syndrome* (Figs. 5-7 and 5-8)

- Posterior synechiae

- Iris transillumination defects due to iris chafing (Fig. 5-9)

- Cellular deposits on the IOL surface (Fig. 5-9)

- Malpositioned IOL haptics

- Retained lens material following cataract surgery

- Disruption of the lens capsule

- Vitritis

- Cystoid macular edema

Differential Diagnosis

- Infectious endophthalmitis
  - Subacute or chronic
  - *Propionibacterium acnes* is a gram-positive anaerobic organism that can be sequestered within the lens capsule following cataract surgery, and may cause a chronic low-grade inflammation and a "white plaque" within the capsular bag.

- Herpes simplex and varicella zoster uveitis, both of which may also cause iris transillumination defects

- Sarcoidosis

- Fuch's heterochromic iridocyclitis

- Infectious diseases such as toxoplasmosis, syphilis, sarcoidosis, tuberculosis, and Lyme disease

Diagnostic Evaluation

- The different etiologies for lens-induced uveitis can be differentiated based on patient history, clinical exam, and testing.

- Gonioscopy can identify lens material retained in the angle as well as a malpositioned anterior chamber IOL.

- High resolution B-scan ultrasonography (ultrasound biomicroscopy [UBM]) and/or anterior segment OCT of the anterior segment can assess the position of the lens haptics in cases of suspected IOL-induced uveitis or UGH syndrome.

- Posterior segment B-scan ultrasonography can detect vitritis, retinal detachment, choroidal detachment, and retained lens material.

- A vitreous or aqueous tap can be useful in cases of suspected infectious endophthalmitis.

  ▪ Large "lipid-laden" macrophages in the anterior chamber in cases of phacolytic glaucoma may be seen.

- Laboratory testing should be ordered as indicated to rule out other possible causes of noninfectious uveitis.

Treatment

- In cases of mild inflammation due to small retained cortical lens material, intensive topical, periocular, or oral steroids can manage the inflammatory response.

- In cases of retained nuclear material, or more significant retained cortical material, prompt removal of retained lens material with vitrectomy is indicated.

- Removal of any retained lens material is indicated in cases with persistent inflammation and/or elevated intraocular pressure.

- If there is traumatic disruption of the lens capsule, cataract extraction is necessary. Lens implantation may be deferred in cases where prolonged postoperative inflammation is likely.

- Vitreous tap and injection of intravitreal antibiotics are necessary if there is any suspicion of infectious endophthalmitis. *P. acnes* may require surgical capsulectomy

with irrigation of the capsular bag, or even explantation of the lens-bag complex.

- UGH syndrome can be treated with reposition or explantation of the lens implant. A single-piece IOL in the ciliary sulcus may require explantation.

Prognosis

Early diagnosis and treatment can lead to good visual prognosis. However, cases with prolonged inflammation and/or increased intraocular pressure, permanent visual loss can result from corneal endothelial cell loss, cystoid macular edema, glaucoma, and retinal detachment.

REFERENCES

Borne MJ, Tasman W, Regillo C, et al. Outcomes of vitrectomy for retained lens fragments. *Ophthalmology.* 1996;103(6):971–976.

Chang DF, Masket S, Miller KM, et al. ASCRS Cataract Clinical Committee. Complications of sulcus placement of single-piece acrylic intraocular lenses: recommendations for backup IOL implantation following posterior capsule rupture. *J Cataract Refract Surg.* 2009; 35(8):1445–1458.

Ho LY, Doft BH, Wang L, et al. Clinical predictors and outcomes of pars plana vitrectomy for retained lens material after cataract extraction. *Am J Ophthalmol.* 2009;147(4):587–594.

Rumelt S, Rehany U. The influence of surgery and intraocular lens implantation timing on visual outcome in traumatic cataract. *Graefes Arch Clin Exp Ophthalmol.* 2010;248(9):1293–1297. Epub 2010 Jun 29.

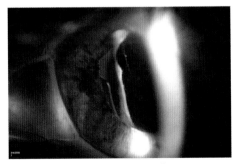

FIGURE 5-6. This person developed uveitis-glaucoma-hyphema syndrome with iris chafing due to sulcus placement of a single-piece intraocular lens. Explantation of the lens with placement of a three-piece lens caused resolution of the symptoms. (Courtesy of Sunir J. Garg, MD.)

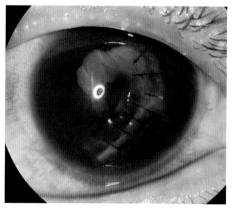

FIGURE 5-7. This person had a perforating corneal injury with rupture of the lens capsule, which caused anterior uveitis. The lens material should be promptly evacuated. (Courtesy of William Benson, MD.)

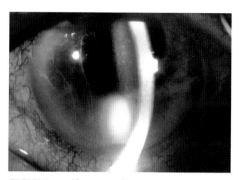

FIGURE 5-8. This person has a visible hyphema with anterior segment inflammation due to malposition of an anterior chamber intraocular lens. (Courtesy of Russell Van Gelder, MD, PhD.)

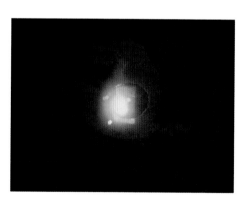

FIGURE 5-9. Iris transillumination defects due to an IOL in the ciliary sulcus are seen in this photograph. (Courtesy of Marc Spirn, MD.)

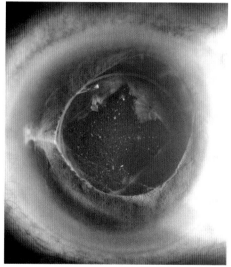

FIGURE 5-10. Chronic postoperative inflammation may result in cellular deposits on the IOL. The deposits may be white or pigmented and range in size from large or fine (as seen in this image). There is vitreous to the wound with peaking of the pupil that is more evident without dilation.

Intermediate Uveitis

Andrea D. Birnbaum and Debra A. Goldstein

Intermediate uveitis (IU) refers to ocular inflammation that localizes primarily to the vitreous and peripheral retina.

Epidemiology and Etiology

- IU most often occurs in children and young adults.

- IU accounts for up to 15% of uveitis cases in adults, with higher percentages reported at tertiary referral centers, and accounts for up to 28% of uveitis cases in children.

- There is no gender predilection.

- HLA associations reported, specifically with HLA-DR15, HLA-DR17, and HLA-A28.

Symptoms

- Blurred vision, floaters

- Pain and photophobia rarely develop as those signs usually occur in association with anterior segment inflammation. When these symptoms develop, they are more common in young children.

Signs

The American Uveitis Society (AUS) describes intermediate uveitis as ocular inflammation localized primarily to the vitreous. Associated findings may include:

- Snowballs and snowbanks (Figs. 6-1 and 6-2)

- Cystoid macular edema (CME) (Fig. 6-3A–C)

- Peripheral vascular sheathing (Fig. 6-3D)

  - Patients may develop peripheral retinal and/or anterior segment neovascularization and vitreous hemorrhage as a result of peripheral ischemia.

- It is bilateral in 75% of patients.

- Spill-over of inflammatory cells into the anterior chamber

- Scant keratic precipitates may be present.

- Band keratopathy may occur in chronic cases.

- Cataract

- Elevated intraocular pressure/glaucoma

Differential Diagnosis

- A helpful mnemonic is SIMPLE:
  - Sarcoidosis
  - Inflammatory bowel disease
  - Multiple sclerosis (MS)
  - Pars planitis is a subset of intermediate uveitis usually seen in children and young adults that is idiopathic and has no extraocular manifestations. This should be diagnosed only when other etiologies have been ruled out. It accounts for up to 50% of cases of IU.
  - *Lymphoma* (primary intraocular lymphoma; Figs. 6-4 and 6-5)
  - *Etc.*: juvenile idiopathic arthritis, and infections (syphilis, Lyme disease, tuberculosis, Whipple's disease, toxocariasis, human T-cell lymphoma virus type I [HTLV-1], hepatitis C, *Bartonella* infection [cat-scratch disease])

Diagnostic Evaluation

- Serum tests
  - ACE and lysozyme for sarcoidosis
  - Specific treponemal test (FTA-ABS or MHA-TP)
  - QuantiFERON-TB Gold for tuberculosis
  - Lyme titers in patients with exposure to ticks in endemic areas
  - Toxocariasis titers in patients with unilateral disease
- Skin testing: purified protein derivative (PPD) for tuberculosis
- Imaging studies
  - Chest radiograph or CT scan for sarcoidosis and tuberculosis
  - MRI of the brain for MS and intraocular lymphoma
- Fluorescein angiography to evaluate for CME and peripheral vascular leakage and nonperfusion.
- Optical coherence tomography (OCT) for CME, epiretinal membrane, and macular atrophy.
- B-scan ultrasonography if significant band keratopathy or cataract is present.
- Gonioscopy should be considered as patients may rarely develop anterior segment neovascularization as a result of peripheral retinal ischemia.

Treatment

- Infections and malignancies should be treated appropriately.
- Many patients with pars planitis who have mild disease, no CME, and good vision can be closely observed. This is one of the few types of chronic uveitis that can be observed.
- Patients with CME, decreased vision, and/or peripheral ischemia with neovascularization require treatment.
  - Short-term systemic steroids as initial treatment for severe, bilateral disease can be used.
  - Periocular corticosteroid injections such as triamcinolone acetonide are very effective for the treatment of IU, and especially for pars planitis. Patients may require multiple injections over a short period of time (1 to 2 months). Prior to use:
    - ▶ Infectious causes must be ruled out.
    - ▶ Consider a trial of topical steroids q.i.d. for at least 2 weeks to evaluate patients for a significant increase in intraocular pressure.
  - Patients must be followed closely with intraocular pressure checks at every visit, regardless of age.

▦ Intraocular steroids can also be used. As with periocular steroid injections, patients should be monitored for increased intraocular pressure and cataract formation. Three commonly used intraocular steroids are:

▸ Intravitreal triamcinolone acetonide

▸ Ozurdex (Allergan, Inc., Irvine, CA)

▸ Retisert (Bausch & Lomb, Rochester, NY)

● Steroid-sparing systemic immunosuppression, such as methotrexate, mycophenolate mofetil, and azathioprine, is useful for cases of bilateral disease, or in cases in which local steroid therapy is not effective/appropriate.

● Laser (or cryotherapy if laser is not possible) to the peripheral retina immediately posterior to the active snowbank has been used with variable success. It is critical for cases of peripheral retinal or anterior segment neovascularization.

● Some investigators advocate pars plana vitrectomy for cases of more severe pars planitis, but there is debate as to the utility of this technique.

Prognosis

● Vision loss is usually secondary to CME.

● Patients can develop cataracts, which may be amblyogenic in children.

● Glaucoma may develop both from inflammation and from chronic steroid use.

Rarely, patients may develop neovascular glaucoma.

● The outcome is dependent upon the disease severity. Patients with active snowbanks typically have more severe CME and a worse visual prognosis.

● Rhegmatogenous retinal detachment may occur in eyes with severe inflammation, particularly when associated with neovascularization of the snowbank.

REFERENCES

Henderly DE, Haymond RS, Rao NA, et al. The significance of the pars plana exudate in pars planitis. *Am J Ophthalmol.* 1987;103(5):669–671.

McCannel CA, Holland GN, Helm CJ, et al. Causes of uveitis in the general practice of ophthalmology. UCLA Community-Based Uveitis Study Group. *Am J Ophthalmol.* 1996;121(1):35–46.

Oruc S, Duffy BF, Mohanakumar T, et al. The association of HLA class II with pars planitis. *Am J Ophthalmol.* 2001;131(5):657–659.

Park SE, Mieler WF, Pulido JS. Peripheral scatter photocoagulation for neovascularization associated with pars planitis. *Arch Ophthal.* 1995;113:1277–1280.

Potter MJ, Myckatyn SO, Maberley AL, et al. Vitrectomy for pars planitis complicated by vitreous hemorrhage: visual outcome and long-term follow-up. *Am J Ophthalmol.* 1978;86:762–774.

Rodriguez A, Calonge M, Pedroza-Seres M, et al. Referral patterns of uveitis in a tertiary eye care center. *Arch Ophthalmol.* 1996;114:593–599.

Smith JA, Mackensen F, Sen HN, et al. Epidemiology and course of disease in childhood uveitis. *Ophthalmology.* 2009;116(8):1544–1551.

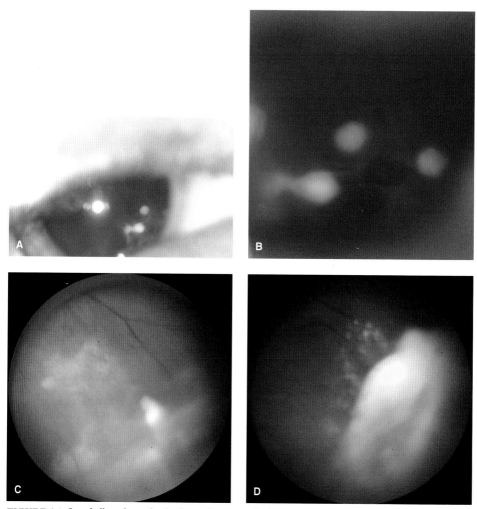

FIGURE 6-1. Snowballs and snowbank of pars planitis. **A.** Slit-lamp photograph of patient with dense snowballs in the anterior vitreous. RetCam photos were taken during an examination under anesthesia and allow for better visualization of the large snowballs (**B**) and thick, active pars plana snowbank (**C, D**).

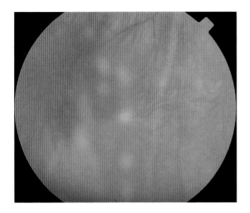

FIGURE 6-2. This person has moderate inferior snowballs characteristic of intermediate uveitis.

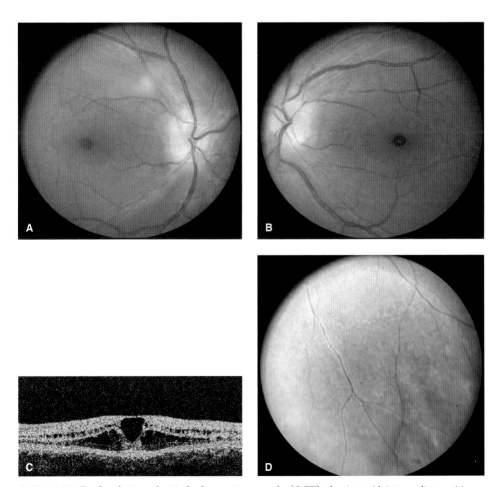

FIGURE 6-3. Fundus photos and optical coherence tomography (OCT) of patient with intermediate uveitis. **A, B.** This patient has hyperemic discs and cystoid macular edema (CME) in both eyes. Note the snowballs obscuring the view of the superotemporal arcade in the right eye. **C.** An OCT of the right eye demonstrates large cystic changes in the macula. **D.** A peripheral photograph of the left eye demonstrates the periphlebitis characteristic of intermediate uveitis.

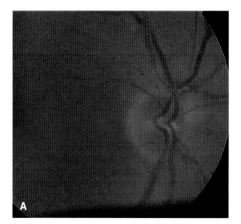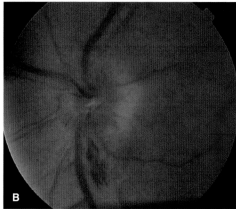

FIGURE 6-4. Central nervous system lymphoma should be considered, especially when older patients present with IU. Disc photos of patient with lymphoma. The right eye is unremarkable (**A**), while the left eye has disc edema with a hemorrhage coming off the disc inferiorly (**B**).

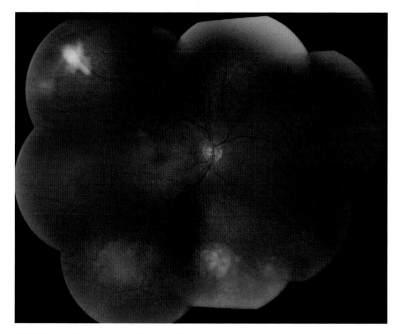

FIGURE 6-5. This 64-year-old man had biopsy-proven intraocular lymphoma that was initally diagnosed as pars planitis. Although mild vitreous haze is present, the inferior snowballs, as well as the temporal infiltrate, are subretinal, which, in combination with the patient's age, should raise suspicion for lymphoma. (Courtesy Sunir J. Garg, MD)

Posterior Uveitis and Collagen Vascular Diseases

SARCOIDOSIS-ASSOCIATED UVEITIS

H. Nida Sen and Robert Nussenblatt

Sarcoidosis is a multisystem granulomatous disorder that most commonly affects the lungs, skin, lymph nodes, eyes, central nervous system (CNS), reticuloendothelial system, the heart, and bones.

Epidemiology and Etiology

• Sarcoidosis occurs most commonly in African Americans and Caucasians of Northern European descent.

• The incidence and prevalence varies among different geographic regions and ethnic groups:

  ▪ In the United States, the prevalence among African Americans is 35 to 82 in 100,000 persons, while in Caucasians it is 8 to 11 in 100,000 persons.

  ▪ In Scandinavia, the prevalence is 64 in 100,000 persons.

• Most common organs involved are the lungs (90% to 95%), followed by skin (15% to 20%), lymph nodes (15% to 40%) and eyes (12% to 20%).

• Systemic sarcoidosis typically affects young adults, while ocular sarcoidosis appears to have a bimodal presentation.

• Ophthalmic involvement occurs in up to 50% of patients with systemic sarcoidosis, but most series suggest the rate is around 25%.

  ▪ Ocular involvement is more common among women compared to men, and in African Americans compared to Caucasians.

  ▪ Patients typically have a bilateral (98%), granulomatous anterior uveitis. This is the presenting sign of sarcoidosis in 10% to 20% of patients.

  ▪ The most common intraocular involvement is anterior uveitis (two-thirds of patients).

  ▪ The most common site of extraocular involvement is the lacrimal gland.

• Although the etiology is unknown, sarcoidosis is believed to be immune-mediated. Both a genetic predisposition (familial

This contribution to the work was done as part of the authors' official duties as NIH employees and is a work of the United States Government.

aggregation, HLA-B8, HLA-DRB1) and environmental factors (environmental allergens and infectious agents) have been suggested.

Symptoms

- Blurry vision, floaters

- Redness, photophobia, ocular discomfort

- Respiratory symptoms (shortness of breath) and constitutional symptoms (fever, fatigue, night sweats, and weight loss)

Signs (**Figs.** 7-1 to 7-7)

- In 2006, the 1st International Workshop on Ocular Sarcoidosis developed criteria for the diagnosis of ocular sarcoidosis, which include seven ocular signs considered suggestive of ocular sarcoidosis (**Table 7-1**).

  ▪ Mutton fat (granulomatous) keratic precipitates (KPs), anterior chamber cells and flare, and iris or angle nodules (granulomas). Busacca nodules are in the iris stroma and Koeppe nodules are on the pupillary margin.

    ▸ The KPs may also be nongranulomatous.

  ▪ Nodules on the trabecular meshwork and/or tent-shaped peripheral anterior synechiae

  ▪ Vitreous cells, vitreous haze, snowballs sometimes with a "string of pearls" appearance, and snowbanks.

  ▪ Multifocal, cream-colored, peripheral chorioretinal lesions (Dalen-Fuchs nodules), either active or atrophic

  ▪ Retinal vasculitis, perivenous sheathing (candle wax drippings, also known as taches de bougie), and/or a retinal macroaneurysm in an inflamed eye.

  ▪ Optic disk or choroidal granulomas

  ▪ Bilaterality

- Other ophthalmic findings include:

  ▪ Lacrimal gland enlargement

  ▪ Subconjunctival granulomas

  ▪ Optic neuritis

▪ Heerfordt's syndrome (uveo-parotid fever): anterior uveitis, parotid gland enlargement, facial palsy, and fever

- Retinal neovascularization, sometimes with a sea fan appearance.

Differential Diagnosis

- The major systemic signs include:

  ▪ Respiratory dysfunction

  ▪ Skin macules and papules, including erythema nodosum and lupus pernio

  ▪ Cranial nerve palsies

  ▪ Ataxia and cognitive dysfunction

  ▪ Cardiomyopathy and arrhythmias

- Vogt-Koyanagi-Harada (VKH) syndrome

- Sympathetic ophthalmia

- Multifocal choroiditis

- Primary intraocular lymphoma (retinal lymphoma)

- Tuberculosis

- Syphilis

- Lyme disease

- Blau syndrome and juvenile idiopathic arthritis in children

Diagnostic Evaluation

- Definitive diagnosis requires tissue biopsy showing noncaseating granulomas. The granulomas appear as whorls of epithelioid cells surrounding multinucleated Langhans giant cells.

- Systemic evaluation and imaging studies: chest radiograph and/or high-resolution chest CT to identify hilar lymphadenopathy gallium scan (not recommended for routine screening); pulmonary function tests (reduction in diffusing capacity); bronchoalveolar lavage (elevated cd4/cd8 ratio); biopsy of the involved tissue; and/or brain MRI if neurosarcoidosis is suspected.

TABLE 7-1. Diagnostic Criteria for Ocular Sarcoidosis from the International Workshop on Ocular Sarcoidosis, Tokyo, 2006

Definite ocular sarcoidosis	Biopsy-supported diagnosis with compatible uveitis
Presumed ocular sarcoidosis	Biopsy not done; bilateral hilar lymphadenopathy with compatible uveitis
Probable ocular sarcoidosis	Biopsy not done; chest radiograph normal; 3 suggestive ocular signs and 2 positive investigational tests
Possible ocular sarcoidosis	Biopsy negative; 4 suggestive ocular signs and 2 positive investigations

(From Herbort CP, Rao NA, Mochizuki M. International criteria for the diagnosis of ocular sarcoidosis: results of the first International Workshop on Ocular Sarcoidosis (IWOS). *Ocul Immunol Inflamm.* 2009;17:160–169.)

- Laboratory testing: Angiotensin-converting enzyme (ACE) is elevated in 75% of patients, lysozyme, hypercalcemia, hypercalciuria, anemia, elevated erythrocyte sedimentation rate (ESR)/C-reactive protein (CRP), anergy, elevated alkaline phosphatase.

- Fluorescein angiography can reveal retinal vascular leakage, early blockage and late staining of choroidal granulomas, retinal pigment epithelial (RPE) window defects, and cystoid macular edema (CME).

- None of the above is specific or diagnostic by itself; therefore, it is a clinical diagnosis, which is supported by imaging and laboratory testing. Tissue biopsy is required for definitive diagnosis.

Treatment

- Corticosteroids are the mainstay of therapy for both ocular and systemic sarcoidosis, and intravenous pulse steroids may be needed in some very severe cases.

- Sarcoidosis is often responsive to steroids; however, chronic uveitis often requires immunomodulatory therapy. Methotrexate, cyclosporine, mycophenolate mofetil, and infliximab have all been used successfully in ocular sarcoidosis.

- Local treatment with topical drops, periocular steroids, and intraocular steroid implants can also be considered in select cases.

Prognosis

- The prognosis is good if treated early.

- African Americans tend to have more acute and severe disease, whereas Caucasians tend to have chronic, asymptomatic disease.

- Chronic posterior or panuveitis, glaucoma, CME, older age at presentation, and delay in presentation to a sarcoid/uveitis subspecialist may confer a poor visual prognosis.

- Ocular complications can include glaucoma, cataract, CME, optic disk edema, occlusive vasculopathy, retinal or optic disk neovascularization, vitreous hemorrhage, and retinal detachment.

REFERENCES

Baughman RP, Teirstein AS, Judson MA, et al. Case Control Etiologic Study of Sarcoidosis (ACCESS) research group. Clinical characteristics of patients in a case control study of sarcoidosis. *Am J Respir Crit Care Med.* 2001;164(10 Pt 1):1885–1889.

Dana MR, Merayo-Lloves J, Schaumberg DA, et al. Prognosticators for visual outcome in sarcoid uveitis. *Ophthalmology.* 1996;103(11):1846–1853.

Herbort CP, Rao NA, Mochizuki M. International criteria for the diagnosis of ocular sarcoidosis: results of the first International Workshop on Ocular Sarcoidosis (IWOS). *Ocul Immunol Inflamm.* 2009;17(3):160–169.

Lobo A, Barton K, Minassian D, et al. Visual loss in sarcoid-related uveitis. *Clin Experiment Ophthalmol.* 2003;31(4):310–316.

Nussenblatt RB and Whitcup SM. *Uveitis: Fundamentals and Clinical Practice.* Philadelphia: Mosby; 2010: 278–288.

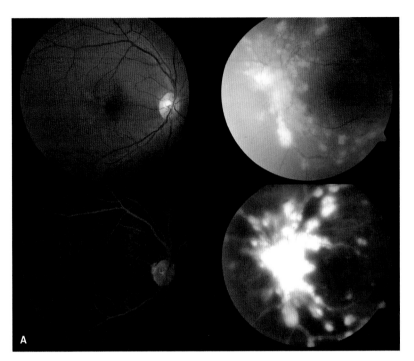

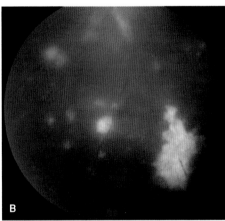

FIGURE 7-1. A. This patient with severe sarcoidosis has posterior uveitis with granulomas and intense exudates surrounding the vessels. Note the asymmetric involvement between the right and left eyes. The fluorescein angiogram of the left eye (lower right) demonstrates leakage and staining in the late frames. **B.** Exudates surrounding the vessels, also known as "candle-wax drippings" or "taches de bougie," are seen inferiorly.

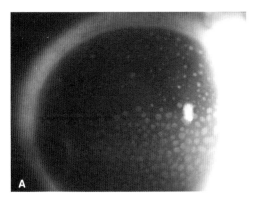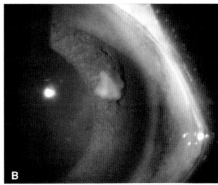

FIGURE 7-2. **A.** There are large, granulomatous-appearing (mutton-fat) keratic precipitates in this patient with sarcoidosis. **B.** Busacca nodules in the iris stroma are typically associated with diseases causing granulomatous uveitis such as sarcoidosis.

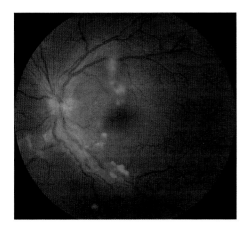

FIGURE 7-3. "Candle-wax drippings" along the major arcade vessels. (Courtesy of Sunir Garg, MD.)

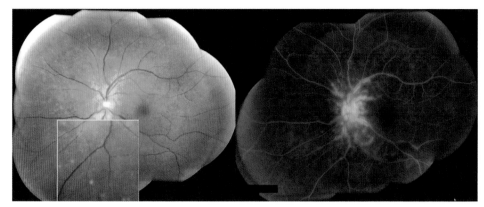

FIGURE 7-4. Sarcoidosis patient with intermediate uveitis with snowballs and retinal vascular sheathing inferiorly (magnified), as well as retinal vasculitis with leakage on fluorescein angiogram. Note that the extent of retinal vascular leakage is significantly more impressive than expected based on the fundus exam.

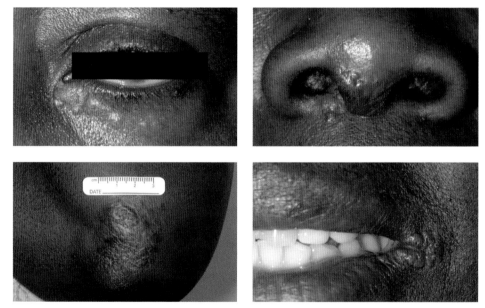

FIGURE 7-5. There are multiple skin nodules due to sarcoidosis in an African American patient with liver and ocular sarcoidosis. The inferior periorbital skin, the nose, elbow, and perioral skin are involved.

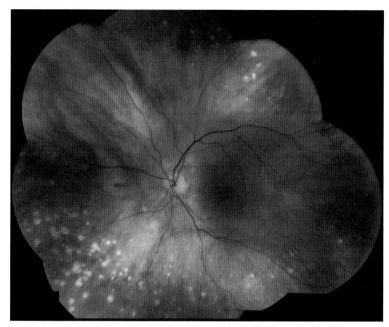

FIGURE 7-6. There are the typical punched-out chorioretinal lesions in a 65-year-old Caucasian patient with ocular sarcoidosis. These lesions are believed to be representative of atrophic Dalen-Fuchs nodules.

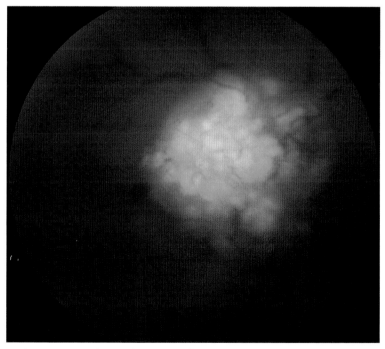

FIGURE 7-7. Optic nerve granuloma in the right eye of a 42-year-old African American patient with sarcoidosis.

SYMPATHETIC OPHTHALMIA

Rishi R. Doshi, S. R. Rathinam, and Emmett T. Cunningham, Jr.

Sympathetic ophthalmia is a bilateral granulomatous panuveitis that occurs when ocular surgery or ocular trauma to one eye (the exciting eye) incites inflammation both in the traumatized eye as well as in the fellow (sympathizing) eye.

Etiology and Epidemiology

- It has an estimated incidence of 0.03 in 100,000; the incidence is higher after vitreoretinal surgery (1 in 1152 procedures) compared to other ocular surgeries and surgery has surpassed trauma as the most common inciting event.

- Previously sequestered ocular antigens from the uvea, retina, or choroidal melanocytes stimulate an autoimmune response.

- Historically, men and children were more commonly affected due to higher rates of trauma, but currently it occurs equally in both men and women with an increased incidence in elderly patients due to higher rates of surgery.

- It may occur after endophthalmitis, with an incidence from 1% to 11%.

- 80% of cases occur within 3 months of surgery/trauma and 90% occur within 1 year, but it has been reported to occur anytime between 1 week to 66 years after injury.

- There is an increased prevalence in patients with HLA-DR4 and HLA-A11.

Symptoms

- Patients often have a prodrome of tearing, photophobia, and blurry vision (loss of accommodation), which may progress to severe vision loss, pain, floaters, and photopsias in both eyes.

Signs (Figs. 7-8 to 7-12)

- Both eyes have inflammation with:
  - Anterior uveitis (55%); granulomatous KPs, iris thickening and synechiae, low or high intraocular pressure (from ciliary body shutdown or angle closure), vitritis (47%); disk edema (20%); serous retinal detachment (12%); choroiditis (8%); and macular edema (5%)
  - Dalen-Fuchs nodules are yellow-white midequatorial RPE lesions composed of epithelioid cells and histiocytes (30% to 70%).
  - Late findings may include sunset glow fundus, optic atrophy, choroidal neovascularization, and phthisis.
  - Systemic findings may include cerebrospinal fluid pleocytosis, hearing disturbances, alopecia, poliosis, and vitiligo (but these are much more typical of VKH).

Differential Diagnosis

- VKH (no history of penetrating trauma or surgery)
- Tuberculosis
- Sarcoidosis
- Syphilis
- Intraocular lymphoma

Diagnostic Evaluation

- On fluorescein angiography, patients have multiple pinpoint areas of hyperfluorescence with late leakage, choroidal lesions that block early and stain late, and late disk staining.

- Optical coherence tomography can show multifocal serous retinal detachments.

- B-scan ultrasonography demonstrates choroidal thickening and serous retinal detachments.

- Histopathology characteristically demonstrates a diffuse granulomatous nonnecrotizing panuveitis with thickening of choroid and early sparing of choriocapillaris.

Treatment

- First-line therapy is high-dose oral cortico-steroids (1 to 2 mg/kg/day), with a slow taper.

- Topical corticosteroids and cycloplegic/mydriatic agents can help alleviate some of the more acute symptoms.

- Corticosteroid-sparing immunosuppressive agents are typically required, as most patients need long-term treatment.

- A fluocinolone acetonide implant (Retisert) may be useful in select cases.

- Enucleation of the exciting eye within 2 weeks of the inciting event may decrease the risk of sympathetic ophthalmia; once sympathetic ophthalmia occurs, enucleation should be considered only in a blind, painful eye.

Prognosis

- It is a vision-threatening disease, with only slightly more than half of treated patients retaining visual acuity ≥20/40. One-fourth of patients have vision worse than 20/200.

- Complications include cataract and glaucoma.

- Predictors of a poor outcome include a traumatic etiology, active, uncontrolled intra-ocular inflammation, and an exudative retinal detachment.

- Long-term visual loss may result from chorioretinal scars, chronic macular edema, and choroidal neovascularization

REFERENCES

Castiblanco CP, Adelman RA. Sympathetic ophthalmia. *Graefes Arch Clin Exp Ophthalmol.* 2009;247:289–302.

Galor A, Davis JL, Flynn HW, et al. Sympathetic ophthalmia: Incidence of ocular complications and vision loss in the sympathizing eye. *Am J Ophthalmol.* 2009; 148:704–710.

Kilmartin DJ, Dick AD, Forrester JV. Prospective surveillance of sympathetic ophthalmia in the United Kingdom and Republic of Ireland. *Br J Ophthalmol.* 2000;84:259–263.

Rathinam SR, Rao NA. Sympathetic ophthalmia following postoperative bacterial endophthalmitis: a clinicopathologic study. *Am J Ophthalmol.* 2006;141(3): 498–507.

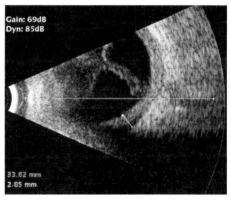

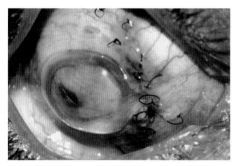

FIGURE 7-8. Phthisis bulbi following a ruptured globe in a patient with sympathetic ophthalmia.

FIGURE 7-9. B-scan ultrasound showing a chronic retinal detachment and choroidal thickening in a patient with sympathetic ophthalmia.

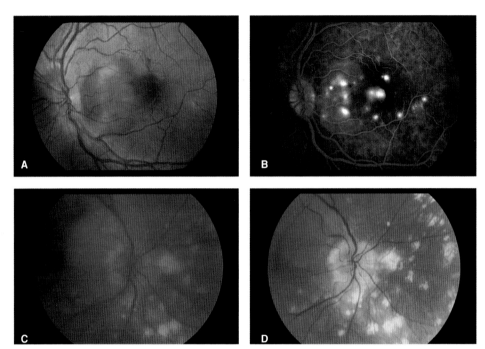

FIGURE 7-10. Characteristic posterior segment findings in two patients who developed sympathetic ophthalmia weeks after uncomplicated pars plana vitrectomy. Color fundus photograph (**A**) and midphase fluorescein angiogram (**B**) from the same patient 2 months following vitrectomy shows a macular serous detachment with multiple, pin-point areas of leakage through the retinal pigment epithelium. (**C**) Color fundus photographs taken approximately 6 months following vitrectomy shows moderate vitreous inflammation and active chorioretinal infiltrates. (**D**) Photograph of the same patient taken approximately 18 months following vitrectomy, after the patient's inflammation had been controlled with high dose systemic corticosteroids followed by noncorticosteroid immunosuppressive agents. Although histopathologically unverified, many would describe these infiltrates clinically as Dalen-Fuchs nodules. (Reproduced from Doshi RR, Arevalo JF, Flynn HW Jr, et al. Evaluating exaggerated, prolonged, or delayed postoperative intraocular inflammation. *Am J Ophthalmol.* 2010, with permission of Elsevier.)

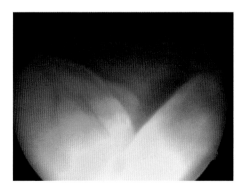

FIGURE 7-11. Bullous serous retinal detachment in a patient with sympathetic ophthalmia.

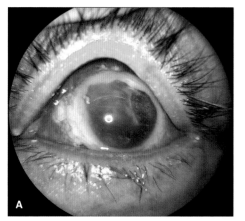

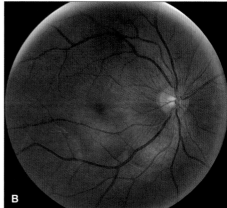

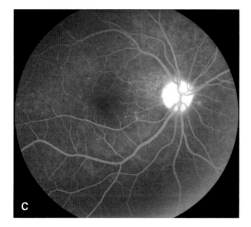

FIGURE 7-12. **A.** This patient underwent ruptured globe repair following blunt trauma. **B.** Several months later, the patient returned complaining of photophobia and blurred vision in the previously healthy right eye. There is disk hyperemia, mild macular striations due to subretinal fluid, and deep, choroidal yellow plaques characteristic of sympathetic ophthalmia. **C.** The fluorescein angiogram demonstrates disk hyperfluorescence and pinpoint leakage and staining from the areas of choroiditis. (Courtesy Allen Chiang, MD, and Andre Witkin, MD.)

VOGT-KOYANAGI-HARADA SYNDROME

Nupura Krishnadev, Robert Nussenblatt, and H. Nida Sen

Vogt-Koyanagi-Harada (VHK) syndrome, or uveomeningitis, is a bilateral granulomatous panuveitis with skin, meningeal, and auditory-vestibular involvement.

Epidemiology and Etiology

- More commonly seen in patients from Japan and Latin America. It also occurs in African Americans and in persons with Native American ancestry.
- It is most common in the second to fourth decade of life.
- There is a slight female preponderance.
- VKH has a genetic predisposition, and has been associated with HLA-DR4, HLA-DRw53, and HLA-DRB1*0405.
- It tends to occur in the spring and fall.
- Unlike sympathetic ophthalmia, patients with VKH have no history of penetrating ocular trauma or surgery.

Symptoms

- Blurry vision, floaters
- Headache, vertigo, neck stiffness
- Dysacusis and tinnitus
- Skin changes: vitiligo, (skin depigmentation), poliosis (hair whitening), and alopecia in the later stages (Fig. 7-13)

Signs

- The American Uveitis Society (AUS) and the International Uveitis Society have established criteria for diagnosis. The AUS criteria for complete VKH are shown in **Table 7-2**.

This contribution to the work was done as part of the authors' official duties as NIH employees and is a work of the United States Government.

Differential Diagnosis

- Sympathetic ophthalmia (these patients have a history of penetrating trauma)
- Bullous central serous chorioretinopathy (these patients have no inflammation)
- Posterior scleritis (eyes have scleral thickening on B-scan ultrasonography)
- Sarcoidosis
- Syphilis
- Lyme disease
- Ocular lymphoma
- Uveal metastasis

Diagnostic Evaluation (Figs. 7-14 to 7-18)

- Fluorescein angiography: Early in the angiogram, there are multiple pinpoint areas of hyperfluorescence at the level of the RPE, which pool in the later frames. Late staining of the disk is often present.
- B-scan ultrasonography: Demonstrates nonspecific choroidal thickening and serous retinal detachments but can be helpful to rule out posterior scleritis and neoplastic disorders.
- Lumbar puncture: The majority of patients will have pleocytosis (but usually this is not needed).
- Laboratory tests to rule out other diseases such as sarcoid and syphilis as needed.

Treatment

- These patients need prompt and aggressive systemic therapy. Corticosteroids are the first-line agent, with some patients requiring 100 mg of prednisone daily, with a slow taper.
- Most patients will need immunosuppression for 1 year.
- If higher doses of prednisone are used for more than 2 to 3 months, steroid-sparing agents such as cyclosporine, tacrolimus, azathioprine, and mycophenolate mofetil should be considered.

TABLE 7-2. Diagnostic Criteria for VKH

1. No history of penetrating ocular trauma
2. No evidence of other ocular disease
3. Bilateral ocular involvement
   a. Early
      i. Diffuse choroiditis presenting as
         1. Focal areas of subretinal fluid, *or*
         2. Bullous serous retinal detachments
      ii. If equivocal fundus findings, then must have both of below:
         1. IVFA showing delayed choroidal perfusion, pinpoint leakage, pooling within the subretinal space, and optic nerve staining
         2. Ultrasound with diffuse choroidal thickening without posterior scleritis
   b. Late
      i. History suggestive of above, or both ii and iii below, or multiple signs from iii:
      ii. Ocular depigmentation
         1. Sunset glow fundus, *or*
         2. Sugiura sign
      iii. Other ocular signs
         1. Nummular chorioretinal depigmented scars, *or*
         2. RPE clumping, *or*
         3. Recurrent or chronic anterior uveitis
4. Neurologic/auditory findings
   a. Meningismus, *or*
   b. Tinnitus, or
   c. CSF pleocytosis
5. Integumentary (skin) findings
   a. Alopecia, *or*
   b. Poliosis, *or*
   c. Vitiligo

Complete VKH requires criteria 1 to 5
Incomplete VKH requires 1 to 3, and either 4 or 5
Probable VKH requires 1 to 3 (isolated ocular disease)

Adapted from Read RW, Holland GN, Rao NA et al. Revised Diagnostic Criteria for Vogt-Koyanagi-Harada disease: report of an International Committee on Nomenclature. *Am J Ophthalmol.* 2001;131:647–652.

Prognosis

- The prognosis is generally good with prompt and aggressive therapy.

- In addition to the development of cataracts and glaucoma, subretinal fibrosis, and choroidal neovascular membranes may occur.

REFERENCES

Rao NA, Gupta A, Dustin L, et al. Frequency of distinguishing clinical features in Vogt-Koyanagi-Harada disease. *Ophthalmology.* 2010;117(3):591–599, 599.e1. Epub 2009 Dec 24.

Read RW, Holland GN, Rao NA, et al. Revised diagnostic criteria for Vogt-Koyanagi-Harada disease: Report of an International Committee on Nomenclature. *Am J Ophthalmol.* 2001;131:647–652.

Yamaguchi Y, Otani T, Kishi S. Tomographic features of serous retinal detachment with multilobular dye pooling in acute Vogt-Koyanagi-Harada disease. *Am J Ophthalmol.* 2007;144(2):260–265. Epub 2007 May 29.

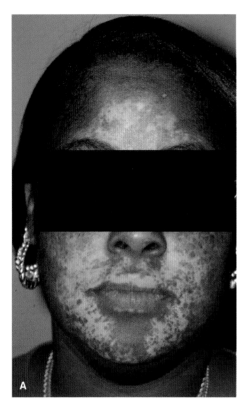

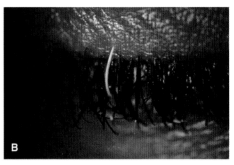

FIGURE 7-13. **A.** Vitiligo. This African American patient with VKH had extensive areas of skin depigmentation. **B.** Poliosis. A single white eyelash (poliosis) was found in this African American patient with VKH.

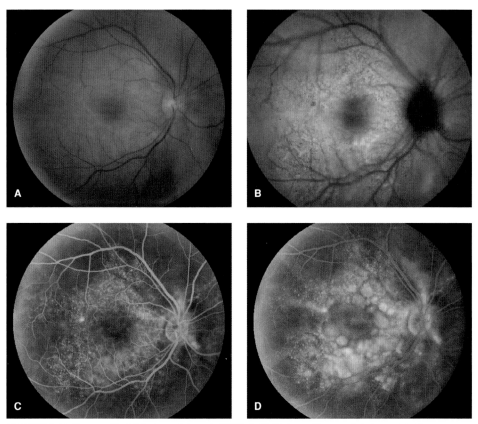

FIGURE 7-14. Serous retinal detachments in early VKH. **A.** Multiple small serous detachments in the right macula of an African American male presenting with a 5-day history of blurred vision. **B.** Fundus autofluorescence shows alterations in the RPE. **C.** Fluorescein angiogram (FA) in the early arteriovenous phase reveals the classic finding of multiple areas of pinpoint leakage. **D.** The late phase of the FA demonstrates pooling of fluorescein in the areas of serous retinal detachments.

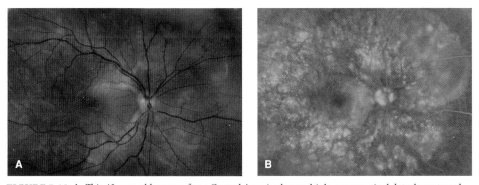

FIGURE 7-15. **A.** This 43-year-old woman from Central America has multiple serous retinal detachments and deep yellow lesions consistent with choroiditis. **B.** The FA shows multiple pinpoint areas of leakage with pooling of dye in the areas of serous retinal detachment. There is also staining of the optic disk. (Courtesy Sunir Garg, MD, and MidAtlantic Retina, the Retina Service of Wills Eye Institute.)

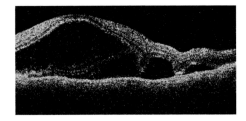

FIGURE 7-16. Optical coherence tomography (OCT) demonstrates a serous retinal detachment with subretinal septae, a finding suggestive of VKH. (Courtesy MidAtlantic Retina, The Retina Service of Wills Eye Institute.)

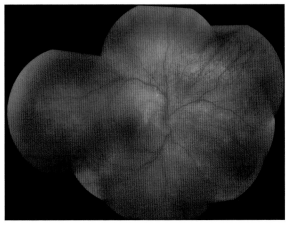

FIGURE 7-17. Sunset glow fundus in late VKH. The orange-red color of the fundus, due to loss of choroidal melanocytes in this patient with Native American ancestry, can develop 2 to 6 months after disease onset. Changes in the RPE are also visible.

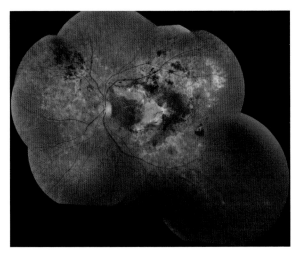

FIGURE 7-18. Subretinal fibrosis in late VKH. Note the extensive fibrosis and pigmentary changes in an advanced case of VKH with a history of poorly controlled uveitis.

OCULAR COMPLICATIONS OF RHEUMATOID ARTHRITIS

Bhupesh Bagga and Virender S. Sangwan

R heumatoid arthritis (RA) is a chronic inflammatory autoimmune disease that predominantly affects the peripheral joints. Patients with rheumatoid arthritis can also have extra-articular systemic and ocular involvement.

Epidemiology and Etiology

● RA is distributed worldwide, with a prevalence between 0.3% and 1.5%.

● Women develop RA more often than men by a 3:1 ratio.

● Although the disease can occur at any point, the incidence increases with advancing age.

● Activated T cells and antigen-antibody complexes cause a microvasculitis that affects joint synovial tissues as well as extra-articular tissues. Immune complex deposition and activation of complement plays a pivotal role in the systemic and ocular pathophysiology.

Symptoms

● Patients may complain of a foreign body sensation, and photophobia. A red eye due to episcleritis and dry eye are both common in RA.

● Patients with scleritis complain of a deep, boring, periocular pain that radiates to the brow and temple.

Signs

● Ocular (**Figs. 7-19 to 7-23**)

▪ Keratoconjunctivitis sicca (dry eye): Rapid tear film breakup time and devitalized corneal epithelium on staining are seen. Schirmer testing demonstrates decreased tear production.

▪ Sterile corneal infiltrates, and corneal edema, opacification, vascularization, and/ or thinning with marginal furrowing can occur.

▪ Peripheral ulcerative keratitis is a more aggressive form of perilimbal vasculitis.

▪ Episcleritis is characterized by dilated episcleral vessels.

▪ Patients with scleritis have a dilated superficial and deep episcleral vascular plexus that imparts a violaceous hue to the sclera. Unlike in episcleritis, the dilated vessels lose their normal radial architecture.

▪ Diffuse anterior scleritis is a more common form and has a better prognosis than other types of scleritis including nodular scleritis, anterior necrotizing scleritis, necrotizing scleritis without inflammation (scleromalacia perforans), and posterior scleritis.

● Systemic

▪ Patients initially develop fatigue, morning stiffness, and myalgias. The typical finding is polyarthritis that primarily affects the hands, feet, and cervical vertebrae.

▪ Patients may also develop anemia, pericarditis, pleuritis, glomerulonephritis, neuropathy, and vasculitis of the skin (**Fig. 7-24**).

Differential Diagnosis

● Sjögren's syndrome

● Reiter's syndrome

● Enteropathic arthritis, including Crohn's disease and reactive arthritis

● Psoriatic arthritis

● Systemic lupus erythematosus

● Sarcoidosis

● Wegener's granulomatosis

- Dermatomyositis
- Polyarteritis nodosa

Diagnostic Evaluation

- Specific markers: Rheumatoid factor (RF), antinuclear antibodies (ANA), antineutrophil cytoplasmic antibody (ANCA), anti-SS-A, anti-SS-B antibodies, and antibodies to cyclic citrullinated peptides
- Nonspecific markers: Complete blood count, chest radiograph, ESR, CRP, liver function tests, kidney function tests

Treatment

- Systemic disease: Three major classes of drugs are used: NSAIDs, disease-modifying antirheumatic drugs (DMARDs), and corticosteroids.
- *Ocular disease*
  - For cases of dry eye, artificial tear substitutes and lubricating ointments, topical steroids, or topical cyclosporin A 2% drops should be used. Temporary punctal plugs and/or permanent punctal occlusion with cautery or permanent tarsorrhaphy are also useful modalities for maintaining adequate ocular lubrication.
  - Keratitis: Topical and oral corticosteroids and topical 2% cyclosporin A drops may play a role in the treatment of RA-associated keratitis, particularly nonulcerative keratitis and infiltrative PUK. However, more severe cases may require systemic immunosuppression.
  - Scleritis: In mild cases, NSAIDS can be used along with, or instead of, low-dose oral steroids. Moderate to severe disease, including necrotizing scleritis and PUK, require systemic treatment. If patients cannot achieve disease remission with less than 10 mg of prednisone daily, steroid-sparing agents should be used. Antimetabolites (methotrexate, azathioprine, and mycophenolate mofetil), calcineurin inhibitors (cyclosporin, and tacrolimus), and biologic agents (infliximab, adalimumab, and rituximab) have all been used with varying degrees of success. Although etanercept has good efficacy for the treatment of systemic RA, it is less efficacious for the treatment of the ocular disease than are the other biologic agents.

  - Nodular scleritis may be treated with injection of triamcinolone over the lesion, and some authors have reported success in treating certain types of anterior scleritis with periocular steroid injections.

Prognosis

If treated early, long-term remission can often be obtained. Acute exacerbations of the disease can be avoided with regular monitoring and titration of the dose of the immunosuppressive agent.

REFERENCES

Albini TA, Zamir E, Read RW, et al. Evaluation of subconjunctival triamcinolone for nonnecrotizing anterior scleritis. *Ophthalmology.* 2005;112(10):1814–1820.

Chauhan S, Kamal A, Thompson RN, et al. Rituximab for treatment of scleritis associated with rheumatoid arthritis. *Br J Ophthalmol.* 2009;93(7):984–985.

Gangaputra S, Newcomb CW, Liesegang TL, et al. Systemic Immunosuppressive Therapy for Eye Diseases Cohort Study. Methotrexate for ocular inflammatory diseases. *Ophthalmology.* 2009;116(11):2188–2198.

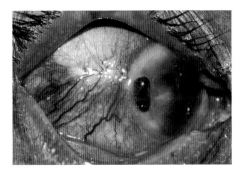

FIGURE 7-19. Diffuse scleritis is characterized by deep, tortuous, dilated scleral vessels. There is also peripheral corneal melting with iris prolapse in this case. (Courtesy of S. R. Rathinam.)

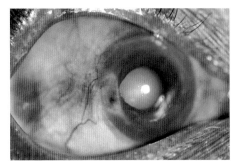

FIGURE 7-20. There is peripheral ulcerative keratitis in a patient with active, previously undiagnosed rheumatoid arthritis. (Courtesy of S. R. Rathinam.)

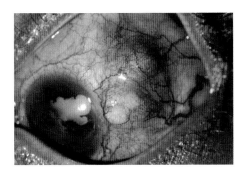

FIGURE 7-21. There are several large, injected nodules as well as diffuse scleritis in this patient with nodular scleritis. Posterior synechiae and a cataract are present. (Courtesy of S. R. Rathinam.)

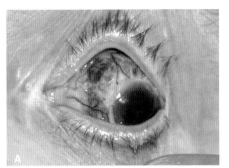

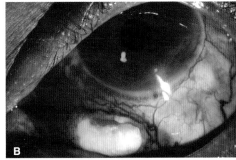

FIGURE 7-22. **A.** Significant scleral thinning with uveal prolapse. The lack of injection is typical of scleromalacia perforans. (Courtesy of Sunir J. Garg.) **B.** Significant scleral thinning with an inferior scleral melt. Compared with patients with necrotizing scleritis, patients with scleromalacia perforans have relatively little scleral redness and often have minimal to no discomfort. (Courtesy of S. R. Rathinam.)

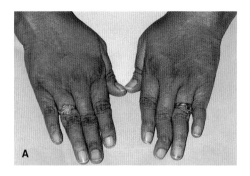

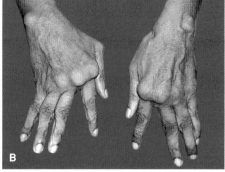

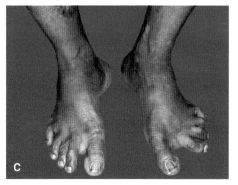

FIGURE 7-23. **A, B.** Rheumatoid arthritis is a polyarthritis which affects the small joints of the hands and feet more frequently than larger joints. The synovial inflammation leads to joint destruction. These patients have the typical finger joint deformities seen in patients with rheumatoid arthritis. Prompt and aggressive therapy can dramatically reduce this debilitating aspect of RA. **C.** Similar joint destruction can also occur in the feet. (Courtesy of S. R. Rathinam.)

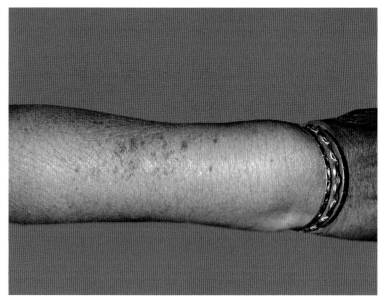

FIGURE 7-24. This patient has vasculitis of the skin, which can be seen in some patients with rheumatoid arthritis. (Courtesy of S. R. Rathinam.)

BEHÇET'S DISEASE

H. Nida Sen

Behçet's disease (BD), or Adamantiades-Behçet's disease, is a chronic, relapsing multisystem inflammatory disorder of unknown etiology that is characterized by intraocular inflammation, oral and mucosal ulcerations, and skin lesions.

Epidemiology and Etiology

- It is more commonly seen in patients from the Mediterranean basin and Japan, along the route of the ancient "silk road." It also occurs in persons with Native American ancestry.

    - In the United States, the prevalence is 8.6 in 100,000 persons, and is as high as 25 to 400 in 100,000 in Mediterranean countries.

- Ocular involvement occurs in approximately 70% of patients with Behçet's disease and is typically bilateral (>70%). Posterior/panuveitis is the most common form of uveitis in these patients.

    - Ocular disease can be the presenting symptom in 10% to 35% of patients and is characterized by recurrent, explosive exacerbations of intraocular inflammation.

- It typically affects young adults (mean age at onset is 25 to 35 years), but it may also occur in children.

- Men are slightly more affected than women.

- Behçet's is a multifactorial disease: Genetic factors, environmental factors, infectious agents, and immunologic mechanisms all have been suggested.

- Affected patients are thought to have a genetic predisposition, and it has been associated with HLA-B51.

Symptoms

- Redness, blurry vision, floaters
- Oral ulcers, genital ulcers, skin changes

Signs

- The International Society for Behçet's Disease and the Japanese Behçet's Disease Research Committee developed criteria for the diagnosis (**Table 7-3**).

- Systemic manifestations: oral ulcers are the most common manifestation occurring in 98% of patients, followed by skin lesions (90%), and genital ulcers (77% to 85%).

- Ocular signs usually manifest as an explosive anterior uveitis typically with a hypopyon. Vitritis, necrotizing retinitis, retinal vasculitis, retinal hemorrhages, retinal edema, vitreous hemorrhage, capillary dropout, retinal neovascularization, and vitreous hemorrhage also occur.

    - Rare ocular manifestations include episcleritis, filamentary keratitis, conjunctivitis and extraocular muscle paralysis secondary to neuro-Behçet's disease.

    - Between episodes, the ocular exam may be unremarkable.

Differential Diagnosis

- HLA-B27–associated anterior uveitis with hypopyon
- Pseudohypopyon
- Viral retinitis (specifically CMV, VZV, HSV)
- Toxoplasmosis
- Ocular lymphoma
- Lupus retinal vasculitis
- Polyarteritis nodosa (PAN)
- Sarcoidosis
- Wegener's granulomatosis–associated vasculitis

Diagnostic Evaluation (Figs. 7-25 to 7-33)

- Fluorescein angiography demonstrates early blockage in areas of retinitis with late staining, staining and leakage of retinal vessels in the mid to late phases, and areas of capillary drop-out.

• Indocyanine green (ICG) angiography demonstrates areas of hyper- and hypofluorescence.

• Presence of HLA-B51 is supportive of the diagnosis, but not diagnostic.

• A positive pathergy test and elevated ESR, CRP, and white blood count (WBC) are also suggestive of the diagnosis, but not diagnostic.

• Histopathology demonstrates leukocytoclastic and monocytic occlusive vasculitis.

Treatment

• Prompt and aggressive systemic therapy with corticosteroids as the first-line agent is critical. Initially, some patients may need IV pulse steroids to control acute inflammation.

• Most patients will need immunosuppressive agents, which typically include cyclosporine, azathioprine, mycophenolate mofetil, alkylating agents (i.e., Cytoxan), infliximab, interferon-alpha, or a combination of these agents.

• The main goal of treatment is to decrease the frequency and severity of the inflammatory episodes.

Prognosis

• The visual prognosis depends upon the involvement of the posterior segment, timeliness of therapy, and sustained control of inflammation.

■ Younger age at onset, poor vision at presentation, posterior segment disease, persistent inflammatory activity, posterior synechiae, elevated intraocular pressure, and hypotony are poor prognostic indicators.

• With prompt and aggressive therapy, structural complications and visual impairment can be minimized.

• Complications are frequent and occur in 60% to 90% of patients. In addition to the development of cataracts and glaucoma, posterior synechiae, macular edema, epiretinal membrane, retinal neovascularization, vitreous hemorrhage, retinal and/or optic atrophy, branch retinal vein occlusion, branch retinal artery occlusion, and retinal detachment can occur.

• Significant vision loss (<20/200) occurs in 20% to 30% of patients within 5 years of disease onset.

REFERENCES

International Study Group for Behçet's Disease, Criteria for diagnosis of Behçet's disease, *Lancet* 335 (1990): 1078–1080.

Kaçmaz RO, Kempen JH, Newcomb C, et al. Systemic Immunosuppressive Therapy for Eye Diseases Cohort Study Group. Ocular inflammation in Behçet disease: incidence of ocular complications and of loss of visual acuity. *Am J Ophthalmol.* 2008;146(6):828–836.

Nussenblatt RB, Whitcup SM. *Uveitis: Fundamentals and Clinical Practice.* 4th ed. Philadelphia: Mosby Elsevier; 2010.

Tugal-Tutkun I, Onal S, Altan-Yaycioglu R, et al. Uveitis in Behçet disease: an analysis of 880 patients. *Am J Ophthalmol.* 2004;138(3):373–380.

Verity DH, Wallace GR, Vaughan RW, et al. Behçet's disease: from Hippocrates to the third millennium. *Br J Ophthalmol.* 2003;87:1175–1183.

TABLE 7-3. Diagnostic Criteria for Behçet Disease

International Study Group Criteria for Behçet's Disease	Modified Japanese Behçet's Disease Research Committee Criteria
• Recurrent oral ulcers (≥3 times/year) *and* • 2 of the below criteria: • Recurrent genital ulcers • Ocular disease (uveitis) • Skin lesions (erythema nodosum, pseudofolliculitis, papulopustular lesions, acneiform lesions) • Positive pathergy test (skin prick test)	*Major criteria* • Recurrent oral aphthous ulcers • Genital ulcerations • Ocular disease • Skin disease (erythema nodosum, cutaneous hypersensitivity thrombophlebitis) *Minor criteria* • Arthritis • GI disease (intestinal ulcers) • Epididymitis/testicular vasculitis • Vascular disease (occlusive vasculitis, aneurysms) • CNS disease (neuropsychiatric symptoms, parenchymal lesions, vascular thrombosis, vasculitis, meningitis/encephalitis) *Complete type:* All 4 major criteria *Incomplete type:* 3 major OR 2 major + 2 minor criteria OR typical ocular disease +1 major (or 2 minor) criteria *Suspect type:* 2 major criteria (other than ocular) *Possible type:* 1 major criteria

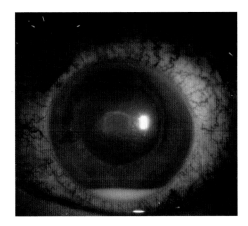

FIGURE 7-25. Color photograph showing acute anterior uveitis with a hypopyon.

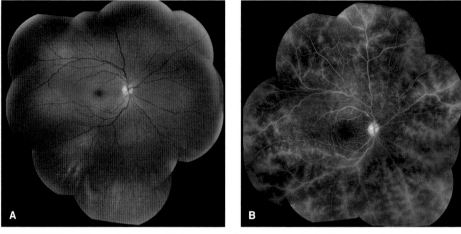

FIGURE 7-26. **A.** 25-year-old female of Italian ancestry had early posterior involvement by Behçet disease. **B.** There is diffuse staining and leakage from the retinal vasculature in the late frames of the angiogram.

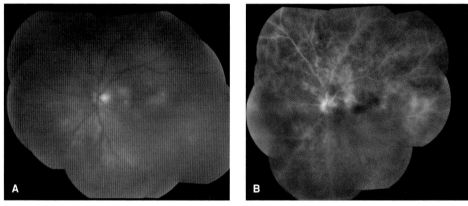

FIGURE 7-27. Retinal vasculitis and macular retinitis with early blockage of fluorescein in areas of retinitis. There is diffuse retinal vascular leakage.

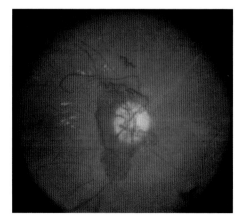

FIGURE 7-28. Severe retinal vasculitis and ischemia resulted in neovascularization of the optic disk. Note the widespread areas of vascular dropout/nonperfusion.

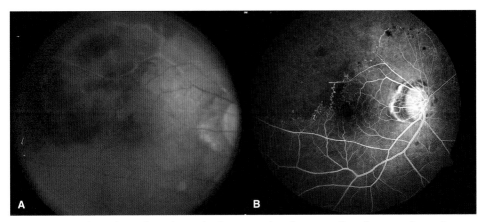

FIGURE 7-29. Advanced retinal vasculitis with sclerotic vessels and severe capillary dropout and extensive retinal ischemia with retinal hemorrhages.

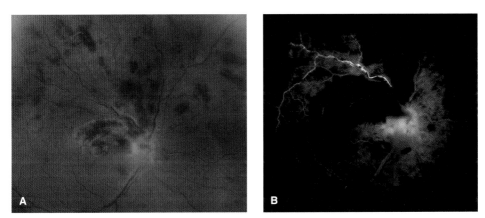

FIGURE 7-30. This 41-year-old woman developed severe vision loss due to arteritis along the superotemporal arcade. She also had oral and genital ulcers. The active vasculitis resolved with treatment, but a permanent visual field defect remained. (Courtesy of Robert Sergott, MD, and Sunir Garg, MD.)

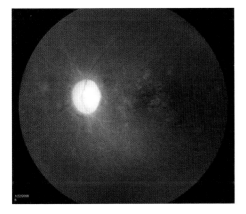

FIGURE 7-31. A 39-year-old Korean man with complete Behçet's disease. The left eye shows end-stage disease with diffuse retinal, vascular, and optic nerve atrophy.

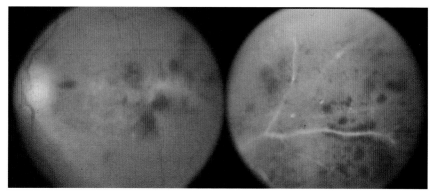

FIGURE 7-32. This patient developed severe occlusive retinal vasculitis with retinal hemorrhages.

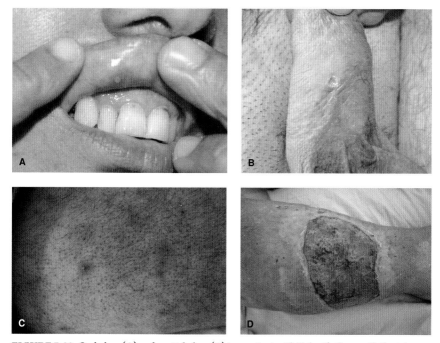

FIGURE 7-33. Oral ulcer (**A**) and genital ulcer (**B**) in a patient with Behçet's disease. **C.** Pustular acneiform skin lesions can also occur in Behçet's disease. **D.** Note the severe venous stasis ulcer in a patient with venous insufficiency secondary to Behçet's disease. (Courtesy of Nilgun Senturk, MD, Turkey.)

SYSTEMIC LUPUS ERYTHEMATOSUS

Robert W. Wong, S. R. Rathinam, and Emmett T. Cunningham, Jr. ▧

Systemic lupus erythematosus (SLE), or lupus, is a chronic, systemic, autoimmune disease characterized by the production and deposition of pathologic autoimmune complexes and autoantibodies in tissues throughout the body and can affect any organ system.

Etiology and Epidemiology

● Lupus is more common in patients of African or Asian descent.

● It is most common in the second to fifth decades of life.

● There is a strong female preponderance (9:1).

● SLE has been linked to major histocompatability complex genes HLA-A1, -B8, -DR3, and -DQ, and to complement complexes C1q, C2, and C4.

● Drug-induced SLE has been associated with medications, including procainamide, hydralazine, and quinidine.

Symptoms

● Ocular:
  ▫ Dry eye
  ▫ Loss of vision

Signs

● Systemic:
  ▫ As lupus can affect essentially all organs, patients may present with any number of often non-specific complaints.
  ▫ The American College of Rheumatology (ACR) has established consensus criteria of which four or more should be present either serially or simultaneously during any period of observation:

  ▸ Malar rash (see Fig. 7-34)
  ▸ Discoid rash
  ▸ Skin photosensitivity
  ▸ Oral ulcers (painless)
  ▸ Arthritis (pleuritis or pericarditis)
  ▸ Serositis (pleuritis or pericarditis)
  ▸ Renal disorder (nephritis; proteinuria and/or cellular casts)
  ▸ Neurologic disorder (seizures or psychiatric)
  ▸ Hematologic disorder (hemolytic anemia, leukopenia, lymphopenia, thrombocytopenia)
  ▸ Immunologic disorder (anti-DNA, anti-Sm, false-positive syphilis serologies, anti-phospholipid antibodies)
  ▸ Antinuclear antibodies (ANA)

▧ Ocular findings are not included in the ACR diagnostic criteria, but may include:
  ▸ Keratoconjunctivitis sicca
  ▸ Anterior scleritis (see Fig. 7-35)
  ▸ Iritis
  ▸ Retinal vasculitis (Fig. 7-36)
  ▸ Retinal hemorrhage
  ▸ Retinal venous occlusive disease
  ▸ Cotton wool spots
  ▸ Vaso-occlusive retinopathy
  ▸ Serous retinal detachment
  ▸ Uveal effusion
  ▸ Posterior scleritis (Fig. 7-37)
  ▸ Optic neuropathy
  ▸ Orbital inflammation/pseudotumor

▫ The antiphospholipid antibody syndrome also may complicate SLE, causing both systemic as well as retinal thrombosis.

Differential Diagnosis

- Retinal vasculitis:
  - Hypertensive retinopathy
  - Mild or impending vein occlusion
  - Behçet's disease
  - Wegener's granulomatosis
  - Sarcoidosis
  - Syphilis
  - Lyme disease
  - HIV retinopathy
  - Cytomegalovirus (CMV) retinitis
  - Tuberculosis
- Choroidopathy:
  - Central serous retinopathy
  - Vogt-Koyanagi-Harada syndrome
  - Sympathetic ophthalmia
  - Choroidal tumor or metastasis

Diagnostic Evaluation

- Fluorescein angiography: Vascular staining or leakage can be seen with retinitis. Capillary nonperfusion may be seen in ischemic disease. Optic nerve leakage may be seen with optic neuritis. Late pinpoint leakage can be seen when choroidopathy or posterior scleritis is present.
- Laboratory testing
  - Testing for ANA
  - Testing for anti-ds DNA and anti-Sm antibodies
  - Testing to rule out other diseases such as tuberculosis, sarcoidosis, and syphilis

Treatment

- Keratoconjunctivitis sicca may be treated with artificial tear supplementation, punctal occlusion, or with topical cyclosporine.
- Episcleritis may be treated with NSAIDs.
- Scleral, retinal, choroidal, neurologic, or orbital disease should be treated systemically, with corticosteroids as the first-line agent.
- Periocular corticosteroid injection may be used as adjunctive treatment.
- If more than 3 months of treatment is anticipated, noncorticosteroid agents such as antimetabolites and biologic agents should be considered. Hydroxychloroquine, up to 6.5 mg/kg/day, may also be used.

Prognosis

- Generally good with prompt treatment of ocular disease
- The visual prognosis is poor if macular infarction or ischemic optic neuropathy is present.
- Patients with lupus have a 15-year survival rate of 80%. Myocardial infarction and stroke are important causes of mortality.

REFERENCES

D'Cruz DP, Khamashta MA, Hughes GR. Systemic lupus erythematosus. *Lancet.* 2007;369:587–596.

Davies JB, Rao PK. Ocular manifestations of systemic lupus erythematosus. *Current Opinion in Ophthalmology.* 2008; 19:512–518.

Utx VM, Tang J. Ocular manifestations of the antiphospholipid syndrome. *Br J Ophthalmol.* Aug 7. [Epub ahead of print]

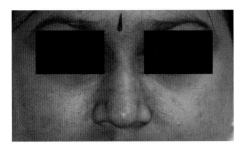

FIGURE 7-34. Malar rash in a patient with systemic lupus erythematosus.

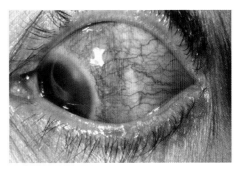

FIGURE 7-35. Anterior scleritis in a patient with systemic lupus erythematosus.

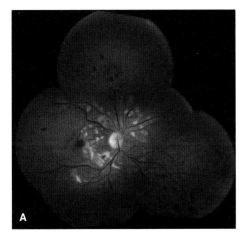

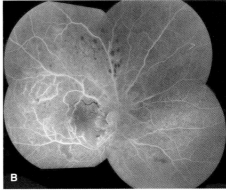

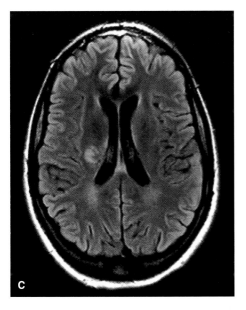

FIGURE 7-36. A 17-year-old girl presented with bilateral vision loss. A targeted workup revealed that she had SLE. **A.** Color fundus photograph of a patient with systemic lupus. There are nerve fiber layer infarcts with scattered retinal hemorrhages. Macular ischemia is also evident. **B.** Fluorescein angiography reveals capillary nonperfusion as well as staining of the retinal vessels in the late frames. The blocking defects are due the retinal hemorrhages. She presented several weeks later with mood, memory, and motor function abnormalities. **C.** MRI of her head found several small cerebral infarcts. (Courtesy of Paul Baker, MD.)

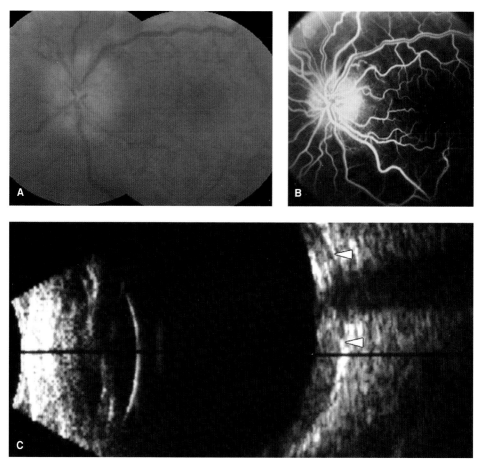

FIGURE 7-37. **A.** Fundus photograph showing optic disk edema and retinal folds in the macula of the left eye. **B.** Fluorescein angiogram showing early disc leakage. **C.** B-scan ultrasound showing thickening of the posterior sclera with juxta-scleral fluid (white arrowheads). (Reproduced with permission from Wong RW, Chan A, Johnson RN, et al. Posterior scleritis in patients with systemic lupus erythematosus. *Retinal Cases & Brief Reports.* 2010;(4): 336–331.)

ANTIPHOSPHOLIPID SYNDROME

Virginia M. Utz and Johnny Tang

Antiphospholipid syndrome (APS) is an autoimmune disease characterized by arterial and venous thrombosis, recurrent fetal loss, and the presence of antibodies directed against phospholipids. The eye is frequently involved and may be the presenting manifestation.

Etiology and Epidemiology

- Pathophysiology
  - APS is due to a heterogeneous group of antibodies directed against negatively charged phospholipids and adaptor proteins that leads to a hypercoagulable state via several pathogenic mechanisms (**Fig. 7-38**).
  - APS may occur in the presence or absence of other autoimmune disorders such as SLE.
- Epidemiology
  - Low levels of antiphospholipid antibodies are present in 2% to 7% of the normal population and increase with age. The risk for thrombosis is low in these individuals.
  - The risk for thrombosis is related to high antiphospholipid titers and previous history of a thrombotic event.
  - The ocular manifestations of APS most commonly affect women around age 40.
- Genetics: APS has been associated with HLA-DR and -DQ as well as with polymorphisms in the β2-glycoprotein I protein.

Symptoms

- Ocular
  - Monocular or binocular blurry vision
  - Amaurosis fugax
  - Transient scotoma

  - Visual field defect
  - Dry eye
  - Redness
  - Pain

Signs

- Systemic (**Table 7-4**)
  - APS can cause thrombosis-related complications in any organ, and can range from an acute ischemic event to chronic ischemia.
  - Deep vein thrombosis is the most common manifestation.
  - Recurrent fetal loss is a hallmark of the disease.
  - Cerebral, renal, pulmonary, and skin ischemia can also occur.
- Ocular
  - Posterior segment changes are the most frequent.
  - Retinal changes include central and branch retinal vein occlusion with retinal hemorrhages, and venous dilation and tortuosity.
  - Central and branch retinal artery occlusion with retinal ischemia
  - Retinal ischemia ranges from mild with retinal telangiectasia and cotton wool spots to severe with peripheral ischemia, and resultant retinal neovascularization and vitreous hemorrhage.
  - Choroidal infarction and ciliochoroidal occlusion can also occur.
  - Rarely will patients develop vitritis.
  - Anterior segment manifestations are unusual but can include keratoconjunctivitis sicca, conjunctival telangiectasia, anterior uveitis, and episcleritis or scleritis.
  - Due to the widespread nature of the emboli, patients may also have

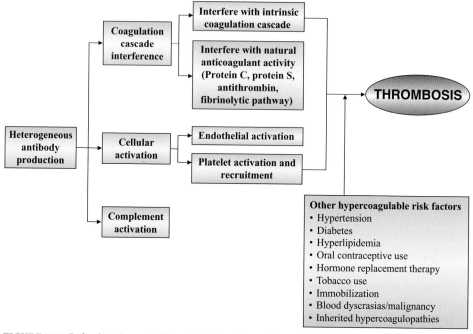

FIGURE 7-38. Pathophysiology of antiphospholipid syndrome. Heterogeneous antibody production with multiple antigenic targets in addition to other host systemic risk factors lead to thrombosis.

TABLE 7-4. Systemic Manifestations of APS

Hematologic	Pulmonary
• Thrombocytopenia	• Pulmonary thrombosis/embolism
• Autoimmune hemolytic anemia	• Secondary pulmonary hypertension
• Hemolytic uremic syndrome	
Central Nervous System	**Dermatologic**
• Stroke or transient ischemic attack	• Livedo reticularis
• Migraine	• Leg ulcers
• Multiple sclerosis–like illness	• Digital gangrene
• Dementia	
Cardiovascular	**Gastrointestinal**
• Heart valve lesions	• Budd-Chiari syndrome
• Coronary artery disease	• Mesenteric ischemia
Renal	**Endocrine**
• Nephropathy	• Adrenal infarction
	• Pituitary gland infarction

neuro-ophthalmologic features such as cranial nerve palsies, nonarteritic ischemic optic neuropathy, secondary idiopathic intracranial hypertension, optic nerve edema, and ischemic infarcts of the visual pathway.

Differential Diagnosis

- The differential diagnosis is quite broad and can include any vaso-occlusive disorder. In patients with no other identifiable underlying predisposing factors, APS should be considered.
- Retinal vascular disease
  - Diabetic retinopathy
  - Branch and central retinal vein occlusion
  - Branch and central retinal artery occlusion
  - Retinal embolization (e.g., talc)
  - Radiation retinopathy
  - Eales' disease
  - Retinopathy of prematurity
  - Familial exudative vitreoretinopathy (FEVR)
- Ocular inflammatory disease
  - Birdshot retinochoroidopathy
  - Serpiginous choroidopathy
  - Toxoplasmosis
  - Sarcoidosis
  - Lyme disease
  - Syphilis
  - Multiple sclerosis
- Systemic
  - Carotid occlusive disease
  - Giant cell arteritis
  - Sickle cell disease (SS/SC/SThal)
  - Sarcoidosis
  - Tuberculosis
  - Nephrotic syndrome

- Inherited hypercoagulopathy (Protein C/S deficiency, antithrombin III deficiency, Factor V Leiden)
- Blood dyscrasias (anemia, thrombocytopenia, leukemia, lymphoma, multiple myeloma)
- Autoimmune occlusive diseases (SLE, polyarteritis nodosa, Thrombotic Thrombocytopenic Purpura/Hemolytic Uremic Syndrome (TTP/HUS), Idiopathic Thrombocytopenic Purpura (ITP))

Diagnostic Evaluation (**Figs. 7-39 and 7-40**)

- The diagnosis of APS requires a history of thromboembolism or recurrent fetal loss within 5 years of a positive serology. Serologic criteria must be confirmed on two or more occasions at least 12 weeks apart as follows:
  - Presence of lupus anticoagulant antibodies, or
  - Presence of moderate to high levels of anticardiolipin and anti–beta-2 glycoprotein I antibodies
- Fluorescein angiography reveals finding consistent with retinovascular disease:
  - Marked delay in the arterial phase and venous return
  - Optic disk edema and leakage
  - Macular edema
  - Leakage from or staining of the vessel walls
  - Extensive peripheral areas of capillary nonperfusion
  - Progressive hyperfluorescence from neovascularization
  - Retinal pigment epithelial window defects

Treatment

- Patients with APS require lifelong anticoagulation with either warfarin or antiplatelet agents in order to reduce the risk of future thromboembolic events (**Fig. 7-41**).

- Reduce modifiable cardiovascular and thromboembolic risk factors such as hypertension, hyperlipidemia, diabetes mellitus, oral anticontraceptive agent use, and tobacco use.

Prognosis

- Generally is good with prompt and aggressive anticoagulant therapy.

- In the absence of anticoagulation, patients with a diagnosis of APS are at a high risk of further thromboembolic complications ranging from 22% to 29% per year.

- Some of the visual loss may be permanent.

REFERENCES

Miyakis S, Lockshin MD, Atsumi T, et al. International consensus statement on an update of the classification criteria for definite antiphospholipid syndrome (APS). *J Thromb Haemost.* 2006;4:295–306.

Ruiz-Irastorza G, Hunt BJ, Khamashta MA. A systematic review of secondary thromboprophylaxis in patients with antiphospholipid antibodies. *Arthritis Rheum.* 2007;57:1487–95.

Tang J, Fillmore G, Nussenblatt RB. Antiphospholipid antibody syndrome mimicking serpiginous choroidopathy. *Ocul Immunol Inflamm.* 2009;17:278–281.

Utz, V, Tang, J. Ocular manifestations of antiphospholipid syndrome. *Br J Ophthalmol.* Aug 2010 (Epub ahead of print).

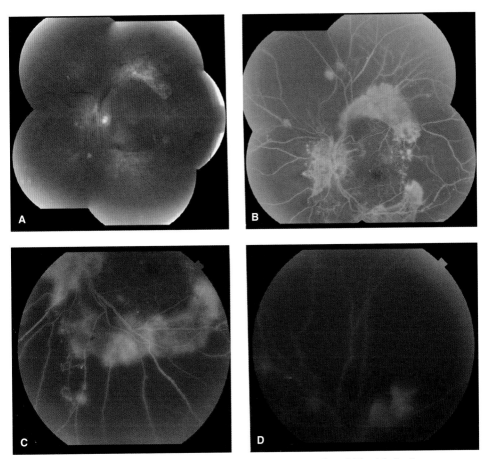

FIGURE 7-39. Posterior pole manifestations of the left eye of a patient with APS. The right fundus was obscured by vitreous hemorrhage. **A.** Color fundus composite photo demonstrating vascular tortuosity, attenuation, and fibrosis involving the temporal arcades. **B.** Composite mid- to late-phase fluorescein angiogram (FA) is significant for extensive nonperfusion, and leakage from the optic disk and retinal vasculature. **C and D.** Peripheral midphase FA shows microvascular remodeling, shunting, and leakage from neovascularization in the setting of peripheral vascular nonperfusion.

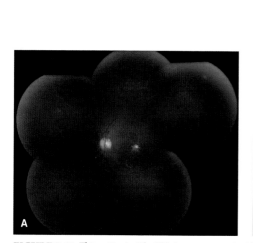
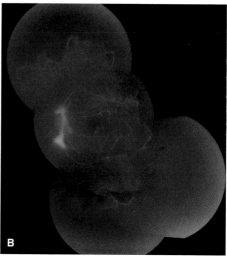

FIGURE 7-40. This patient with APS demonstrates significant peripheral nonperfusion. **A.** There is neovascularization of the disk with inferior vitreous hemorrhage. Hard exudates are present in the macula. There is vascular remodeling temporal to the fovea. **B.** The fluorescein angiogram demonstrates neovascularization of the disk. There is profound peripheral nonperfusion. (Courtesy of Alok Bansal, MD, and Nik London, MD.)

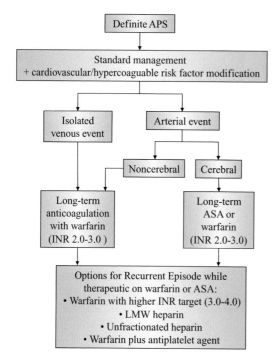

FIGURE 7-41. Treatment algorithm for management of APS. Standard management includes warfarin for a venous thrombus and antiplatelet therapy for a stroke or arterial event.

EALES' DISEASE

Jyotirmay Biswas and
Parthopratim Dutta Majumder

Eales' disease is an idiopathic inflammatory venous occlusive disease that primarily affects the peripheral retina of young individuals.

Etiology and Epidemiology

● The etiology is unknown; however, hypersensitivity to tuberculin protein has been suggested and tubercle bacilli have been identified in pathology specimens. Other immune-mediated mechanisms, such as predominant T-cell involvement, have also been demonstrated through experimental studies.

● Although patients in a number of countries have developed Eales' disease, it is most common in the Indian subcontinent. It typically affects healthy adults who are in their 20s to 30s and it is more common in men. Over half of patients have bilateral disease.

Symptoms

● Patients most commonly describe floaters and blurred vision.

● Patients may have moderate to severe loss of vision due to vitreous hemorrhage and retinal detachment.

● Rarely, patients can have myelopathy, vestibuloauditory dysfunction, or strokes.

Signs

● Active perivasculitis often with sheathing and perivascular retinal hemorrhages involving one or more quadrants.

● Varying degrees of peripheral retinal nonperfusion with remnants of obliterated vessels.

● The peripheral retinal ischemia can result in retinal neovascularization and recurrent vitreous hemorrhage, as well as anterior segment neovascularization. (Figs. 7-42 to 7-44)

● Retinal detachment

● Anterior chamber cell and flare, KPs, and cystoid macular edema may occur.

Differential Diagnosis

● Diabetic retinopathy

● Behçet's disease

● Sickle cell retinopathy

● Branch retinal vein occlusion

● Coats' disease

● Retinopathy of prematurity

● FEVR

● Hyperviscosity syndrome

● Sarcoidosis

● Collagen vascular disease

● Ocular ischemic syndrome

● Talc retinopathy

Diagnostic Evaluation

● No specific testing is used to diagnose Eales' disease. It is a diagnosis of exclusion, and other underlying diseases should be ruled out.

● Most patients are purified protein derivative (PPD) positive.

● Fundus fluorescein angiography may show early staining of vessels with leakage of dye in the late phases. Peripheral retinal ischemia is common.

● B-scan ultrasonography is useful in cases of vitreous hemorrhage to rule out an underlying retinal detachment.

Treatment

● Oral prednisone (1 mg/kg bodyweight), with a taper of 10 mg/wk over 6 to 8 weeks remains the mainstay of therapy in the treatment of active perivasculitis. Intravitreal triamcinolone can also be used to treat the vasculitis.

● Cases of gross capillary nonperfusion, retinal or anterior segment neovascularization, and/or vitreous hemorrhage, require panretinal laser photocoagulation (Fig. 7-45).

● Recent studies have demonstrated a close relationship between the prominent neovascular proliferation in Eales' disease and intense expression of vascular endothelial growth factor. Intravitreal injection of anti–vascular endothelial growth factor agents may be useful, especially in cases with early neovascular glaucoma.

- Pars plana vitrectomy is used to clear vitreous hemorrhage, to remove epiretinal membranes, and to repair retinal detachment (Fig. 7-46).

Prognosis

Early treatment carries a good prognosis, with the majority of patients maintaining 20/40 vision or better.

REFERENCES

Das T, Pathengay A, Hussain N, et al. Eales disease: diagnosis and management. *Eye.* 2010;24: 472–482.

Ishaq M, Feroze AH, Shahid M, et al. Intravitreal steroids may facilitate treatment of Eales' disease (idiopathic retinal vasculitis): an interventional case series. *Eye (Lond).* 2007 Nov;21(11):1403–1405.

Therese KL, Deepa P, Therese J, et al. Association of mycobacteria with Eales' disease. *Indian J Med Res.* 2007;126(1):56–62.

Verma A, Biswas J, Radhakrishnan S, et al. Intra-ocular expression of vascular endothelial growth factor (VEGF) and pigment epithelial-derived factor (PEDF) in a case of Eales' disease by immunohistochemical analysis: a case report. *Int Ophthalmol.* 2010;30(4): 429–434.

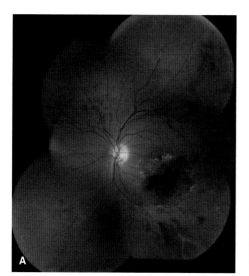
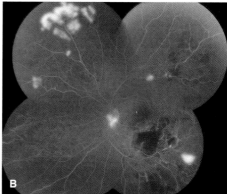

FIGURE 7-42. **A.** Montage fundus photograph of a patient with Eales' disease shows multiple areas of active perivasculitis, peripheral nonperfusion, and superficial retinal hemorrhages. **B.** Fluorescein angiogram montage demonstrates multiple areas of nonperfusion with neovascularization at the border of perfused and nonperfused retina. (Courtesy of Paul Baker, MD.)

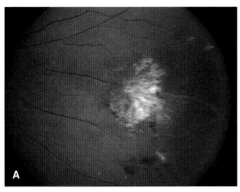

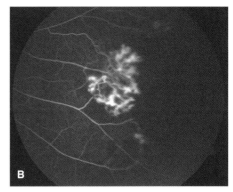

FIGURE 7-43. **A.** Fundus photograph showing peripheral retinal neovascularization at the junction of perfused and nonperfused retina. **B.** Fluorescein angiogram demonstrating the area of neovascularization. (Courtesy of S. R. Rathinam.)

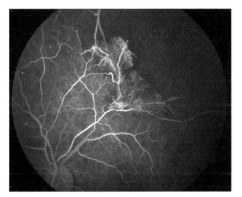

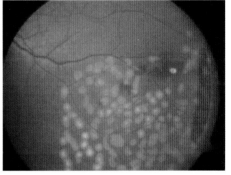

FIGURE 7-44. Fluorescein angiogram demonstrating a large neovascular frond at the junction of perfused and nonperfused retina. (Courtesy of S. R. Rathinam.)

FIGURE 7-45. Fundus photograph showing sector laser photocoagulation to the area of retinal nonperfusion.

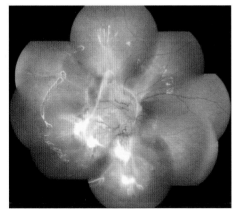

FIGURE 7-46. Montage fundus photograph of a tractional retinal detachment secondary to fibrovascular proliferation. Vitrectomy with membrane peel and pan-retinal laser photocoagulation would be indicated.

GRANULOMATOSIS WITH POLYANGIITIS (WEGENER'S GRANULOMATOSIS)

Keith Wroblewski

Granulomatosis with polyangiitis (also called Wegener's granulomatosis) is an ANCA-associated systemic vasculitis. Although it can affect all organ systems, the classic triad consists of necrotizing granulomas of the upper and lower respiratory tracts, systemic vasculitis, and glomerulonephritis.

Etiology and Epidemiology

- The male to female ratio is roughly equal.
- Most patients are in their late 40s to early 50s at the time of diagnosis.
- Caucasians constitute over 90% of patients.
- Ocular involvement (uveitis, scleritis, retinal vasculitis) occurs in up to 16% of patients.

Symptoms

- The most common symptoms are nonspecific, and include fever, malaise, anorexia, arthralgias, and weight loss.
- As any part of the eye can be affected, patients may have diplopia, pain, redness, tearing, and decreased vision.
- Patients often have chronic sinus congestion, cough, hemoptysis, dyspnea, and chest discomfort.
- Bloody or purulent nasal discharge, as well as ear pain or swollen gums can occur.

Signs (Figs. 7-47 to 7-52)

- Because granulomatosis with polyangiitis can affect any and all organ systems, it can have a myriad of presentations.
- Orbital disease and scleritis are the most common ocular manifestations. Signs may include:

This contribution to the work was done as part of the author's official duties as an NIH employee and is a work of the United States Government.

- Proptosis (orbital pseudotumor), compressive optic neuropathy, nasolacrimal duct obstruction
- Conjunctivitis, episcleritis, scleritis, necrotizing scleritis and scleral perforation, and peripheral ulcerative keratitis
- Anterior, intermediate, or posterior uveitis
- Retinal vascular occlusions with associated neovascularization and vitreous hemorrhage
- Ciliochoroidal effusion with peripheral retinal hemorrhages and nonperfusion
- Peripheral retinal or choroidal mass
- Extraocular
  - Upper respiratory tract: Epistaxis, sinusitis, nasal septal perforation with saddle nose deformity, hearing loss, tinnitus, otitis media, gingivitis or subglottic tracheal stenosis leading to airway obstruction
  - Lower respiratory: Pulmonary nodules, hemorrhagic atelectasis, respiratory failure
  - Renal: Hematuria and proteinuria due to glomerulonephritis with subsequent renal failure
  - Skin: Papules, nodules, hemorrhagic vesicles, and ischemic ulcers
  - CNS: Meningitis, cranial neuropathy, and cerebral vasculitis
  - Cardiac: Pericarditis or coronary vasculitis

Differential Diagnosis

- Polyarteritis nodosa
- Sarcoidosis
- Tuberculosis
- Goodpasture's syndrome
- Churg-Strauss syndrome (a systemic vasculitis associated with peripheral eosinophilia, asthma, and allergic rhinitis)
- Microscopic polyangiitis
- Histoplasmosis

- Orbital cellulitis
- Orbital pseudotumor
- Grave's eye disease
- Mucocutaneous leishmaniasis

Diagnostic Evaluation

It is a clinical diagnosis confirmed by laboratory findings. Although 80% to 90% of patients are ANCA positive, a negative test does not exclude the diagnosis.

- Laboratory testing:
  - c-ANCA: c-Antineutrophil cytoplasmic antibody (c-ANCA or PR3) testing is helpful to not only confirm the diagnosis but also to follow the disease course (prognosis).
  - Nonspecific tests include an elevated ESR, anemia, leukocytosis, thrombocytosis, hypergammaglobulinemia.
  - Serum creatinine and glomerular filtration rate should be checked to evaluate kidney function and all patients suspected of WG should have urinalysis with microscopic analysis of urinary sediment to look for hematuria and proteinuria.
- Radiographic studies:
  - Chest radiograph or chest CT should be used to evaluate pulmonary involvement.
  - Orbital CT can be useful in cases with suspected orbital involvement.
- Tissue biopsy can demonstrate necrotizing granulomatous inflammation with leukocytoclastic vasculitis.
- Ocular testing: Fluorescein angiography can be used to evaluate retinal vascular involvement.

Treatment

- Wegener's granulomatosis has historically had a high mortality rate. Prompt and aggressive therapy with prednisone and agents such as cyclophosphamide, azathioprine, or methotrexate has dramatically reduced the morbidity and mortality associated with this illness.
  - Initial treatment with cyclophosphamide and steroids induces remission in 85% to 90% within 2 to 6 months.
  - Recent trials indicate that rituximab may be an effective alternative to cyclophosphamide.
- Other than in isolated cases of mild anterior uveitis, topical therapy is not sufficient.
- Surgical intervention may be needed for progressive orbital disease, impending scleral perforation, or lacrimal disease.
- Adverse side effects such as hemorrhagic cystitis or malignancy after treatment with cyclophosphamide and septicemia with rituximab can occur.

Prognosis

- With prompt and aggressive treatment, patients rarely die from the disease; however, renal disease and older age portends higher mortality.
- Visual prognosis is good when treated with appropriate systemic therapy, but compressive optic neuropathy, globe perforation, cystoid macular edema, and peripheral ulcerative keratitis can permanently impact vision.

REFERENCES

Leavitt RY, Fauci AS, Bloch DA, et al. The American College of Rheumatology 1990 criteria for the classification of Wegener's granulomatosis. *Arthritis Rheum.* 1990;33(8):1101–1107.

Leveille AS, Morse PH. Combined detachments in Wegener's granulomatosis. *Br J Ophthal.* 1981; 65: 564–567.

Perry SR, Rootman J, White VA. The clinical and pathologic constellations of Wegener's granulomatosis of the orbit. *Ophthalmology.* 1997;104:683–694.

Spalton DJ, Graham EM, Page NG, et al. Ocular changes in limited forms of Wegener's granulomatosis. *Br J Ophthal.* 1981;65:553–563.

Stone JH, Merkel PA, Spiera R, et al. Rituximab versus cyclophosphamide for ANCA-associated vasculitis. *N Engl J Med.* 2010;363(3):221–232.

Woo TL, Francis IC, Wilczek GA, et al. Australasian orbital and adnexal Wegener's granulomatosis. *Ophthalmology.* 2001;108(9):1535–1543.

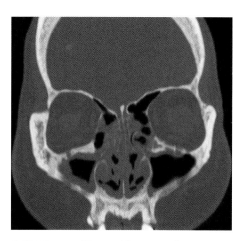

FIGURE 7-47. CT scan of the sinuses shows severe, bilateral, mucosal thickening, boney erosion of the nasal septum, and perturbation of the turbinate anatomy.

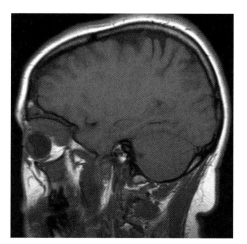

FIGURE 7-48. T1-weighted MRI image of the head shows an isointense superior orbital mass that is causing inferior and posterior globe displacement. (Courtesy Diva Salomao, MD, Mayo Clinic, Rochester, MN.)

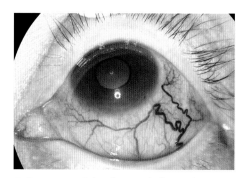

FIGURE 7-49. Color photograph shows scleritis with large, dilated vessels. There is mild peripheral ulcerative keratitis (PUK) inferiorly.

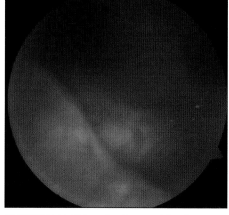

FIGURE 7-50. This patient has a peripheral choroidal mass due to Wegener's granulomatosis.

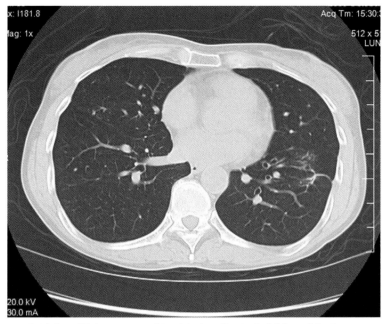

FIGURE 7-51. Axial chest CT shows increased interstitial marking in the left lower lobe that can progress to large cavitary lesions.

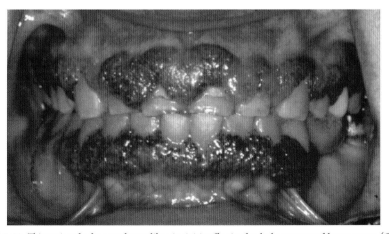

FIGURE 7-52. This patient had a strawberry-like gingivitis affecting both the upper and lower gums. (Courtesy of Armed Forces Institute of Pathology.)

KAWASAKI'S DISEASE

Leon Charkodian and Sunil K. Srivastava

Kawasaki's disease, also known as Kawasaki's syndrome and mucocutaneous lymph node syndrome, is an acute, self-limited vasculitic pediatric syndrome classically involving the blood vessels, mucous membranes, skin, and lymph nodes. It is characterized by a necrotizing vasculitis of medium-sized vessels and is the leading cause of an acquired cardiomyopathy in children.

Etiology and Epidemiology

- It is a disease of childhood, typically occurring in individuals under the age of 5 years.
- The peak prevalence in the United States is between ages 18 and 24 months.
- It is most common in Asian populations, particularly in people of Japanese ancestry.
- There is a slight male preponderance (approximately 1.5:1).
- The etiology is unknown, though it is thought to be an autoimmune inflammatory process, possibly due to exposure to an infectious antigen.

Symptoms

- Abrupt onset of fever (>39°C) of at least 5 days in duration
- Irritability, often out of proportion to physical findings
- Lack of improvement with antibiotics and/or antipyretics

Signs

- Bilateral nonsuppurative conjunctival injection (85%)
- Pharyngeal edema, fissured/swollen lips, strawberry tongue (90%)
- Polymorphous, nonvesicular rash, often generalized (80%)
- Erythema, edema, and desquamation of extremities (75%)
- Cervical lymphadenopathy, often unilateral (40%)
- A diagnosis of classic Kawasaki's disease requires at least four of the above major criteria along with fever of at least 5 days in duration.
- Coronary artery aneurysms (10% to 18%) may occur, developing 2 to 6 weeks after initial fever.
- An additional predominant ocular finding is anterior uveitis with or without KPs.
- Nonspecific findings may precede fever and include malaise, nausea, vomiting, decreased oral intake, tachycardia, cough, diarrhea, rhinorrhea, orchitis, urethritis, myositis, pericarditis, abdominal pain, and joint pain.

Differential Diagnosis

- Scarlet fever
- Juvenile idiopathic arthritis
- Erythema multiforme/toxic epidermal necrolysis/Stephens-Johnson syndrome
- Toxic shock syndrome
- Pharyngitis
- Bacteremia/sepsis
- Meningitis/encephalitis
- Tick-borne diseases
- Staphylococcal scalded skin syndrome
- Leptospirosis
- Mercury toxicity

Diagnostic Evaluation

- Initial laboratory testing: ESR and CRP
- If ESR is <40 mm/hr and CRP is <3 mg/dL, then supportive care is typically given.
- If ESR is >40 mm/hr and CRP is >3 mg/dL, then additional testing is indicated:
  - WBC count: abnormal if >12,000
  - Albumin: abnormal if <3 g

▪ ALT: abnormal if elevated for age

▪ Urinalysis: abnormal if pyuria is present

▪ Platelets: abnormal if >450,000 after 7 days of illness

▪ Hematocrit: abnormal if anemic for age

● If three or more of these additional laboratory tests are abnormal, the child should receive an echocardiogram and pharmacologic treatment.

● If fewer than three of the additional laboratory tests are abnormal, an echocardiogram alone is performed. If positive, pharmacologic treatment should be given. If negative but fever persists, an echocardiogram may be repeated. If negative and fever abates, Kawasaki's disease is unlikely.

Treatment

● Intravenous gamma globulin is now the mainstay of treatment (typically 2 g/kg infused over 12 hours). Treatment is initiated 5 to 7 days after onset of fever.

● Aspirin is typically given, though its benefit in addition to intravenous gamma globulin is unclear. The dose is 80 to 100 mg/kg/day divided q.i.d. for 2 weeks, then 3 to 5 mg/kg once daily for 6 to 8 additional weeks. Aspirin therapy is continued longer if coronary vessel abnormalities are present.

● Patients are admitted to an inpatient service for monitoring and treatment, along with cardiac consultation.

● Ibuprofen should be avoided, as it antagonizes aspirin's antiplatelet activity.

Prognosis

● If patients do not develop coronary artery aneurysms, the disease usually resolves without sequelae.

● Patients who develop coronary artery aneurysms require prolonged monitoring and treatment. Coronary artery bypass grafting and possibly cardiac transplantation may be indicated for giant aneurysms resistant to pharmacologic therapy.

REFERENCES

Puglise JV, Rao NA, Weiss RA, et al. Ocular features of Kawasaki's disease. *Arch Ophthalmol.* 1982;100(7):1101–1103.

Rowley AH, Shulman ST. Pathogenesis and management of Kawasaki disease. *Expert Rev Anti Infect Ther.* 2010;8(2):197–203.

Smith LB, Newburger JW, Burns JC. Kawasaki syndrome and the eye. *Pediatr Infect Dis J.* 1989;8(2):116–118.

RELAPSING POLYCHONDRITIS

S. R. Rathinam

Relapsing polychondritis is a multisystem connective tissue disease that causes recurrent episodes of inflammation of the cartilaginous tissues of the nose, ear lobes, respiratory tract, and joints, as well as of proteoglycan-rich tissues including the media of the arteries, conjunctiva, and sclera.

Etiology and Epidemiology

- The cause is unknown. Immune complex deposition, T-cell–mediated changes, and autoantibodies to collagen types II, IX, and XI, which are found in the cornea and sclera, may be responsible for the ocular complications.
- Relapsing polychondritis occurs in all races, and is more common during third to fifth decades of life with a slight female predominance.

Symptoms

- Intermittent fever, weight loss, fatigue, and skin rash
- Abrupt onset of nasal and ear pain, swelling, and redness
- Ocular redness and pain
- Joint pain
- Coughing, hoarseness of voice, shortness of breath

Signs (Figs. 7-53 to 7-55)

- Inflammation of the pinna of the ear, with pain, redness, and swelling, is present in the vast majority of patients.
- Sudden hearing loss, vertigo, tinnitus
- Recurrent episodes of eyelid edema, episcleritis, scleritis, peripheral ulcerative keratitis, iritis, and rarely retinopathy may occur. Patients may also develop ocular muscle paresis or optic neuritis.

- Nasal inflammation causes pain, redness, and a stuffy and/or runny nose. Chronic inflammation can cause a saddle-nose deformity.
- Voice hoarseness, epiglottitis, and laryngo-tracheal-bronchial stricture
- Inflammation of the aortic ring can cause aortic regurgitation, aortic dissection, and cardiac conduction defects. Patients may develop mitral valve regurgitation.
- Arthritis, most commonly of the hands and knees, can eventually cause joint deformity.
- Glomerulonephritis with associated renal failure and anemia
- Nonspecific skin rashes

Differential Diagnosis

- Patients may have concomitant connective tissue diseases such as:
  - Rheumatoid arthritis
  - Behçet's disease
  - Wegener's granulomatosis
  - Polyarteritis nodosa
  - Systemic lupus erythematosus
- Infectious causes:
  - Orbital cellulitis
  - syphilis
  - leprosy
  - Lyme disease

Diagnostic Evaluation

- It is a clinical diagnosis, but biopsy of involved cartilage is helpful. The diagnostic criteria consist of at least three of the following clinical features:
  - Bilateral auricular chondritis
  - Nasal chondritis
  - Respiratory tract chondritis
  - Nonerosive seronegative inflammatory polyarthritis
  - Ocular inflammation

- Cochlear and/or vestibular dysfunction
- Or one of the above with compatible histologic features from a cartilage biopsy
- Consider chest imaging, EKG/ECG, ESR, and serologies as needed to narrow the differential diagnosis.

Treatment

- Prednisone (1 mg/kg body weight daily) alone or in combination with oral methotrexate (15 to 20 mg weekly) or azathioprine (2 to 3 mg/kg body weight daily) is effective.
- A number of other drugs, including dapsone, mycophenolate mofetil, and infliximab have been used with success. ESR, urinalysis, and pulmonary function tests can also be used to follow treatment response.

Prognosis

- Prognosis depends on the organ involvement and response to treatment.

- To prevent significant morbidity and mortality, early diagnosis and aggressive treatment is important.
- Significant cardiovascular or renal involvement is associated with a poorer outcome overall.

REFERENCES

Gergely P, Poor G. Relapsing polychondritis. *Best Practice & Research Clinical Rheumatology.* 2008;18(5): 723–738.

McAdam CM, O'Hanlan MA, Bluestone R, et al. Relapsing polychondritis: prospective study of 23 patients and a review of the literature. *Medicine Baltimore.* 1976;55: 193–215.

Michet CJ Jr, McKenna CH, Luthra HS, et al. Relapsing polychondritis. Survival and predictive role of early disease manifestations. *Annals of Internal Medicine.* 1986;104:74–78.

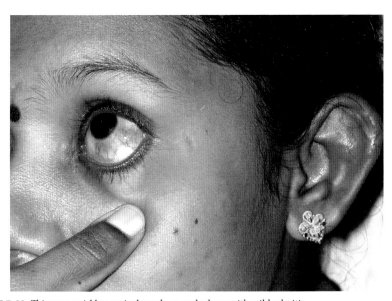

FIGURE 7-53. This young girl has auricular redness and edema with mild scleritis.

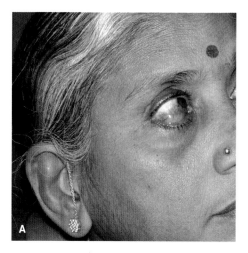

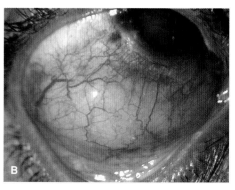

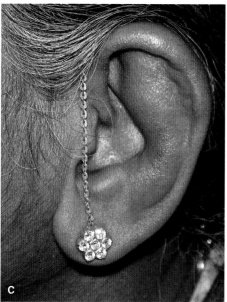

FIGURE 7-54. A. Severe auricular edema of the right ear along with scleritis of the right eye. **B.** On higher magnification, the scleritis is associated with peripheral corneal infiltrates. **C.** The left ear shows inflammation of the pinna with edema and erythema. The ear lobe is spared, which is typical of this disease.

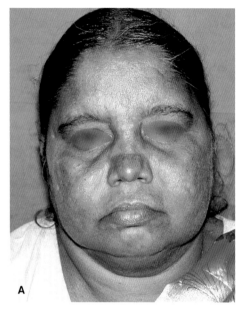

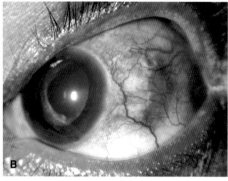

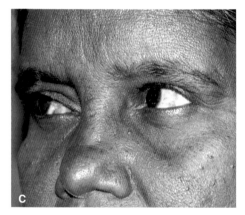

FIGURE 7-55. **A.** This person has developed a "saddle-nose" deformity due to long-standing chondritis. She has cushingoid "moon facies" secondary to prolonged steroid treatment. (Her eyes have been blurred for patient privacy.) **B.** There is scleral necrosis with resultant thinning of the left eye due to chronic scleritis. **C.** Several months later, the active scleritis of the left eye has resolved, but the scleral thinning remains. She has recurrent active scleritis in the right eye. The nasal deformity is more apparent from the side view.

SCLERODERMA

S. R. Rathinam ▨

Scleroderma is a chronic, multisystem autoimmune disease, clinically characterized by progressive fibrosis. Pathologically, it is characterized by chronic inflammation, microvascular injury, and excessive extracellular matrix production and deposition of type I and type III collagens. It also affects the eye, lungs, heart, kidneys, and gastrointestinal tract.

Etiology and Epidemiology

- Scleroderma is a connective tissue disorder of unknown etiology. It occurs worldwide in all races, but people of African descent are affected more frequently.
- Women are four times more likely to be affected than men.
- The peak onset occurs between 30 and 50 years.

Symptoms

- Systemic: fatigue, dysphagia, progressive dyspnea, and arthralgia.
- CNS symptoms can also occur.
- Ocular: redness and pain

Signs (Figs. 7-56 to 7-60)

- Systemic
  - Scleroderma is the major diagnostic criterion and is characterized by tight, shiny skin with a characteristic loss of hair and loss of ability to make a skin fold.
  - Induration of the skin on the fingers, face, neck, and trunk.
  - Sclerodactyly (sclerosis of the fingers and toes)
  - Microstomia due to perioral involvement

  - Ischemic digital ulcers and/or digital pitting scars
  - Decreased sweating
  - Arthritis, joint contractures
- Ocular
  - Keratoconjunctivitis sicca: The most common ocular manifestation, and may be severe
  - Episcleritis, scleritis, scleral pits, and peripheral corneal ulcer
  - Eyelid skin fibrosis, which can cause lid stiffness, and shallowing of the fornices
  - Nonspecific alterations of the retinal pigment epithelium
  - Telangiectasis of the eyelids and other parts of the face
  - Children may develop similar signs as adults. In addition, they may develop anterior uveitis. They also may have linear scleroderma of the face called "en coup de sabre," which looks like a sword cut across the frontoparietal lobe and may involve the periorbital area, including the eye.

Differential Diagnosis

- Other collagen vascular disorders
- Sjögren syndrome

Diagnostic Evaluation

- The diagnosis is mainly clinical; however, anticentromere antibodies (ACAs), anti-topoisomerase antibodies, and anti-RNA polymerase III antibodies are reported to be specific autoantibodies associated with distinct clinical subsets of scleroderma.

Treatment

- Systemic treatment: Corticosteroids are the first-line drugs; oral prednisone (1 mg/kg body weight daily) alone or in combination with oral methotrexate (10 to 15 mg weekly) or azathioprine (2 to 3 mg/kg body weight daily) is often successful.

- Ocular treatment: Lubricants and punctal occlusion for dry eye

Prognosis

- Pulmonary involvement, including interstitial lung disease and/or pulmonary hypertension, develops in up to 80% of patients and is currently the leading cause of death in scleroderma.

- Ocular prognosis is good if systemic treatment is started early.

REFERENCES

Subcommittee for Scleroderma. Criteria of the American Rheumatism Association Diagnostic and Therapeutic Criteria Committee, Preliminary criteria for the classification of systemic sclerosis (scleroderma). Subcommittee for scleroderma criteria of the American Rheumatism Association Diagnostic and Therapeutic Criteria Committee. *Arthritis Rheum.* 1980;23:581–590.

Tailor R, Gupta A, Herrick A, et al. Ocular manifestations of scleroderma. Survey of *Ophthalmology.* 2009; 54(2):292–304.

Zannin ME, Martini G, Athreya BH, et al. Ocular involvement in children with localized scleroderma: a multicentre study. *Br J Ophthalmol.* 2007;91:1311–1314.

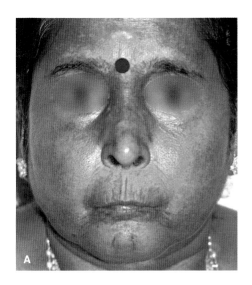

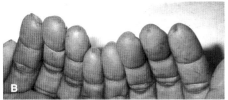

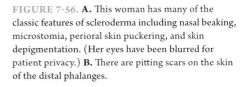

FIGURE 7-56. **A.** This woman has many of the classic features of scleroderma including nasal beaking, microstomia, perioral skin puckering, and skin depigmentation. (Her eyes have been blurred for patient privacy.) **B.** There are pitting scars on the skin of the distal phalanges.

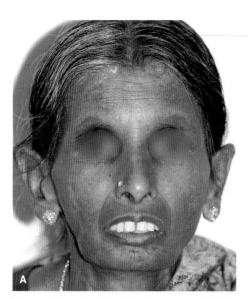

FIGURE 7-57. **A.** This 70-year-old woman has loss of facial skin creases and tight skin. (Her eyes have been blurred for patient privacy.) **B.** She also has flexion contractures of the finger joints and bony resorption of the terminal phalanges.

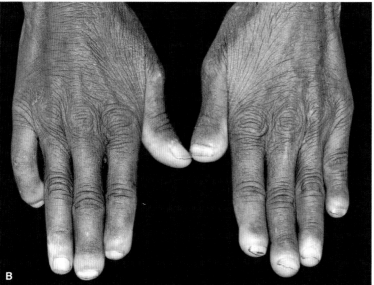

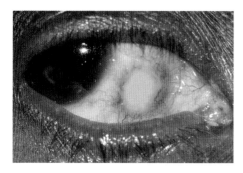

FIGURE 7-58. There is an area of scleral melting nasal to the cornea.

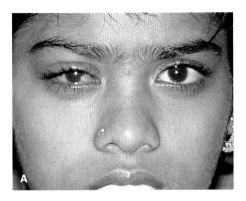

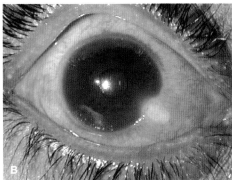

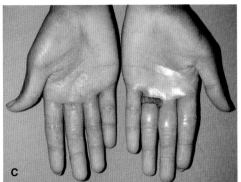

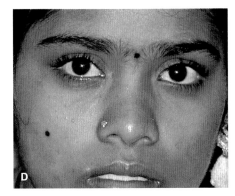

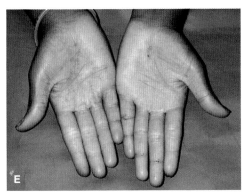

FIGURE 7-59. **A.** This girl has absence of facial skin creases, and she has marked conjunctival injection, mild scleritis, and a nasal corneal ulcer. **B.** Higher magnification of the right eye. **C.** There is sclerodactyly with typical thickened shiny skin of the fingers with marked edema. **D.** After prompt treatment with systemic steroids, there is marked improvement of both her systemic and ocular condition. **E.** The sclerodactyly has greatly improved as a result of systemic treatment.

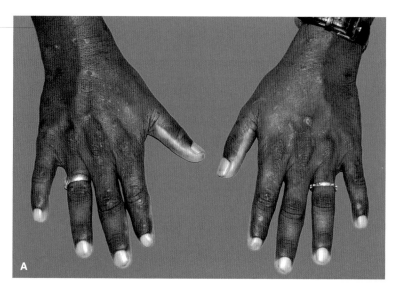

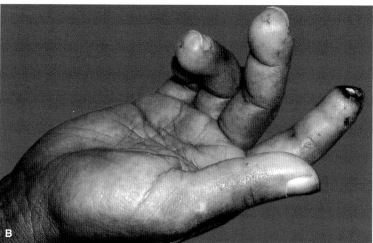

FIGURE 7-60. **A.** There are numerous digital pits on the dorsal surface of the hand, as well as resolving areas of induration. **B.** There is an ischemic digital ulcer on the tip of the index finger, and digital pitting on the tip of the ring finger.

DERMATOMYOSITIS AND POLYMYOSITIS

S. R. Rathinam ▦

Polymyositis is a multisystem autoimmune disorder characterized by inflammation and degeneration of the striated muscles. When it is associated with a skin rash, it is referred as dermatomyositis, in which the muscle, skin, and surrounding connective tissues are also affected.

Etiology and Epidemiology

- Polymyositis has been thought to be an immune-mediated syndrome caused by defective cellular immunity directed toward myofibers, however more recent work suggests a role for an antigen-driven response as well.

- Viral infections, malignancies, or connective tissue disorders all have been implicated as triggering factors. Dermatomyositis has been thought to be a humoral attack against the capillaries and small arterioles resulting in microinfarction, atrophy, and calcification of muscle and subcutaneous tissue; recent work suggests that it is a multimechanism disorder.

- These diseases occur most often in children between 5 and 15 years of age and in adults between 50 and 70 years.
- Women are affected twice as often as men.
- It is prevalent throughout the world.

Symptoms

- Difficulty getting up from a chair or climbing up steps

- Fatigue, myalgias, arthralgias, and muscle cramps

- Red eye, tearing

Signs (Figs. 7-61 to 7-64)

- Polymyositis
  - ▦ Proximal muscle weakness and tenderness
  - ▦ Nondestructive arthritis
  - ▦ Cardiomyositis
  - ▦ Interstitial lung disease
  - ▦ Raynaud's phenomenon
  - ▦ Diffuse cutaneous, subcutaneous, and sometimes muscular calcification
  - ▦ The eye muscles are spared and the facial muscles are involved only in severe disease.

- Dermatomyositis
  - ▦ The rash consists of a heliotrope (i.e., blue-purple) discoloration on various parts of the body including the eyelids.
  - ▦ Patients may have erythematous, scaly, elevated skin lesions called Gottron rash. Patients may also have widespread scaling, hyperpigmentation, and depigmentation of the skin.
  - ▦ Ocular involvement is usually confined to the eyelids. Some patients may have a well-circumscribed atrophic lid scar. Corneal scarring can result from the eyelid disease. Retinal vascular disease is rare.

Differential Diagnosis

- Muscular dystrophies
- Thyroid hormone disorders
- Drug-induced myopathy (statin drugs or chloroquine/hydroxychloroquine)

Diagnostic Evaluation

- Elevation of enzymes including creatinine phosphokinase, aldolase, SGOT, SGPT, and lactate dehydrogenase
- MRI and muscle biopsy
- Some serum autoantibodies like myositis-associated antibodies, and myositis-specific antibodies are found in approximately 40% of patients.
- Muscle strength testing and pulmonary function testing can be useful to follow disease progression.

Treatment

- Corticosteroids are the first-line drug. Prednisolone (1 mg/kg body weight daily) alone or in combination with oral methotrexate (10 to 15 mg weekly) or azathioprine (2 to 3 mg/kg body weight daily) is effective.

- Intravenous immunoglobulin (IVIG), mycophenolate mofetil, taciolimus, and rituximab have shown some benefit in preliminary studies.

Prognosis

- Spontaneous remission has been reported in one-fifth of cases. Early treatment maintains the muscle strength and reduces the relapse rate. In the long term, myositis has a major effect on quality of life.

- Patients with polymyositis may have other diseases such as Sjögren's disease or scleroderma.

- Cancer is found in up to 15% of patients with dermatomyositis.

REFERENCES

Akikusa JD, Tennankore DK, Levin AV, et al. Eye findings in patients with juvenile dermatomyositis. *J Rheumatology.* 2005;32(10):1986–1991.

Allanore Y, Vignaux O, Arnaud L, et al. Effects of corticosteroids and immunosuppressors on idiopathic inflammatory myopathy related myocarditis evaluated by magnetic resonance imaging. *Ann Rheum Dis.* 2006; 65:249–252.

Dalakas MC. Immunotherapy of myositis: issues, concerns and future prospects. *Nat Rev Rheumatol.* 2010;6(3):129–137.

Hengstman GJ, van den Hoogen FH, van Engelen BG. Treatment of the inflammatory myopathies: update and practical recommendations. *Expert Opin Pharmacother.* 2009;10(7):1183–1190.

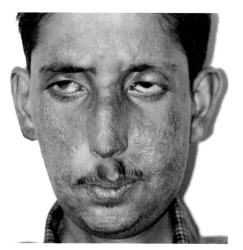

FIGURE 7-61. Scarring and pigmentation over the cheeks, and hyperpigmented patches are seen on the skin of nose and ear lobes.

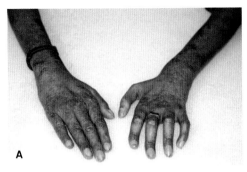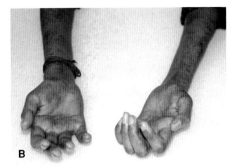

FIGURE 7-62. **A.** This patient has the characteristic heliotrope rash (blue-purple) and edema on the dorsum of hands, with a scaly, erythematous eruption on the knuckles (Gottron rash). **B.** Note the muscle atrophy of the forearms and palms.

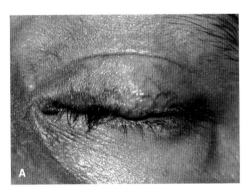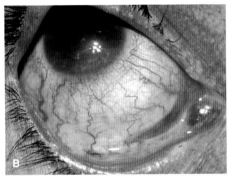

FIGURE 7-63. **A.** This patient has telangiectasis of the upper eyelid skin. This telangiectasia can appear as a purple line, which may precede a heliotrope rash. **B.** There is chronic meibomianitis and corneal infiltrates.

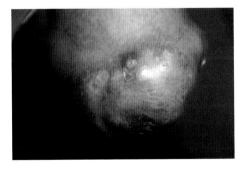

FIGURE 7-64. There is cutaneous calcification at the elbow joint. (Courtesy of Dr. Parthiban, Dermatology, Madurai.)

POLYARTERITIS NODOSA

Julie Lew and *Shree Kurup*

Polyarteritis nodosa (PAN), also known as periarteritis nodosa, is an uncommon multisystem, necrotizing vasculitis that affects medium- and small-sized arteries throughout the body that can result in retinal and choroidal infarcts. PAN most commonly affects the skin, joints, gastrointestinal tract, kidneys, and peripheral nerves. The eye is affected in 10% to 20% of cases, and PAN can affect both the anterior and posterior segments.

Etiology and Epidemiology

- PAN occurs more often in males (60%) than in females (40%).
- Mean age at onset is 45 years.
- It is an immune complex-mediated disease that has also been linked with seropositivity to hepatitis B surface antigen.

Symptoms

- Fever, weight loss, malaise
- Abdominal pain
- Myalgias
- Skin rash including livedo reticularis, nodules, purpura, and Raynaud's phenomenon
- Red, painful eye
- Blurry vision, floaters
- Epididymitis or ovarian pain

Signs

- The American College of Rheumatology (ACR) has defined 10 criteria for classification of PAN. A patient is said to have PAN if at least three of these criteria are present:
  - Weight loss ≥4 kg
  - Livedo reticularis
  - Testicular pain or tenderness
  - Myalgias, weakness, or leg tenderness
  - Mononeuropathy or polyneuropathy
  - Diastolic BP >90 mm Hg
  - Elevated blood urea nitrogen or creatinine
  - Hepatitis B virus
  - Arteriographic abnormality
  - Biopsy of small or medium-sized artery containing polymorphonuclear neutrophils
- Ocular signs (**Figs. 7-65 and 7-66**)
  - Vasculitis affecting the choroidal vessels is the most common ocular finding in PAN. Choroidal and posterior ciliary artery ischemia can cause an ischemic optic neuropathy as well.
  - Central retinal artery occlusion
  - Vascular tortuosity
  - Cotton wool spots
  - Hard exudates
  - Marginal corneal ulceration and keratitis
  - Scleritis and episcleritis

Differential Diagnosis

- Wegener's granulomatosis
- Syphilis
- Behçet's syndrome
- SLE
- Mixed connective tissue disease
- Dermatomyositis
- Rheumatoid arthritis

Diagnostic Evaluation

- No test is diagnostic of PAN, but a workup should include: Complete blood count, metabolic panel, rheumatoid factor, ESR, ANA, hepatitis B antigen, ANCA, rapid plasma reagin (RPR), and fluorescent treponemal antibody-absorption (FTA-Abs).
- Urinalysis for kidney involvement
- Biopsy of tissue with involved arteries

- Fluorescein angiography if retinal vasculitis is suspected

- Kidney arteriogram if kidney involvement suspected

Treatment

- Systemic corticosteroids are first-line therapy.

- Steroid-sparing agents may be used alone or in combination with steroids for refractory cases. All steroid-sparing agents, including cytotoxic agents such as cyclophosphamide, have been used with some success.

- Azathioprine has been shown to be an effective maintenance therapy to prevent disease relapse.

- Plasmapheresis has also been shown to be beneficial when used as an adjunct therapy with corticosteroids.

Prognosis

- Early immunosuppressive therapy is the key to obtaining a good prognosis.

- The 5-year survival rate increases from 12% to 80% with prompt institution of systemic immunosuppressive therapy.

REFERENCES

Galetta SL. Vasculitis. In: Miller NR, Newman NJ, eds. *Walsh and Hoyt's Clinical Neuro-Ophthalmology.* 5th ed. Vol. 3. Baltimore: Williams & Wilkins; 1998: 3744–3760.

Hsu CT, Kerrison JB, Miller NR, et al. Choroidal infarction, anterior ischemic optic neuropathy, and central retinal artery occlusion from polyarteritis nodosa. *Retina.* 21(4):348–351.

Morgan CM, Foster CS, D'Amico DJ, et al. Retinal vasculitis in polyarteritis nodosa. *Retina.* 1986;6: 205–209.

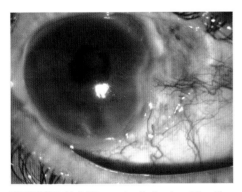

FIGURE 7-65. PAN-associated sclerokeratitis with pannus and scleral thinning.

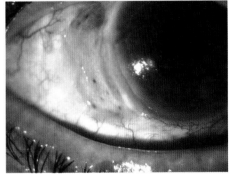

FIGURE 7-66. There is scleral thinning (scleromalacia) due to old necrotizing scleritis (note the area of scleral thinning and avascularity extending 3 to 4 mm from the limbus).

White Dot Syndromes

ACUTE POSTERIOR MULTIFOCAL PLACOID PIGMENT EPITHELIOPATHY

Céline Terrada and Bahram Bodaghi

Don Gass, MD, first described acute posterior multifocal placoid pigment epitheliopathy (APMPPE or AMPPE) in 1968. The clinical presentation is usually characterized by multiple, bilateral, cream-colored, placoid lesions at the level of the outer retina/retinal pigment epithelium (RPE). It is caused by ischemic changes occurring within the choriocapillaris.

Epidemiology and Etiology

- It predominantly occurs in young individuals that are in the second to fourth decades of life.

- It affects men and women equally.

- APMPPE is usually bilateral, but it can be quite asymmetric and the second eye may not become involved for several weeks after the first eye.

- APMPPE is idiopathic, but it has been associated with mumps, secondary syphilis, Lyme disease, streptococcal group A infection and anti–hepatitis B virus vaccination.

- The disease has also been called acute multifocal ischemic choroidopathy.

Symptoms

- Patients complain of visual disturbances, blurred vision, photopsias and scotomas.

- The degree of visual impairment can be variable depending upon the location of the lesions.

- Visual loss is due to macular involvement, and there is usually a gradual improvement in vision over the course of a few weeks.

Signs

- Systemic signs include a flu-like syndrome and headache.

- Episcleritis, scleritis, anterior uveitis, vitreous haze, papillitis, and retinal vasculitis can occur.

- On fundus examination during the acute phase, the lesions are characterized by multiple yellow-white deep plaques, ranging from one-half to one optic disk diameter in size.

- Lesions appear to be at the level of the outer retina and the RPE even though the ischemic alterations involve the choriocapillaris.

- After a few days, healing starts at the center of the plaques, leaving a pigmented scar or mottled RPE.

- New lesions can appear in the posterior pole within the first 3 weeks of disease onset.

- APMPPE may be associated with serous retinal detachments, mimicking Vogt-Koyanagi-Harada (VKH) disease.

Differential Diagnosis

- White dot syndromes: Presumed ocular histoplasmosis syndrome, punctuate inner choroidopathy (PIC), multifocal choroiditis
- Sarcoidosis, syphilis, tuberculosis (TB)
- VKH syndrome
- Sympathetic ophthalmia
- Subretinal fibrosis/uveitis syndrome
- Serpiginous choroiditis
- Birdshot chorioretinopathy

Diagnostic Evaluation (Figs. 8-1 to 8-4)

- Fluorescein angiography
  - Acute stage
    - ▶ Early and intermediate hypofluorescence followed by staining and pooling in the late frames
    - ▶ Delay in choriocapillaris circulation
  - Late stage: Hyperfluorescence in early and late frames without leakage (window defect)
- Indocyanine green angiography (ICGA) shows hypofluorescence during the intermediate and late transit frames.

- Optical coherence tomography (OCT) demonstrates nodular hyperreflectivity at the level of the photoreceptors and RPE.

- Visual field testing objectively identifies the scotomata the patients report.

- Interestingly, the electroretinogram (ERG) and electrooculogram (EOG) are normal.

Treatment

- Usually no treatment is required.

- In patients with macular involvement, systemic corticosteroids can be initiated to hasten visual recovery and immunosuppressive agents are rarely required.

Prognosis

- The prognosis is good with a visual acuity of 20/25 after 6 months although small scotomas may persist.

- Recurrences or exacerbations are rare.

- Macular localization may be more aggressive.

- Subretinal neovascularization remains a rare complication.

REFERENCES

Gass JD. Acute posterior multifocal placoid pigment epitheliopathy. *Arch Ophthalmol.* 1968;80:177–185.

Jones BE, Jampol LM, Yannuzzi LA, et al. Relentless placoid chorioretinitis: a new entity or an unusual variant of serpiginous chorioretinitis? *Arch Ophthalmol.* 2000;118:931–938.

Senanayake SN, Selvadurai S, Hawkins CA, et al. Acute posterior multifocal placoid pigment epitheliopathy associated with erythema nodosum and a flu-like illness. *Singapore Med J.* 2008;49:e333–335.

Souka AA, Hillenkamp J, Gora F, et al. Correlation between optical coherence tomography and autofluorescence in acute posterior multifocal placoid pigment epitheliopathy. *Graefes Arch Clin Exp Ophthalmol.* 2006; 244:1219–1223.

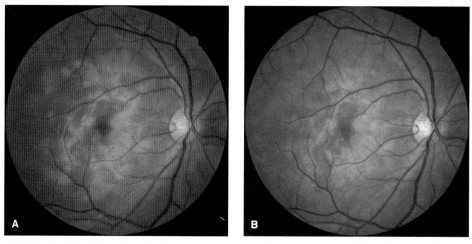

FIGURE 8-1. Color (**A**) and red-free (**B**) fundus photographs show multiple, deep yellow-white placoid lesions.

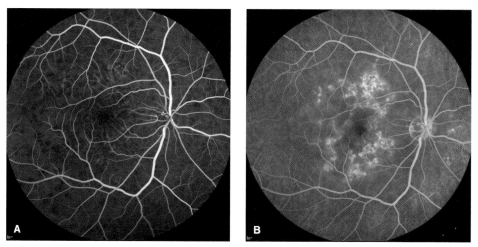

FIGURE 8-2. Fluorescein angiography (FA). The early frame shows hypofluorescence (**A**), and the late frame shows staining and pooling (**B**).

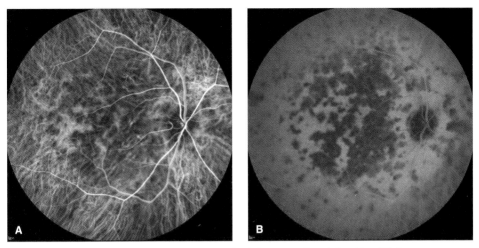

FIGURE 8-3. ICG demonstrates hypofluorescence in both the intermediate (**A**) and late (**B**) frames.

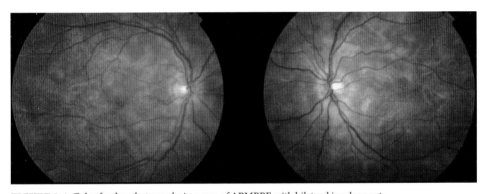

FIGURE 8-4. Color fundus photographs in a case of APMPPE with bilateral involvement.

SERPIGINOUS CHORIORETINOPATHY

Céline Terrada and Bahram Bodaghi

Serpiginous choroidopathy, also known as serpiginous choroiditis, geographic choroidopathy or geographic helicoid peripapillary choroidopathy, is an inflammatory disorder involving the choroid, the choriocapillaris and the RPE. It gets its name due to the serpentine pattern it develops as it progresses from the optic disk.

Epidemiology and Etiology

• Serpiginous choroiditis is a rare cause of posterior uveitis (<5% of cases in uveitis clinics), and usually occurs in the fourth to seventh decades of life.

• The disease is a chronic, progressive, recurrent inflammatory or infectious condition.

• Most patients present with unilateral vision loss, but on examination usually have bilateral disease.

• Males are affected slightly more often.

• The geographic distribution is worldwide.

• The etiology is unknown, but autoimmune and infectious hypothesis have been proposed (herpes viruses and TB).

• There is no human leukocyte antigen (HLA) association.

Symptoms

• Patients without macular alterations and choroidal neovascularization (CNV) present with photopsias and decreased vision.

• Patients with macular involvement or CNV are usually symptomatic and may have metamorphopsia, scotoma and sudden vision loss.

Signs (**Figs. 8-5 to 8-7**)

• The main finding is a peripapillary choroiditis that has a characteristic serpentine appearance. In some cases, it involves the macula while sparing the peripapillary region.

• The lesions are typically not multifocal as opposed to ampiginous or tuberculous serpiginous-like choroiditis.

• The areas of active choroiditis appear gray or white-yellow. They often appear to elevate the overlying retina.

• The active lesions spontaneously resolve after 6 to 8 weeks and result in atrophy of the RPE and choriocapillaris. Inactive lesions appear as pigmented and atrophic scars that are usually connected to the optic disk.

• Patients may have recurrences months to years after the initial lesions and the reactivation occurs at the edges of the previous lesions.

• One-third of affected individuals have mild inflammatory cells in the posterior vitreous. Rarely is inflammation seen in the anterior segment.

• CNV may occur in up to 35% of cases.

• Occasionally patients may have RPE and serous retinal detachments.

Differential Diagnosis

• White dot syndromes: APMPPE or ampiginous choroiditis (which have a multifocal presentation of lesions)

• Tuberculous serpiginous-like choroiditis (TB-SLC): Patients with TB-SLC come from areas in which TB is endemic, have significant vitritis, and usually have multifocal lesions in the periphery and posterior pole. Patients with serpiginous choroiditis have little to no vitritis, have bilateral involvement, and have a larger, more confluent lesion, which extends mainly from the disk and usually is confined to the posterior pole.

• Sarcoidosis

• Syphilis

• VKH syndrome

- Sympathetic ophthalmia
- Subretinal fibrosis/uveitis syndrome

Diagnostic Evaluation

- Fundus photography is helpful to follow disease progression.
- Fluorescein angiography (FA)
  - If no CNV is present:
    - ▶ Areas of acute choroiditis demonstrate early hypofluorescence with blockage and diffuse late staining and leakage of dye.
    - ▶ Inactive, atrophic lesions appear as a window effect with a late hyperfluorescent border. Disappearance of the hyperfluorescent border suggests a recurrence.
  - CNV in these cases shows the typical signs of a classic CNV: well-defined early hyperfluorescence with leakage in the late phase.
- ICGA
  - Hypoperfusion of the choroid is more extensive than shown by FA. It appears as a primary inflammatory choriocapillaropathy.
  - Lesions not seen on the FA can be apparent on ICGA.
- OCT can identify:
  - Macular edema in rare cases
  - Areas of retinal atrophy (which appears to be secondary to atrophy of the RPE and choriocapillaris)
  - Visual fields can be useful to identify scotomas, which can be absolute and/or relative. The visual field deficit can vary over time.
- It is important to exclude TB with a tuberculin skin test (PPD), chest radiograph, and/or interferon-gamma releasing assays (e.g., QuantiFERON), especially before any immunosuppressive therapy is instituted.

Treatment

- Patients with an active inflammatory component benefit from treatment.
  - Corticosteroids: High-dose systemic steroids, as well as periocular steroids, can be used to control acute inflammation.
  - Immunomodulatory or immunosuppressive agents
    - ▶ May be considered in refractory cases or for individuals intolerant to corticosteroids
    - ▶ Mycophenolate mofetil, azathioprine, cyclosporine A and cyclophosphamide have been used in severe cases, and some investigators have recommended triple therapy with azathioprine, cyclosporine and oral prednisone.
    - ▶ Treatment must be adapted to the severity of each situation and must take into account the potential side effects.
- Active disease with CNV: Corticosteroids and immunosuppressive agents are usually used along with other adjunctive measures.
  - Extrafoveal: Focal laser
  - Juxtafoveal: Anti–vascular endothelial growth factor (VEGF) therapy, photodynamic therapy, focal laser
  - Subfoveal: Anti-VEGF therapy, photodynamic therapy
  - Peripapillary: Focal laser for small lesions, anti-VEGF therapy

Prognosis

- The prognosis depends on macular involvement and complications including CNV formation.
- Unilateral or bilateral severe visual loss may be observed in 25% of cases.

REFERENCES

Akpek EK, Jabs DA, Tessler HH, et al. Successful treatment of serpiginous choroiditis with alkylating agents. *Ophthalmology.* 2002;109:1506–1513.

Cardillo-Piccolino F, Grosso A, Savini E. Fundus autofluorescence in serpiginous choroiditis. *Graefes Arch Clin Exp Ophthalmol.* 2009;247:179–185.

Gupta V, Gupta A, Rao NA. Intraocular tuberculosis: an update. *Surv Ophthalmol.* 2007;52:561–587.

Lim WK, Buggage RR, Nussenblatt RB. Serpiginous choroiditis. *Surv Ophthalmol.* 2005;50:231–244.

Song MH, Roh YJ. Intravitreal ranibizumab for choroidal neovascularization in serpiginous choroiditis. *Eye.* 2008.

Vasconcelos-Santos DV, Rao PK, Davies JB, et al. Clinical features of tuberculous serpiginouslike choroiditis in contrast to classic serpiginous choroiditis. *Arch Ophthalmol.* 2010;128:853–858.

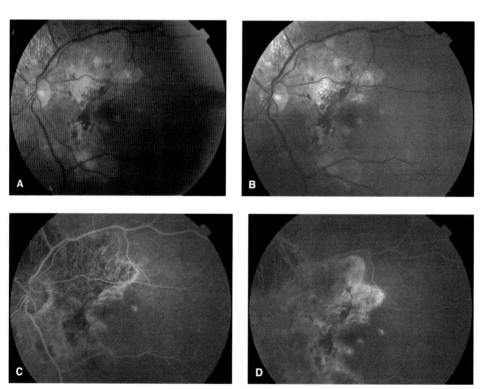

FIGURE 8-5. Color fundus photograph (**A**) and red-free photo (**B**) show the sequelae of choroiditis. Note the geographic pigmented and atrophic scars connected to the optic disk. **C.** The early frame of the fluorescein angiogram shows hypofluorescence likely due to limited perfusion. **D.** The late frame demonstrates staining and with a hyperfluorescent border, characteristic of inactive serpiginous.

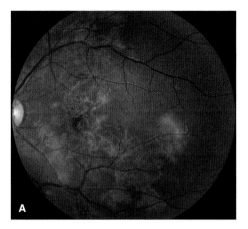

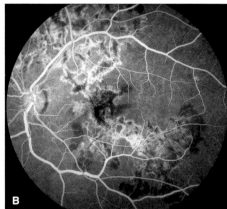

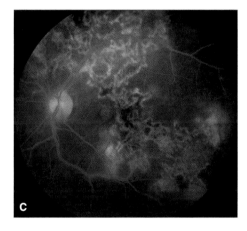

FIGURE 8-6. This patient with a previous diagnosis of serpiginous chorioretinopathy came in with further vision changes. **A.** The color photograph reveals darker areas consistent with earlier scarring, as well as yellow areas of active chorioretinitis. **B.** The early frame of the fluorescein angiogram reveals RPE window defects in the area of previous scarring. The new lesions block early. **C.** The new lesions stain in the late frames of the angiogram. (Courtesy of MidAtlantic Retina, the Retina Service of Wills Eye Institute.)

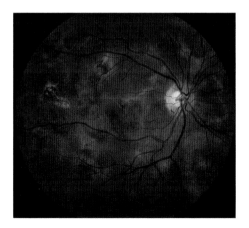

FIGURE 8-7. A 27-year-old woman had serpiginous choroiditis that progressed despite numerous immunosuppressive agents. Her vision was 20/400 in this eye. (Courtesy of Sunir Garg, MD.)

MULTIPLE EVANESCENT WHITE DOT SYNDROME

Céline Terrada and Bahram Bodaghi

Multiple evanescent white dot syndrome (MEWDS) is a rare, acute, multifocal inflammatory retinochoroidopathy. It spontaneously resolves with an excellent visual outcome.

Epidemiology and Etiology

- It occurs mainly in young, healthy young women in the second to fourth decades of life.
- The etiology remains unknown, however an infectious etiology has been suspected, as one-third of patients have a viral prodrome.
- Patients often have mild myopia.

Symptoms

- Photopsias, often in the temporal visual field
- Blurry vision, with visual acuity ranging from 20/20 to 20/400
- Central microscotoma

Signs (Figs. 8-8 to 8-10)

- Multiple small dots in the fundus at the level of the outer retina and the RPE
- An orange granularity of the fovea
- No anterior segment inflammation, but some patients have a mild vitritis
- A mild afferent pupillary defect may occur
- Optic disk edema
- Usually monophasic, unilateral and self-limited

Differential Diagnosis

- Inflammatory white dot syndromes
- Acute idiopathic blind spot enlargement syndrome (AIBSE)
- Acute zonal occult outer retinopathy (AZOOR)

Diagnostic Evaluation

- White dots
  - FA demonstrates both early and late hyperfluorescence of the dots and late staining of the optic disk
  - ICG
    - ▶ Intermediate/late hypofluorescent spots scattered throughout the posterior pole and mid-periphery.
    - ▶ The lesions are more numerous on ICGA than seen clinically or on FA.
    - ▶ Intermediate transient pinpoint hyperfluorescence.
  - Fundus autofluorescence
    - ▶ In the acute phase of the disease, there are small areas of hypoautofluorescence around the disk and posterior pole and hyperfluorescent areas corresponding to the white dots. These spots evolve over time and may persist or fade.
    - ▶ The lesions are more numerous than clinically seen.
  - OCT demonstrates defects located at the level of the outer retina and RPE. The areas corresponding to the white spots show interruption or signal attenuation of the photoreceptor inner segment/outer segment band.
- Granularity of the macula
  - FA shows hyperfluorescence throughout the angiogram.
  - ICGA demonstrates intermediate/late hypofluorescence.
  - Fundus autofluorescence shows pinpoint areas of increased or decreased autofluorescence.

Treatment

- Observation as MEWDS spontaneously resolves over a period of several weeks to months with return of normal vision in nearly all patients.

Prognosis

- Very good.

- Mild pigmentary changes may be seen after recovery, and some patients will have persistent visual field or color deficits.

- Submacular CNV may rarely develop.

REFERENCES

Dell'Omo R, Mantovani A, Wong R, et al. Natural evolution of fundus autofluorescence findings in multiple evanescent white dot syndrome. *Retina.* 2010; 30:1479–1487.

Gass JD, Hamed LM. Acute macular neuroretinopathy and multiple evanescent white dot syndrome occurring in the same patient. *Arch Ophthalmol.* 1989; 107:189–193.

Jampol LM, Sieving PA, Pugh D, et al. Multiple evanescent white dot syndrome. I. Clinical findings. *Arch Ophthalmol.* 1984;102:671–674.

Mamalis N, Daily MJ. Multiple evanescent white dot syndrome. A report of eight cases. *Ophthalmology.* 1987;94:1209–1212.

Nguyen MH, Witkin AJ, Reichel E, et al. Microstructural abnormalities in MEWDS demonstrated by ultrahigh resolution optical coherence tomography. *Retina.* 2007; 27:414–418.

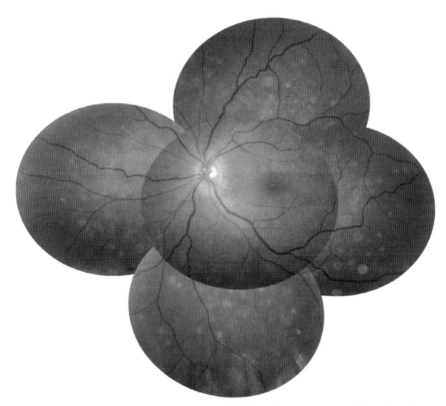

FIGURE 8-8. Color photograph showing numerous small, yellow-white spots scattered throughout the posterior pole in a patient with MEWDS.

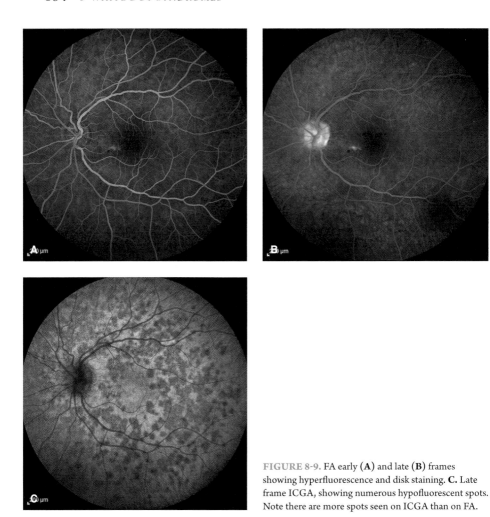

FIGURE 8-9. FA early (**A**) and late (**B**) frames showing hyperfluorescence and disk staining. **C.** Late frame ICGA, showing numerous hypofluorescent spots. Note there are more spots seen on ICGA than on FA.

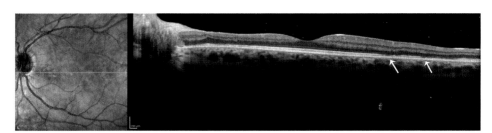

FIGURE 8-10. SD-OCT in MEWDS patient illustrating interruption or signal attenuation of the photoreceptor inner segment/outer segment band (arrows).

MULTIFOCAL CHOROIDITIS/SUBRETINAL FIBROSIS SYNDROME

Céline Terrada and Bahram Bodaghi ▥

Multifocal choroiditis and panuveitis syndrome (MFCP) was described by Dreyer and Gass in 1984. It is a rare, idiopathic, inflammatory choroidal disease, mimicking presumed ocular histoplasmosis syndrome (OHS), which affects otherwise healthy young adults. MFCP, PIC, MEWDS and AIBES may constitute different clinical presentations of the same disease but this hypothesis has not been validated.

Epidemiology and Etiology

- The disease usually affects Caucasian adults (80% of cases).

- MFCP usually occurs in the third to fourth decades of life, and affects women more than men (approximately 3:1), and most patients have some degree of myopia.

- The disease is bilateral in approximately 80% of cases, but it can be asymmetric or unilateral at presentation.

- It occurs worldwide.

- There are usually no other systemic findings.

- There is no well-defined HLA-association. It may be virally induced.

Symptoms

- Patients describe photopsias, floaters, and/or an enlarged blind spot; rarely some patients may remain asymptomatic.

- With macular involvement or submacular choroidal neovascular membrane formation, patients describe metamorphopsia, subjective scotomas and/or sudden central vision loss.

Signs

- Anterior chamber flare and cells are variable in intensity but are usually mild.

- Vitreous haze is common and is useful to distinguish MFC from ocular histoplasmosis.

- Multiple choroidal lesions (20 to 100) are randomly distributed throughout the posterior pole and mid-periphery. Active lesions have a "creamy" appearance, while older lesions appear atrophic and can become pigmented at their edges. The lesions appear to be at the level of the RPE and choroid.

- The lesion size ranges from 50 to 350 μm in diameter. They can enlarge and become coalescent.

- CNV is present in 30% of cases. CNV is characterized by the presence of subretinal fluid, subretinal hemorrhage and subretinal exudate.

- Cystoid macular edema (CME), epiretinal membrane (ERM), optic disk edema, enlarged blind spots and peripapillary scarring also occur.

- Subretinal fibrosis may link the atrophic scars and is probably due to subclinical progression of the disease.

Differential Diagnosis

- White dot syndromes

  ▥ Ocular histoplasmosis: Unlike MFC, OHS does not have anterior uveitis or vitritis.

  ▥ Punctate inner choroidopathy: Many feel that this is a variant of MFC. In PIC, the lesions tend to be deeper and more punched out, and these patients have less vitritis.

  ▥ Birdshot retinochoroidopathy: These patients are usually HLA-A29 positive, are older, and have larger and less discrete lesions.

- Sarcoidosis, syphilis, TB
- VKH syndrome
- Sympathetic ophthalmia
- Subretinal fibrosis/uveitis syndrome
- Serpiginous choroiditis

Diagnostic Evaluation (Figs. 8-11 to 8-13)

- FA
  - Acute choroiditis appears as early hypofluorescence with staining in late frames.
  - Late (chronic) choroiditis has early hyperfluorescence that persists in the late frames (window effect).
    - Staining of the optic disk and vessels
    - CME
  - If a CNV is present, there is well-defined early hyperfluorescence with late leakage.
- ICGA
  - Large and small hypofluorescent inflammatory lesions that may cluster around the disk
  - There are more lesions on ICGA than seen clinically.
- Fundus autofluorescence shows hypoautofluorescent scars.
  - The larger lesions (>125 μm) appear as atrophic scars.
  - Interestingly, there are often hundreds of smaller lesions (<125 μm) that are not clinically apparent.
- OCT demonstrates nodular hyperreflectivity at the level of the photoreceptors and RPE.
- Visual field testing objectively identifies the areas of visual field loss and periodic testing may help to monitor disease progression.
- ERG finding are often normal or mildly depressed and are nonspecific. Multifocal ERG can show diffuse depression in addition to focal areas of greater depression, which correspond to the scotomas on the visual field.

Treatment

- Uveitic component
  - Corticosteroids
    - Systemic corticosteroids are effective to control acute inflammation.
    - Periocular and intravitreal injections and sustained-release devices may be useful.
  - Immunomodulatory therapy (IMT)
    - Given the chronic nature of MFC, consideration should be given to IMT, especially in cases of inflammation which cannot be controlled with low-dose steroids or for patients who are intolerant to corticosteroids.
    - Methotrexate, mycophenolate mofetil and azathioprine have been used with success.
    - IMT has been found to greatly reduce the risk of macular complications, including CME, ERM and CNV formation.
- CNV: Corticosteroids and IMT may reduce recurrences by controlling the inflammatory state.
  - Extrafoveal CVNM can be treated with focal laser.
  - Juxta- and subfoveal CNVM have been treated with anti-VEGF agents, photodynamic therapy and intravitreal triamcinolone injection. Submacular surgery may still be useful in cases with vision worse than 20/100 that did not respond to other treatments.
  - Peripapillary CNV may be treated with focal laser for small lesions and anti-VEGF therapy.
  - Spontaneous resolution of the active neovascularization has been reported.

Prognosis

- Seventy-five percent of patients develop permanent visual loss in at least one eye due to subfoveal lesions, CNVM, chronic CME or subretinal fibrosis.

● Therapy with systemic corticosteroids and IMT has improved the prognosis:

▪ Eighty-three percent reduction in risk of macular complications

▪ Ninety-two percent reduction in the risk of developing vision loss to less than 20/200 in the affected eye

REFERENCES

Dreyer RF, Gass DJ. Multifocal choroiditis and panuveitis. A syndrome that mimics ocular histoplasmosis. *Arch Ophthalmol.* 1984;102:1776–1784.

Fine HF, Zhitomirshy I, Freund KB, et al. Bevacizumab (Avastin) and ranibizumab (Lucentis) for choroidal neovascularization in multifocal choroiditis. *Retina.* 2009;29:8–12.

Michel SS, Ekong A, Baltazis S, et al. Multifocal choroiditis and panuveitis: immunomodulatory therapy. *Ophthalmology.* 2002;109:378–383.

Parnell JR, Jampol LM, Yanuzzi LA, et al. Differentiation between presumed ocular histoplasmosis syndrome and multifocal choroiditis with panuveitis based on morphology and photographed fundus lesions and fluorescein angiography. *Arch Ophthalmol.* 2001; 119:208–212.

Thorne JE, Wittenberg S, Jabs DA, et al. Multifocal choroiditis with panuveitis: incidence of ocular complications and loss of visual acuity. *Ophthalmology.* 2006; 113:2310–2316.

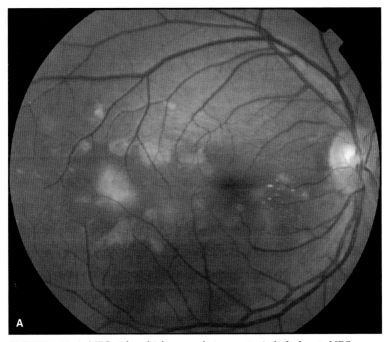

FIGURE 8-11. A. MFC with multiple creamy lesions are typical of subacute MFC.

(*continued*)

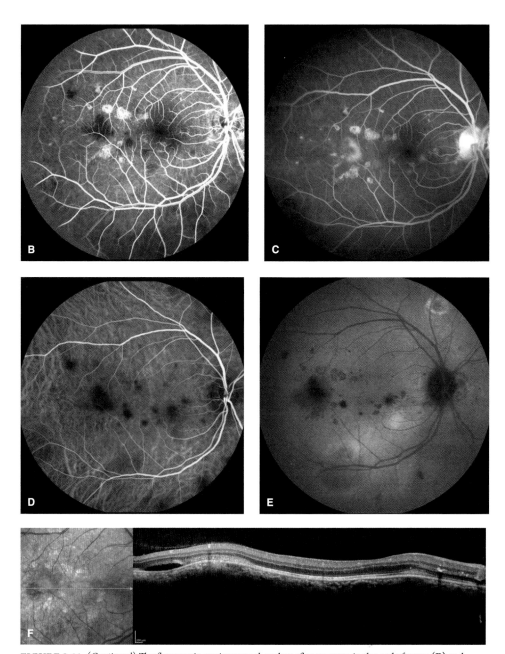

FIGURE 8-11. (*Continued*) The fluorescein angiograms show hypofluorescence in the early frames (**B**) and staining in the late frames (**C**). ICGA shows hypocyanescent lesions both early (**D**) and late (**E**). Often more lesions are present on ICGA than on color photographs or FA. **F.** The OCT shows hyperreflective lesions in the outer retina/RPE. There is subretinal fluid temporal to the fovea.

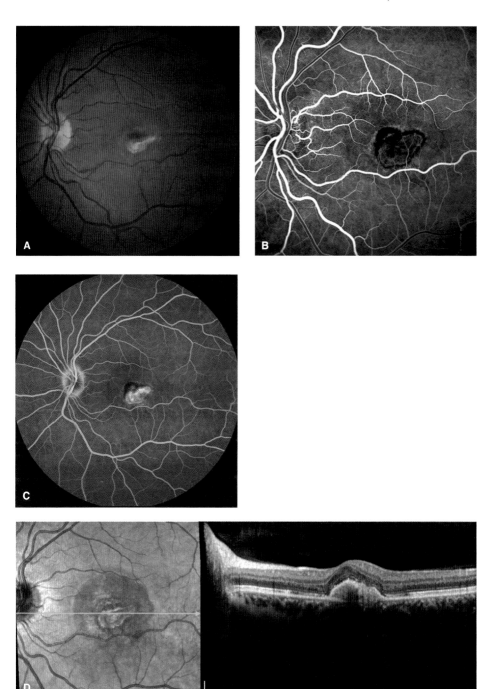

FIGURE 8-12. MFC with subfoveal CNV. **A.** The color fundus photograph shows a subfoveal CNVM. FA shows hyperfluorescence in the early frames (**B**) and staining in the late frames (**C**). **D.** OCT shows a subfoveal CNV.

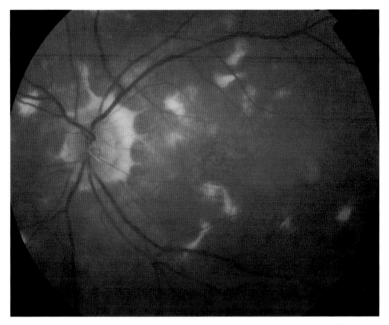

FIGURE 8-13. MFC with subretinal fibrosis. Serial color photographs are helpful to document disease progression.

PUNCTUATE INNER CHOROIDOPATHY

Céline Terrada and Bahram Bodaghi

Punctuate inner choroidopathy (PIC) was first described in 1984. PIC belongs to the MFCP spectrum of diseases, sharing many of the same clinical symptoms and signs, but it does have a few specific characteristics, most notably lesion size.

Epidemiology and Etiology

- Although PIC has a worldwide geographic distribution, it is most prevalent in Caucasian patients, who make up 80% of cases.
- Eighty-five percent of eyes are myopic.
- Most affected patients are in the second to fourth decades of life, which is younger than patients who have MFC.
- PIC is usually unilateral, but it can be bilateral and asymmetric at presentation.
- There is usually no associated systemic condition or HLA association.
- PIC is primarily an inflammatory disorder of the choriocapillaris. It results in nonperfusion of the choriocapillaris with severe secondary ischemia of the outer retina. Subretinal neovascularization is a common complication.

Symptoms

- Patients without direct foveal involvement often notice central photopsias and/or a small scotoma.
- Patients who have direct foveal involvement or subfoveal CNV are usually much more symptomatic and complain of sudden vision loss, metamorphopsia and central scotoma.
- Floaters and photophobia can also occur.

Signs

- These patients have no anterior segment or vitreous inflammation.
- Fundus examination shows multiple (5 to 20), deep gray lesions scattered throughout the posterior pole. They are small, ranging in size from 50 to 200 μm in diameter.
- Lesions are smaller and less pigmented than those seen in MFC.
- Serous retinal detachment may be rarely observed.
- CNV occurs in up to 70% of cases, and presents with subretinal fluid, subretinal hemorrhage and subretinal exudates (most notably in chronic cases). It usually occurs within 1 year of onset of symptoms.
- Subretinal fibrosis may occur in 80% of patients.
- Both CNV and subretinal fibrosis usually occur less than 1 year after the onset of the disease.

Differential Diagnosis

- Ocular histoplasmosis
- Multifocal choroiditis
- Birdshot chorioretinopathy
- Toxoplasmosis, syphilis, TB
- Multifocal chorioretinal lesions in the early stage of endogenous endophthalmitis (candidiasis)
- Sarcoidosis
- VKH syndrome
- Sympathetic ophthalmia
- Subretinal fibrosis/uveitis syndrome
- Primary intraocular lymphoma

Diagnostic Evaluation (Figs. 8-14 to 8-16)

- Fluorescein angiography:
  - Without CNV:
    - ▶ Active lesions demonstrate early hyperfluorescence with late staining or leakage, but most of the clinical lesions are not apparent on FA.
    - ▶ Pooling of dye in the late frames if a serous retinal detachment is associated.

▶ Scars appear as early hypofluorescence with late hyperfluorescence.

▪ With CNV: Early well-defined hyperfluorescence with late leakage.

● ICG angiography

▪ Small hypocyanescent inflammatory lesions at the level of the posterior pole are the characteristic findings.

▪ There are more lesions on ICGA than are seen clinically.

▪ ICGA is the only procedure that can detect the extent of active lesions.

● Fundus autofluorescence shows hypoautofluorescent spots scattered throughout the posterior pole.

● OCT: The features are similar to those observed in multifocal choroiditis (nodular hyperreflectivity at the level of the photoreceptors and RPE) even though the lesions are more severe, especially at the level of the choroid.

● Visual field testing objectively identifies the scotomas the patients report. These deficits are more centrally localized than those seen with MFC.

Treatment

● Acute inflammatory component

▪ Corticosteroids

▶ Systemic corticosteroids are an effective way to control acute inflammation.

▶ Intravitreal injections and sustained release devices may also be useful, both for treatment of CNV as well as for associated macular edema.

▪ Immunomodulatory therapy: PIC may need long-term immunosuppression as it is a chronic disease and secondary CNV is very common.

▶ It should be considered in all patients with refractory inflammation or those who are intolerant of corticosteroids.

▶ Methotrexate, mycophenolate mofetil, azathioprine, and cyclosporine A have all been used with success.

▶ Systemic treatment is associated with a reduction in the risk of macular complications such as CME, ERM and CNV, as well as a reduced risk of vision loss.

● CNV: Corticosteroids and IMT may reduce recurrences by controlling the inflammatory state. The lesion itself can be treated similarly to other CNV.

▪ Extrafoveal: Consider focal laser

▪ Juxta- and subfoveal CNV: Intraocular steroids, photodynamic therapy, anti-VEGF therapy, submacular surgery

▪ Peripapillary: Focal laser (for small lesions), anti-VEGF therapy

▪ Spontaneous resolution of the active neovascularization may occur.

Prognosis

● Patients without CNV, subretinal fibrosis and foveal lesions have a favorable prognosis with the majority maintaining vision greater than 20/40.

● With foveal CNV, subretinal fibrosis or inflammatory lesions, the prognosis is guarded.

● Corticosteroids and IMT are not always successful.

REFERENCES

Brueggeman RM, Noffke AS, Jampol LM. Resolution of punctuate inner choroidopathy lesions with oral prednisone therapy. *Arch Ophthalmol.* 2002;120:996.

Gerstenblith AT, Thorne JE, Sobrin L, et al. Punctate inner choroidopathy: a survey analysis of 77 persons. *Ophthalmology.* 2007;114(6):1201–1204.

Shimada H, Yuzawa M, Hirose T, et al. Pathological findings of multifocal choroiditis with panuveitis and punctuate inner choroidopathy. *Jpn J Ophthalmol.* 2008;52: 282–288.

Watzke RC, Packer AJ, Folk JC, et al. Punctuate inner choroidopathy. *Am J Ophthalmol.* 1984;98:572–584.

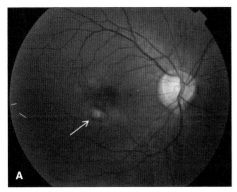
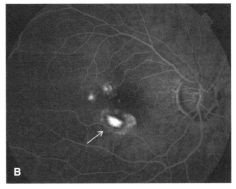

FIGURE 8-14. **A.** A color fundus photograph of a case of bilateral PIC with inactive scars and a secondary CNV in the right eye. **B.** FA confirms the active CNV in the right eye. RPE window defects correspond to the areas of atrophy.

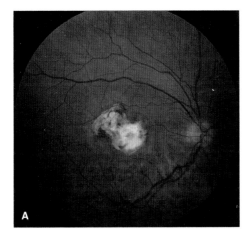

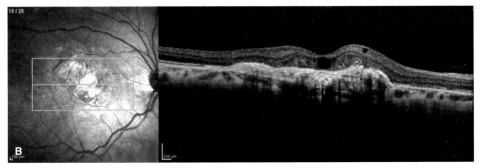

FIGURE 8-15. **A.** This patient with PIC developed a subfoveal CNV that required long-term intravitreal anti-VEGF therapy as well as systemic immunosuppression. **B.** OCT of the CVN demonstrates subretinal fibrosis and overlying CME.

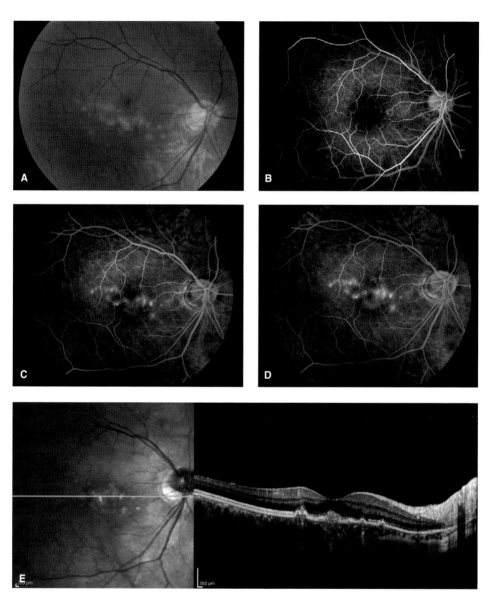

FIGURE 8-16. Unilateral PIC in a 25-year-old patient. **A.** Color photograph shows multiple small, deep gray macular lesions. FA shows early hyperfluorescence (**B**) increasing during the intermediate (**C**) and late (**D**) phases. **E.** OCT demonstrates focal RPE detachments with subretinal deposits and outer retinal alterations. (Courtesy of M.B. Rougier.)

OCULAR HISTOPLASMOSIS SYNDROME

P. Kumar Rao

Ocular histoplasmosis syndrome (OHS) is a choroidopathy presumably due to infection with *Histoplasmosis capsulatum*. Patients may have unilateral or bilateral involvement. Typically, no intraocular inflammation is present.

Etiology and Epidemiology

- Infection with *H. capsulatum* is most commonly found in the Ohio and Mississippi River valleys of the United States, and is uncommon elsewhere in the world. This disorder is presumably caused by inhalation of the organism.

- Up to 12.9% of patients in endemic areas will have ocular findings.

- Most patients become symptomatic in the third to fourth decades of life.

- There appears to be an association with HLA-DRw2 and HLA-B7.

- It is most commonly found in Caucasian patients.

Symptoms

- Initial infection with *H. capsulatum* may present with flu-like symptoms. Most patients are diagnosed during routine eye examinations.

- Patients may present with central vision loss or distortion. Up to 2% of patients with OHS develop vision loss due to CNV.

Signs (**Figs. 8-17 to 8-22**)

- The four main signs of OHS are:

  - Punched out chorioretinal scars, also called "histo spots." These are usually small, round, atrophic, depigmented lesions. They may be scattered throughout the posterior pole, and occasionally appear as linear "histo streaks."

  - Peripapillary atrophy appearing as a depigmented area adjacent to the disk

  - An absence of inflammatory cells in the vitreous or aqueous

  - Subretinal hemorrhage, fluid, or scarring due to submacular choroidal neovascular membrane

Differential Diagnosis

- Multifocal choroiditis
- Sarcoidosis
- TB
- Syphilis
- Birdshot choroiditis
- Age-related macular degeneration

Diagnostic Evaluation

- FA reveals window defects or staining in the area of punched-out chorioretinal scars and leakage in the areas of CNV.

- Skin testing with histoplasmin antigen is usually not indicated.

Treatment

- No treatment is required for the punched out chorioretinal scars.

- There have been a number of different treatments tried for treatment of CNVM in OHS, including anti-VEGF injections, laser photoablation, photodynamic therapy, subretinal surgery and periocular or systemic steroids. Periodic intravitreal injection of anti-VEGF agents show great promise for the treatment of this disease, and may be considered as first-line therapy for subfoveal CNVM.

- Submacular surgery has been shown to be beneficial in patients with vision worse than 20/100. However, with the advent of other treatment modalities, submacular surgery should be considered only when other treatment options have been exhausted.

Prognosis

● Occurrence of CNV greatly influences the final visual outcome.

REFERENCES

Adan A, Mateo C, Navarro R, et al. Intravitreal bevacizumab (Avastin) injection as primary treatment of inflammatory choroidal neovascularization. *Retina.* 2007;27:1180–1186.

Busquets MA, Shah GK, Wickens J, et al. Ocular photodynamic therapy with verteporfin for choroidal neovascularization secondary to ocular histoplasmosis syndrome. *Retina.* 2003;23(3):299–306.

Davidorf FH, Anderson JD. Ocular lesions in the Earth Day, 1970, histoplasmosis epidemic. *Int Ophthalmol Clin.* 1975;15(3):51–63.

Ehrlich R, Ciulla TA, Maturi R, et al. Intravitreal bevacizumab for choroidal neovascularization secondary to presumed ocular histoplasmosis syndrome. *Retina.* 2009;29(10):1418–1423.

Hawkins BS, Bressler NM, Bressler SB, et al. Submacular Surgery Trials Research Group. Surgical removal vs observation for subfoveal choroidal neovascularization, either associated with the ocular histoplasmosis syndrome or idiopathic: I. Ophthalmic findings from a randomized clinical trial: Submacular Surgery Trials (SST) Group H Trial: SST Report No. 9. *Arch Ophthalmol.* 2004;122(11):1597–1611.

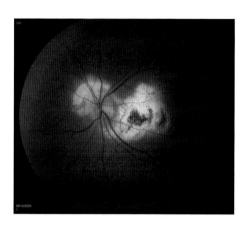

FIGURE 8-17. Color photograph of peripapillary atrophy and associated disciform scar following CNV.

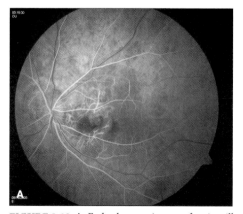
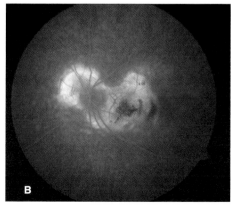

FIGURE 8-18. A. Early phase angiogram of peripapillary and macular atrophy and scar. **B.** Late-phase angiogram revealing hyperfluorescence consistent with staining in the areas of peripapillary and macular atrophy and scarring.

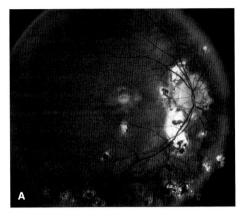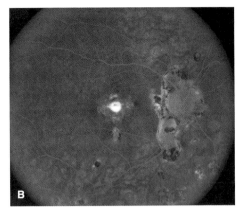

FIGURE 8-19. **A.** Color photo with peripapillary atrophy, multiple, punched out lesions, and a regressed subfoveal CNV. **B.** Late-phase angiogram revealing hyperfluorescence consistent with staining at the edges of peripapillary atrophy and staining of the subfoveal CNVM.

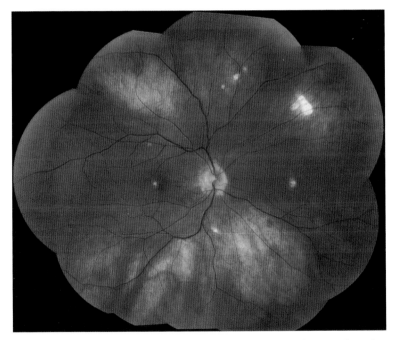

FIGURE 8-20. A color montage demonstrates a clear media, peripapillary atrophy, and a few scattered punched-out lesions in the posterior pole and mid-periphery.

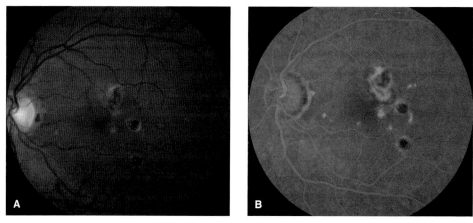

FIGURE 8-21. A. This patient had no vitritis, but did have peripapillary atrophy, focal areas of chorioretinitis of the posterior pole, and a subretinal CNVM superotemporal to the fovea. **B.** The fluorescein angiogram demonstrates areas of RPE window defects (hyperfluorescent), areas of chorioretinal atrophy (hypofluorescent), and staining of the superotemporal CNVM.

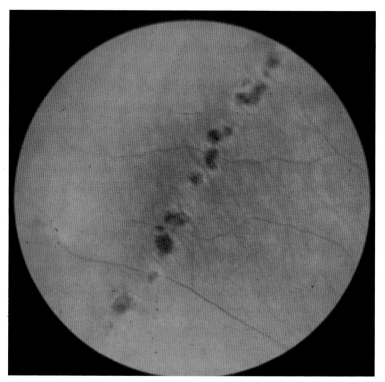

FIGURE 8-22. The patient has linear hyperpigmented spots in the mid-periphery, which are the linear "histo streak."

BIRDSHOT CHORIORETINOPATHY (VITILIGINOUS CHORIORETINITIS)

Matthew A. Cunningham and Steven Yeh

Initially described in 1980 by Ryan and Maumanee and subsequently by Gass in 1981, birdshot chorioretinopathy is an uncommon, idiopathic form of posterior uveitis, typically characterized by multiple hypopigmented choroidal lesions scattered throughout the fundus. It accounts for 6% to 7.9% of cases of posterior uveitis.

Epidemiology and Etiology

- Birdshot chorioretinopathy is a chronic, recurrent, bilateral disease most commonly occurring between the third to seventh decades of life.

- It has a slight female predominance and is more common in Caucasian patients.

- Retinal S-antigen has been suggested as the antigen potentially involved in the pathogenesis of birdshot chorioretinopathy but the precise etiology of birdshot chorioretinopathy is unknown. There is a strong genetic association with HLA-A29.

- Histopathology from individuals with untreated birdshot chorioretinopathy demonstrated foci of lymphocytes (mostly CD8+ T-cells) involving the choroid, the photoreceptors and around retinal blood vessels.

Symptoms

- Patients describe floaters, dyschromatopsia, and/or nyctalopia, subtle loss of central vision and photopsias in an otherwise healthy individual.

- Symptoms may be out of proportion to the clinical findings (i.e. individuals complain of blurred vision despite 20/20 visual acuity).

Signs (Figs. 8-23 to 8-26)

- Quiet conjunctiva and sclera, with minimal to no anterior segment inflammation. Keratic precipitates and posterior synechiae are not seen.

- Vitritis without snowballs or snowbanking

- Deep, indistinct, hypopigmented or cream-colored choroidal lesions in the midperiphery and posterior pole. They have indistinct borders.

  - May occur years after symptoms begin

  - Described by Ryan as "multiple, small, white spots that frequently have the pattern seen with birdshot in the scatter from a shotgun"

  - Oval or round lesions are typical, and they may assume a linear configuration.

  - Usually found clustered around the optic disk, especially nasal and inferior to the optic disk, but may be diffuse and involve the peripheral retina only (although uncommon)

- Other key findings include retinal periphlebitis, which may be better appreciated on fluorescein angiography, optic disk edema and cystoid macular edema, which is the most common cause of visual loss in birdshot chorioretinopathy.

Differential Diagnosis

- Sarcoidosis
- Intraocular lymphoma
- MFCP
- Multifocal evanescent white dot syndrome
- APMPPE
- Posterior scleritis
- Sympathetic ophthalmia
- Syphilis
- TB
- VKH

Diagnostic Evaluation

- HLA-A29 typing: 80% to 90% of bird-shot patients show HLA-A29 positivity versus 7% of control subjects (relative risk of almost 50).
- FA: Used to assess disease activity and sequelae

  ▪ Birdshot lesions demonstrate early hypofluorescence and late hyperfluorescence.

  ▪ Retinal and optic nerve neovascularization, retinovascular leakage, optic disk edema and macular edema may be seen.

- ICGA

  ▪ Active lesions demonstrate hypofluorescence in the early and intermediate phases and isofluorescence or hyperfluorescence during the late phase.

  ▪ Chronic, inactive lesions may show hypofluorescence in all phases.

  ▪ More lesions may be seen on ICG angiography than with FA or on clinical exam.

- ERG

  ▪ May be abnormal despite excellent visual acuity

  ▪ May appear normal early in the disease process, but amplitudes and implicit times may become abnormal as the disease progresses; scotopic b-wave response is typically affected prior to photopic b-wave

- Visual fields

  ▪ Visual field deficit may not correlate to the distribution of birdshot lesions.

  ▪ Central scotomata, paracentral scotomata, diffuse peripheral constriction or generalized depression may be seen.

- OCT is useful to determine the extent of cystoid macular edema, and to follow response to treatment.

Treatment

- Periocular and systemic corticosteroids remain the mainstay of therapy for acute inflammation.
- Steroid-sparing immunomodulatory agents are usually required in order to maintain long-term control of the disease. Patients with cystoid macular edema, ERG abnormalities, or visual field abnormalities, should be considered for treatment even though they may have good central acuity.

  ▪ Cyclosporine has been shown to be effective in decreasing inflammation and stabilizing or improving visual acuity. It is the most commonly used corticosteroid-sparing agent for birdshot chorioretinopathy.

  ▪ Good results with antimetabolites (methotrexate, azathioprine, mycophenolate mofetil) and alkylating agents (chlorambucil, cyclophosphamide) also have been reported. The antimetabolites have a good, long-term safety profile.

  ▪ Daclizumab (humanized anti-IL-2 receptor) also appears effective for long-term disease remission.

- Sequelae of birdshot chorioretinopathy (i.e., cystoid macular edema, and choroidal neovascularization) may require local or systemic therapy in addition to control of the choroidal inflammation.

Prognosis

- Long-term preservation of visual function and decreased or stabilization of inflammation is possible with systemic immunosuppression.
- Retinal function, both subjective and objective, may improve following immunosuppressive therapy.
- Sequelae of birdshot chorioretinopathy, including CME and choroidal neovascularization, may lead to visual loss if not treated promptly.

- Optic atrophy, macular or foveal atrophy, retinal neovascularization and central/branch retinal vein occlusions may contribute to visual morbidity.

REFERENCES

Becker MD, Wertheim MS, Smith JR, et al. Long-term follow-up of patients with birdshot retinochoroidopathy treated with systemic immunosuppression. *Ocul Immunol Inflamm.* 2005;13(4):289–293.

Le Hoang P, Girard B, Deray G, et al. Cyclosporine in the treatment of birdshot retinochoroidopathy. *Transplant Proc.* 1988;20(suppl):128–130.

Monnet D, Brézin AP, Holland GN, et al. Longitudinal cohort study of patients with birdshot chorioretinopathy. I. Baseline clinical characteristics. *Am J Ophthalmol.* 2006;141(1):135–142.

Nussenblatt RB, Mittal KK, Ryan S, et al. Birdshot retinochoroidopathy associated with HLA-A29 antigen and immune responsiveness to retinal S-antigen. *Am J Ophthalmol.* 1982;94:147–158.

Rothova A, Berendschot TT, Probst K, et al. Birdshot chorioretinopathy: long-term manifestations and visual prognosis. *Ophthalmology.* 2004;111:954–959.

Zacks DN, Samson CM, Loewenstein J, et al. Electroretinograms as an indicator of disease activity in birdshot retinochoroidopathy. *Graefes Arch Clin Exp Ophthalmol.* 2002;240:601–607.

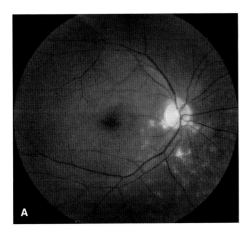

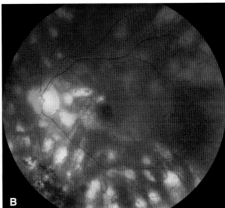

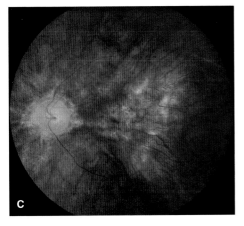

FIGURE 8-23. **A.** Inferonasal and peripapillary oval, cream-colored lesions with mild retinal pigment epithelial atrophy inferonasally in a patient with birdshot chorioretinopathy. **B.** Multiple oval areas of chorioretinal atrophy in a patient with longstanding birdshot chorioretinopathy. **C.** Optic atrophy and macular atrophy in a patient with poorly controlled birdshot chorioretinopathy.

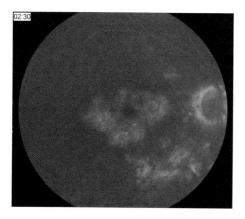

FIGURE 8-24. CME is the most common cause of a decline in visual acuity in birdshot chorioretinopathy. A FA shows CME with hyperfluorescence along the inferotemporal arcade.

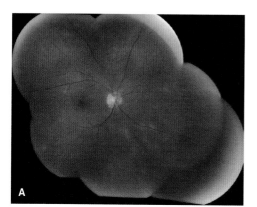

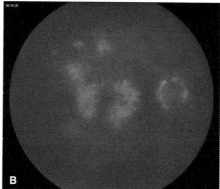

FIGURE 8-25. A. This patient had mild birdshot chorioretinopathy. Note the mild vitritis overlying the superotemporal arcade. Inferonasally, there is mild vasculitis present along the vascular arcade, and the lesions are less distinct. Indirect ophthalmoscopy with a 20D lens may allow easier detection of these lesions compared to the higher magnification of slit lamp exam. **B.** There is significant CME on the fluorescein angiogram, but the lesions themselves are more subtle in appearance. (Courtesy of Paul Baker, MD.)

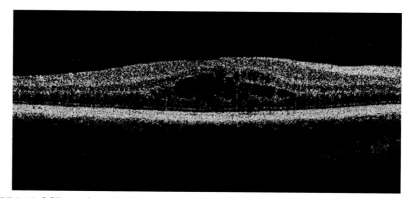

FIGURE 8-26. OCT scan shows CME in a patient with birdshot. Local and systemic immunosuppressive therapy is typically required to maintain disease control and improve visual function.

ACUTE ZONAL OCCULT OUTER RETINOPATHY

Annal D. Meleth ▥

I nitially described by Don Gass, MD, acute zonal occult outer retinopathy (AZOOR) is a syndrome of outer retinal dysfunction associated with visual field and ERG abnormalities, which is most common in women in their fourth decade of life.

Epidemiology and Etiology

● It is rare and usually affects younger women.

● Women are affected more than men, in a 3:1 ratio.

● Twenty percent to 30% may have an associated systemic autoimmune disease.

▥ It can develop in patients with a history of other white dot syndromes, including MEWDS, MFC, acute macular neuroretinopathy (AMN), AIBSES and PIC.

● Dr. Gass postulated an infectious trigger, but this has yet to be established.

Symptoms

● Photopsias

● Acute progressive visual field loss over a period of weeks to months

● The visual acuity is variably affected.

● AZOOR is typically bilateral, but may be asymmetric. If initially unilateral, the other eye can become involved within weeks to months.

Signs

● Typically, there are no clinically visible changes during the acute phase.

● Over the ensuing few weeks to months after onset, patients may develop:

▥ An afferent pupillary defect

▥ Vitritis

▥ RPE atrophy/abnormal RPE pigmentation

Differential Diagnosis

● Dr. Gass termed these diseases the AZOOR complex of diseases. These include:

▥ MEWDS

▥ PIC

▥ MFC

▥ AIBSE

● Cancer-associated retinopathy

● Melanoma-associated retinopathy

● Autoimmune retinopathy

● Optic neuritis

● Chiasmal lesions

● Diffuse unilateral subacute necrosis (DUSN)

● Syphilis

Diagnostic Evaluation (Fig. 8-27)

● FA is typically normal in the acute phase but can show CME and perivenous sheathing if present.

● Autofluorescence is usually normal early in the disease course. Patients can develop a peripapillary halo of hypoautofluorescence with a hyperautofluorescent border. Other patients have hypoautofluorescence in the periphery, and less commonly in the posterior pole.

● Visual field characteristically shows enlargement of the blind spot with arcuate extension into temporal quadrants.

● ERG is abnormal early in the disease. There is prolonged implicit time on 30-Hz flicker, and an abnormal b-wave amplitude on photopic responses.

● Multifocal ERG also shows outer retinal dysfunction.

● OCT can show hyperreflectivity in the outer retina as well as generalized disruption of the normal retinal layers.

This contribution to the work was done as part of the author's official duties as an NIH employee and is a work of the United States Government.

Treatment

- No treatment has been proven to improve the visual outcome, although steroids, nonsteroidal immunosuppressive agents, antivirals and antifungal agents have been tried, with mixed success.

Prognosis

- Three-fourths of patients will have stabilization of field loss within 6 months. If recovery occurs, it is typically incomplete.

- Two-thirds of patients recover 20/40 vision but 18% become legally blind.

- Approximately 30% of patients experience recurrence of the disease.

REFERENCES

Francis PJ, Marinescu A, Fitzke FW, et al. Acute zonal occult outer retinopathy: towards a set of diagnostic criteria. *Br J Ophthalmol.* 2005;89:70–73.

Gass JD. Acute zonal occult outer retinopathy: Donders Lecture: The Netherlands Ophthalmological Society. *Retina.* 2003;23(6 Suppl):79–97.

Gass JD, Agarwal A, Scott IU. Acute zonal occult outer retinopathy: a long-term follow-up study. *Am J Ophthalmol.* 2002;134(3):329–339.

Monson DM, Smith JR. Acute zonal occult outer retinopathy. *Surv Ophthalmol.* 2010. [Epub ahead of print]

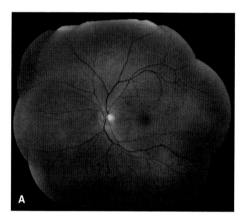

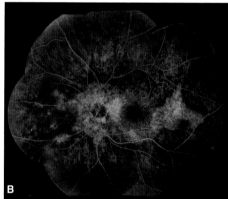

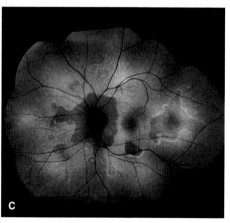

FIGURE 8-27. Left fundus of a 35-year-old woman with an enlarged blind spot and photopsias on initial presentation. **A.** Fundus photograph demonstrates mild pigment changes in the peripapillary region and temporal macula. **B.** FA shows window defects in the areas of RPE atrophy. **C.** Fundus autofluorescence better demonstrates areas of RPE atrophy with a hyperautofluorescent halo.

ACUTE MACULAR NEURORETINOPATHY

Jaclyn L. Kovach and Janet L. Davis

Acute macular neuroretinopathy (AMN) is a rare condition characterized by acute paracentral scotomas that correspond to flat, reddish, wedge-shaped intraretinal lesions that usually surround the fovea.

Etiology and Epidemiology

- It occurs predominantly in young women.
- It can be unilateral or bilateral.
- Possible vascular or viral etiologies have been suggested as AMN is often preceded by a viral illness or flu-like syndrome.
- Changes in outer retina in affected regions
- Associated factors include oral contraceptive use, contrast media, epinephrine, trauma, headache and hypotensive episodes.

Symptoms

- Paracentral scotomas
- Normal to mildly decreased visual acuity

Signs (Fig. 8-28)

- Multiple, sharply defined, somewhat confluent, flat, wedge-shaped intraretinal lesions in a flower-petal arrangement around the central macula
- Lesions are round to oval and reddish to brown in color and can appear to point toward the fovea.
- Retinal hemorrhages can occur.

Differential Diagnosis

- APMPPE
- Acute retinal pigment epitheliitis
- Idiopathic central serous chorioretinopathy

Diagnostic Evaluation

- Lesions are best appreciated with red-free light.
- Humphrey visual field and Amsler grid testing demonstrates a scotoma in affected areas.
- FA is usually normal.
- Spectral domain OCT: Reduced signal corresponding to the photoreceptor inner and outer segment junction and the photoreceptor outer segments.
- Scanning laser ophthalmoscopy enhances lesion visibility with red and infrared light.
- Multifocal ERG has a localized depression in waveform amplitudes in the area corresponding to the lesions.

Treatment

- No definitive treatment is yet available.

Prognosis

- The disease is self-limiting, but a number of patients may have scotomas that persist for months or years.

REFERENCES

Bos PJ, Deutman AF. Acute macular neuroretinopathy. *Am J Ophthalmol.* 1975;80(4):573–584.

Gillies M, Sarks J, Dunlop C, et al. Traumatic retinopathy resembling acute macular neuroretinopathy. *Aust N Z J Ophthalmol.* 1997;25(3):207–210.

Neuhann IM, Inhoffen W, Koerner S, et al. Visualization and follow-up of acute macular neuroretinopathy with the Spectralis HRA+OCT device. *Graefes Arch Clin Exp Ophthalmol.* 2010;248(7):1041–1044.

Turbeville SD, Cowan LD, Gass JD. Acute macular neuroretinopathy: a review of the literature. *Surv Ophthalmol.* 2003;48(1):1–11.

Watzke RC, Shults WT. Annular macular neuroretinopathy and multifocal electroretinographic and optical coherence tomographic findings. *Retina.* 2004;24(5):772–775.

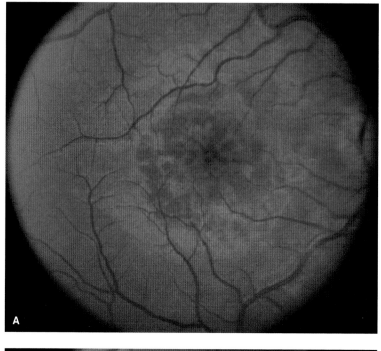

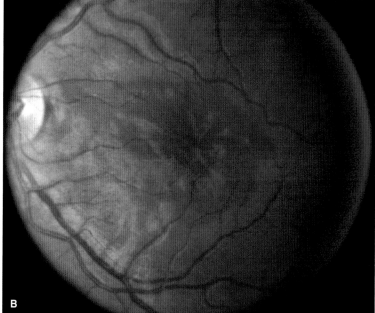

FIGURE 8-28. **A.** Fundus photo of the right eye shows partly confluent, reddish, intraretinal lesions in a petaloid pattern coalescing around the fovea. **B.** Fundus photo of the left eye shows similar reddish-brown lesions centered around the fovea.

UNILATERAL ACUTE IDIOPATHIC MACULOPATHY

Jaclyn L. Kovach and Janet L. Davis

U nilateral acute idiopathic maculopathy (UAIM) causes severe, unilateral vision loss secondary to an exudative maculopathy with rapid, spontaneous resolution of the exudative changes and restoration of vision over weeks to months.

Etiology and Epidemiology

- It occurs in young adults.
- Many patients have a viral prodrome.
- There is a possible association with the coxsackievirus, pregnancy and HIV.
- It is rarely bilateral.

Symptoms

- Sudden, severe unilateral loss of central vision
- Central scotoma
- Some patients have a viral prodrome.

Signs (**Figs. 8-29 and 8-30**)

- Patients have an irregular macular neurosensory retinal detachment with an underlying yellow, white or gray plaque at the level of the RPE.
- It can look like a choroidal neovascular membrane.
- Patients can develop a choroidal neovascular membrane as the acute lesion resolves.
- Vitreous cells, intraretinal hemorrhages, papillitis, eccentric macular lesions, subretinal exudation may also occur.
- As the unilateral exudative detachment resolves, subretinal atrophic and pigmentary changes and a possible bull's-eye maculopathy often occur.

Differential Diagnosis

- Idiopathic choroidal neovascularization
- Serous detachment of the RPE
- Central serous chorioretinopathy
- VKH
- Serpiginous choroidopathy
- Posterior scleritis
- APMPPE
- Placoid syphilitic retinitis
- Vitelliform maculopathy associated with cuticular drusen

Diagnostic Evaluation

- Fluorescein angiography: In the early frames, there can be irregular areas of both hypo- and hyperfluorescence. The late frames show hyperfluorescence secondary to window defects and late staining of the lesion, as well as pooling of the dye within the subretinal space.
- OCT demonstrates hyperreflectivity and thickening of the RPE layer and possible subretinal fluid in the acute phase. There can be defects of the RPE with increased penetration into the choroid in the late phase of the disease.
- EOG: Decreased Arden ratio
- ERG: The full field ERG is normal, but the multifocal ERG shows reduced amplitudes.

Treatment

- No treatment is usually required as patients have spontaneous resolution.
- Systemic corticosteroids can hasten resolution, but do not appear to achieve a better final visual outcome.
- Choroidal neovascular membranes can be treated as is the standard, including with anti-VEGF agents.

Prognosis

- Overall it is excellent, unless secondary CNV occurs.

REFERENCES

Beck AP, Jampol LM, Glaser DA, et al. Is coxsackievirus the cause of unilateral acute idiopathic maculopathy? *Arch Ophthalmol.* 2004;122(1):121–123.

Freund KB, Yannuzzi LA, Barile GR, et al. The expanding clinical spectrum of unilateral acute idiopathic maculopathy. *Arch Ophthalmol.* 1996;114(5): 555–559.

Haruta H, Sawa M, Saishin Y, et al. Clinical findings in unilateral acute idiopathic maculopathy: new findings in acute idiopathic maculopathy. *Int Ophthalmol.* 2010;30(2):199–202.

Lam BL, Lopez PF, Dubovy SR, et al. Transient electro-oculogram impairment in unilateral acute idiopathic maculopathy. *Doc Ophthalmol.* 2009;119(2):157–161.

Yannuzzi LA, Jampol LM, Rabb MF, et al. Unilateral acute idiopathic maculopathy. *Arch Ophthalmol.* 1991; 109(10):1411–1416.

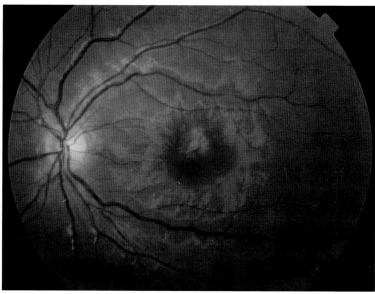

FIGURE 8-29. Fundus photo of the left macula shows subretinal exudate with a subtle overlying neurosensory retinal detachment.

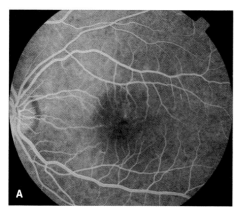 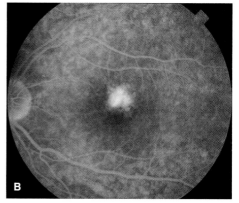

FIGURE 8-30. A. FA reveals early hypo- and hyperfluorescence. **B.** The later frame of the angiogram shows irregular foveal hyperfluorescence. (Courtesy of Byron Lam, MD. Reprinted with permission from Springer; Lam BL, Lopez PF, et al. Transient electro-oculogram impairment in unilateral acute idiopathic maculopathy. *Doc Ophthalmol.* 2009;119(2):157–161.)

ACUTE RETINAL PIGMENT EPITHELIITIS

Jason Hsu

Acute retinal pigment epitheliitis (ARPE) is a rare, transient macular disorder that is characterized by small dark spots or fine pigment stippling surrounded by a halo of hypopigmentation, which is often yellowish in appearance.

Etiology and Epidemiology

- The etiology of ARPE is unclear, although a viral etiology is suspected.

- Patients tend to be young, healthy adults in the second to fourth decades with no history of preceding illness or viral prodrome.

- Hepatitis C and IV bisphosphonate use have been reported in patients with clinical presentations consistent with ARPE.

- ARPE has been postulated to be an inflammatory condition occurring at the level of the RPE.

- Recent OCT findings of ARPE support an alternate theory suggesting that the initial disturbance may involve the photoreceptors with a secondary postinflammatory response by the RPE.

Symptoms

- Patients present with acute onset of unilateral blurred vision, metamorphopsia, or central scotoma, although a few bilateral cases have been reported.

Signs

- Visual acuity typically ranges from 20/20 to 20/100.

- Amsler grid or visual field testing demonstrates central metamorphopsia or central scotoma, respectively.

- The typical macular lesions are discrete, tiny clusters of hyperpigmented dots at the level of the RPE that are surrounded by a yellow-white hypopigmented halo (**Figs. 8-31 and 8-33**).

- Rarely, a mild vitritis may be noted.

Differential Diagnosis

- Acute macular neuroretinopathy

- Acute posterior multifocal placoid pigment epitheliopathy

- Central serous chorioretinopathy

- Viral retinitis

  - Rubella

  - Herpes simplex virus

  - Measles virus

  - CMV

Diagnostic Evaluation (Fig. 8-32)

- FA reveals early hyperfluorescence with occasional blockage of the choroidal fluorescence from the pigment mottling.

- OCT may vary over time.

  - Acutely, abnormal dome-shaped hyperreflectivity is seen involving the outer nuclear layer and photoreceptors with disruption of the inner segment/outer segment hyperreflective band.

  - Soon after, involvement of the RPE-choriocapillaris band can be noted with backscattering noted beneath the lesion.

  - In the resolution phase, the outer retinal hyperreflectivity subsides though some backscattering may persist.

- ERG is normal.

- EOG may be abnormal in the acute phase suggesting a more widespread dysfunction at the level of the RPE than what is clinically seen.

Treatment

- Supportive, as this is a self-limited disease.

Prognosis

- Complete, spontaneous resolution of symptoms occurs in most patients within 6 to 12 weeks.

- Recurrences have been reported but are rare.

- A few patients have been reported who later developed central serous chorioretinopathy.

REFERENCES

Chittum ME, Kalina RE. Acute retinal pigment epitheliitis. *Ophthalmology*. 1987;94:1114–1119.

Eifrig DE, Knobloch WH, Moran JA. Retinal pigment epitheliitis. *Ann Ophthalmol*. 1977;9:639–642.

Friedman MW. Bilateral recurrent acute retinal pigment epitheliitis. *Am J Ophthalmol*. 1975;79:567–570.

Gilhotra JS, Gilhotra AK, Holdaway M, et al. Acute retinal pigment epitheliitis associated with intravenous bisphosphonate. *Br J Ophthalmol*. 2006;90:798–799.

Hsu J, Fineman MS, Kaiser RS. Optical coherence tomography findings in acute retinal pigment epitheliitis. *Am J Ophthalmol*. 2007;143:163–165.

Krill AE, Deutman AF. Acute retinal pigment epitheliitis. *Am J Ophthalmol*. 1972;74:193–205.

Luttrull JK, Chittum ME. Acute retinal pigment epitheliitis. *Am J Ophthalmol*. 1995;120:389–391.

Piermarocchi S, Corradini R, Midena E, et al. Correlation between retinal pigment epitheliitis and central serous chorioretinopathy. *Ann Ophthalmol*. 1983;15:425–428.

Quillen DA, Zurlo JJ, Cunningham D, et al. Acute retinal pigment epitheliitis and hepatitis C. *Am J Ophthalmol*. 1994;118:120–121.

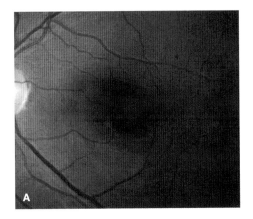

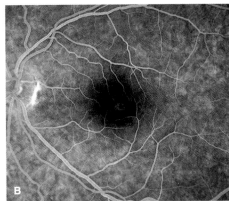

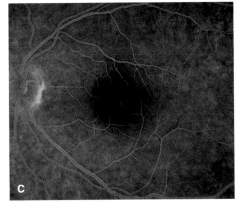

FIGURE 8-31. A. Fundus photograph of a patient presenting within 24 hours of the onset of symptoms with pigment stippling surrounded by foveal hypopigmentation. **B.** Mid-phase fluorescein angiogram of the patient in Figure 1 showing an area of hyperfluorescence corresponding to the area of hypopigmentation. **C.** Late-phase fluorescein angiogram showing decreased hyperfluorescence consistent with transmission hyperfluorescence.

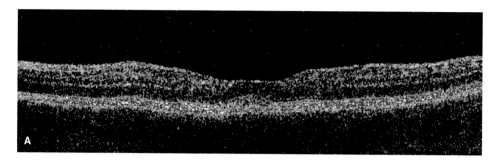

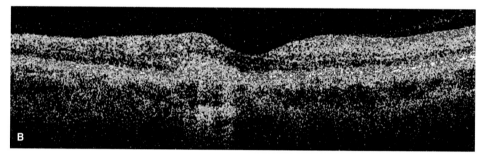

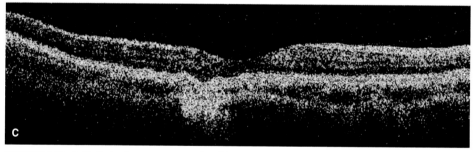

FIGURE 8-32. **A.** Optical coherence tomography of the patient in Figure 8-30 shows a dome-shaped area of hyperreflectivity involving the photoreceptors and outer nuclear layer with disruption of the photoreceptor inner segment-outer segment hyperreflective band. **B.** Optical coherence tomography shows a dome-shaped area of hyperreflectivity involving the retinal pigment epithelium, photoreceptors, and outer nuclear layer with moderate backscattering. **C.** Four weeks later, optical coherence tomography demonstrates normalization of the previous hyperreflectivity, although prominent backscattering remains.

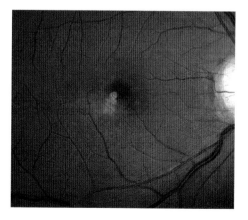

FIGURE 8-33. Two days after the onset of symptoms in another patient, the fundus photograph demonstrates fine pigment stippling surrounded by discrete, yellowish hypopigmentation with additional surrounding areas of subtle hypopigmentation.

Infectious Posterior Uveitis

VIRAL INFECTION

HERPETIC

*Karina Julian, Bahram Bodaghi,
and Phuc LeHoang* ▇

Herpes viruses infecting the retina manifest themselves differently depending upon the interaction between the virus and the host immune system. Most of them are known as necrotizing retinopathies, but nonnecrotizing forms should also be considered in atypical cases of chronic posterior uveitis.

• Necrotizing retinopathies are by far the most frequent clinical picture, with a spectrum of severity ranging from the acute retinal necrosis syndrome (almost always seen in healthy individuals) to the progressive outer retinal necrosis syndrome, (PORN), and cytomegalovirus (CMV) retinitis, both of which mainly affect severely immunocompromised patients.

• Nonnecrotizing herpetic retinopathies are less frequent and have a number of different manifestations, including vitritis, occlusive vasculitis, papillitis, or macular edema.

ACUTE RETINAL NECROSIS SYNDROME

Acute retinal necrosis (ARN) syndrome is characterized by peripheral necrotizing retinitis, retinal vasculitis, a prominent inflammatory reaction in the vitreous, and a granulomatous anterior uveitis.

Epidemiology and Etiology

• ARN is a rare disease, occurring in 1 per 1.6 to 2.0 million people per year in Western countries.

• In most cases, ARN is caused by varicella zoster virus (VZV); however, herpes simplex viruses 1 (HSV-1) and 2 (HSV-2) also cause ARN.

■ HSV-2 is more prevalent in children and adolescents, while HSV-1 mainly occurs in young adults. VZV is usually found in the elderly.

Symptoms

• Acute, painless visual loss with floaters

• 65% of cases are unilateral at presentation; 33% of cases are bilateral (BARN, bilateral acute retinal necrosis)

• Conjunctival and ciliary injection of varying intensity

Signs (Figs. 9-1 to 9-6)

- Anterior granulomatous uveitis, which rarely can be associated with hypopyon or hyphema

- Intense vitritis

- Patchy or confluent areas of white or cream-colored retinal necrosis initially affecting the peripheral retina and then extending centripetally

- Occlusive vasculopathy

- Papillitis of varied intensity

- Immunocompetent, otherwise healthy young or middle-aged patients, with or without a remote history of herpes virus infection or herpetic encephalitis (an established risk factor for ARN)

- ARN is a *medical emergency*. It is rapidly progressive and second eye involvement will naturally occur in almost 70% of patients in the absence of treatment. More than 50% of patients develop a rhegmatogenous retinal detachment (RRD) due to retinal atrophy secondary to necrosis and vitreous contraction.

Differential Diagnosis

- ARN needs to be differentiated from other nonviral necrotizing retinopathies, infectious or not (**Table 9-1**):

  - Extensive *Toxoplasma* retinochoroidopathy

  - Syphilitic retinitis

  - Fungal endogenous endophthalmitis

  - Primary intraocular lymphoma (PIOL)

  - Retinitis associated with Behçet's disease

  - CMV retinitis (occurs only in severely immunocompromised patients)

Diagnostic Evaluation

- ARN is primarily a clinical diagnosis.

- Because the natural disease course is usually devastating, ancillary tests confirm the etiology and/or eliminate nonviral causes, but they should never cause a delay in empirical treatment.

- Two different assays are performed in ocular samples (aqueous humor or vitreous):

  - Polymerase chain reaction (PCR) for direct detection of viral DNA is highly sensitive with 80% to 96% positivity in both immunocompetent and immunocompromised hosts.

  - Indirect detection of antibodies directed against virus proteins has 50% to 70% positivity in immunocompetent patients.

- In cases of suspected meningitis, a brain MRI and a lumbar puncture should be performed without delay as simultaneous herpetic meningitis or encephalitis is possible.

Treatment

- The primary treatment is medical. Traditionally, this has been administered in an inpatient setting during the acute phase; however, outpatient management has been reported recently but remains somewhat controversial.

  - The primary treatment is antiviral therapy, which is used to control viral replication and to reduce the risk of bilateralization. Intravitreal injections can be used in cases that are imminently threatening the macula or optic nerve.

  - Anti-inflammatory therapy is used to minimize the deleterious effects associated with inflammation. Viral replication must be controlled with antiviral medications before administration of systemic corticosteroids.

  - Antithrombotic therapy should be considered in order to reduce vascular complications.

TABLE 9-1. Necrotizing Retinopathies

	Acute Retinal Necrosis	Extensive Toxoplasmosis	Syphilis	Fungal Endogenous Endophthalmitis	PIOL	Behçet's Disease	CMV Retinitis
Predisposing conditions	None History of herpes encephalitis or other herpes virus infection	Elderly patients Immuno-compromised	AIDS	Immunosuppression IV drug users Diabetes	Elderly patients	Young adults, Silk road disease	Immuno-compromised (e.g., HIV)
Clinical picture	Vitritis Midperipheral whitish necrosis with hemorrhage, extends rapidly	Pigmented scars Dense vitritis	Papillitis, vasculitis, retinal necrosis	Chorioretinitis Dense vitritis	Infiltrative retinal lesions	Vasculitis, Retinitis, Papillitis, vitritis	Yellow-white necrosis with hemorrhage, slowly progressive
Diagnosis	Clinical, PCR, detection of antibodies	PCR and Goldmann-Witmer coefficient are useful for the diagnosis	TPHA, VDRL, FTA-abs	Culture and PCR	Cytology High IL-10/IL-6 ratio is highly suggestive	Diagnostic criteria defined by the International Study Group for Behçet disease	Clinical, PCR, HIV serology

- Laser retinopexy may reduce the occurrence of a RRD, but its efficacy remains controversial.

- Patients with vitreous hemorrhage secondary to retinal neovascularization or for RRD should have pars plana vitrectomy, with or without silicone oil tamponade. Early vitrectomy with intravitreal injection of antiviral medications and laser retinopexy can be performed to prevent RRD, although no improvement in final visual acuity has been reported.

- Treatment medications are outlined in **Table 9-2**.

Prognosis

- Despite early recognition and institution of prompt therapy, the final visual outcome is generally poor.

- RRD and ischemic optic neuropathy (with subsequent optic nerve atrophy) preclude good final visual acuity.

REFERENCES

Aizman A, Johnson MW, Elner SG. Treatment of acute retinal necrosis syndrome with oral antiviral medications. *Ophthalmology.* 2007;114:307–312.

Balansard B, Bodaghi B, Cassoux N, et al. Necrotizing retinopathies simulating acute retinal necrosis syndrome. *Br J Ophthalmol.* 2005;89(1):96–101.

Ganatra JB, Chandler D, Santos C, et al. Viral causes of the acute retinal necrosis syndrome. *Am J Ophthalmol.* 2000;129(2):166–172.

Holland, GN. Standard diagnostic criteria for the acute retinal necrosis syndrome. Executive Committee of the American Uveitis Society. *Am J Ophthalmol.* 1994; 117(5):663–667.

Tibbetts MD, Shah CP, Young LH, et al. Treatment of acute retinal necrosis. *Ophthalmology.* 2010;117(4):818–824.

Wong R, Pavesio CE, Laidlaw DA, et al. Acute retinal necrosis: the effects of intravitreal foscarnet and virus type on outcome. *Ophthalmology.* 2010;117(3):556–560.

TABLE 9-2. Medical Treatment of ARN

	Active Drug	Dosages
Antivirals	Acyclovir	10 mg/kg/8 h (1500 mg/m^2) IV or 800 mg PO 5 times/day
	Foscarnet	90 mg/kg/12 h IV or/and intravitreal injections
	Ganciclovir	5 mg/kg/12 h IV or/and intravitreal injections
	Valganciclovir	900 mg/day b.i.d.
Anti-inflammatory drugs	Methylprednisolone	500 mg daily IV for 3 days
	Prednisone	0.5–1 mg/kg/day with a gradual taper
Antithrombotic drugs	Standard heparin	
	Aspirin (acetylsalicylic acid)	100 mg/day

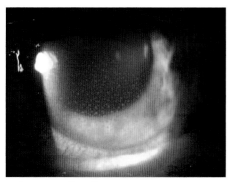

FIGURE 9-1. Granulomatous anterior uveitis in a patient with ARN syndrome.

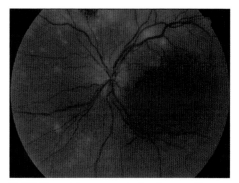

FIGURE 9-2. There are multiple white to yellow-white foci of peripheral retinal necrosis in a case of ARN syndrome. These occur in a circumferential fashion.

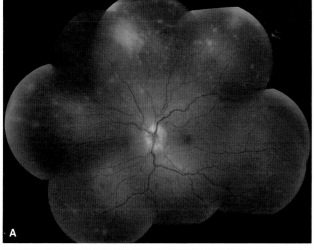

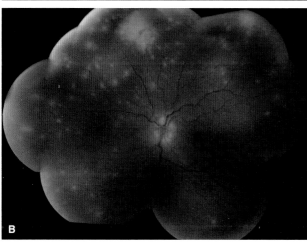

FIGURE 9-3. This 48-year-old patient presented with sudden onset of blurred vision and floaters. **A.** There are numerous focal white areas of retinitis and vasculitis in the periphery along with optic disk edema. **B.** Three days after the institution of therapy, the areas of retinitis appear slightly larger and better defined. Some scattered peripheral retinal hemorrhages are visible.

(*continued*)

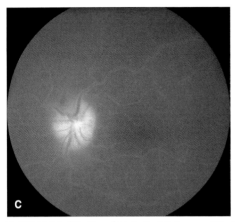

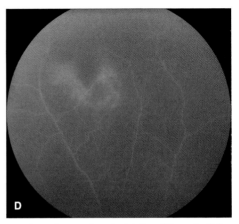

FIGURE 9-3. (*Continued*) **C.** In the late frames of the fluorescein angiogram, there is staining of the optic disk. **D.** The larger, superior patch of retinitis appears hypofluorescent centrally with a ring of late staining. (Courtesy of Paul Baker, MD.)

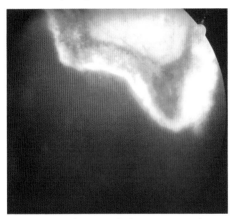

FIGURE 9-4. This person had extensive toxoplasma retinochoroiditis masquerading as ARN.

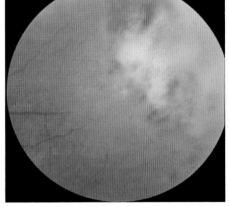

FIGURE 9-5. Pseudo-ARN syndrome with dense vitritis, retinal necrosis, and hemorrhages in a case of primary intraocular lymphoma.

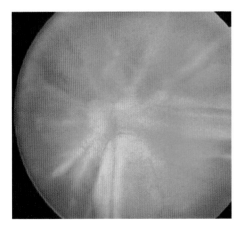

FIGURE 9-6. This patient with extensive ARN developed a retinal detachment.

PROGRESSIVE OUTER RETINAL NECROSIS

Progressive outer retinal necrosis (PORN) is the major form of necrotizing herpetic retinitis affecting immunocompromised patients. Early diagnosis and aggressive antiviral therapy is mandatory, but the visual prognosis generally remains poor.

Epidemiology and Etiology

- PORN is the most severe clinical form of herpetic retinitis. Although it appears to affect the outer retina, all retinal layers can become involved.

- VZV is the most common agent identified in patients with PORN, but a few cases of HSV-1–associated PORN have been described.

- Patients are usually deeply immunocompromised. Most of them suffer from AIDS; however, it has also been described in patients who have had bone marrow transplantation and also those treated with high-dose systemic corticosteroids.

- PORN represents an ophthalmologic and *medical emergency*, as it usually is bilateral and progresses rapidly, and CNS involvement is possible. PORN usually has a poor visual outcome.

Symptoms

- Painless decrease of visual acuity
- Abrupt loss of central vision in those cases with initial macular involvement
- Constriction of visual fields

Signs (Figs. 9-7 to 9-9)

- Multifocal, poorly demarcated, deep retinal opacities of various sizes, without granular borders, scattered throughout the posterior pole and the midperipheral retina. The retinitis spreads outwardly and peripherally, becoming confluent within a few days.

- Retinal vasculitis and optic neuritis occur in less than 20% of cases.

- The aqueous humor and the vitreous have minimal to no inflammation.

- Extremely rapid progression to total retinal necrosis over the course of a few days.

- The disease is bilateral at presentation in 70% of cases, and 80% will become bilateral within the first month.

- There is a history of recent or ongoing VZV infection in 75% of cases.

Differential Diagnosis

- CMV retinitis remains the most common opportunistic infection in AIDS, but the clinical picture and course is very different and it usually does not represent a diagnostic dilemma.

- ARN syndrome is also a diagnosis to exclude. ARN occurs in otherwise healthy patients, affects the retinal vasculature, and is associated with vitritis (**Table 9-3**).

- Toxoplasma retinochoroiditis when affecting the elderly or immunosuppressed hosts may also produce a similar clinical picture.

Diagnostic Evaluation

- The classic clinical picture should suggest the diagnosis and prompt empirical treatment should be administered before ancillary tests are performed.

- Aqueous humor PCR should be performed for viral DNA identification and antibody production in order to confirm the pathogenic agent and eliminate other nonviral etiologies.

- Brain MRI and lumbar puncture should be performed in every case of PORN, because extremely immunosuppressed patients have an increased risk of encephalitis.

Treatment (**Table 9-4**)

- Patients with PORN must be treated in an inpatient setting.

TABLE 9-3. Clinical Characteristics of ARN and PORN Syndromes

	ARN	PORN
Host immune status	Immunocompetent or immunocompromised	Immunocompromised, mainly AIDS
Etiologic agent	VZV, HSV-1, HSV-2	Mainly VZV
Retinal vasculitis	Present	Rare
Intraocular inflammation (KPs, AC cells, vitritis)	Present and very important	Rare
Bilaterality	25% at presentation	70% at presentation
Progression	Centripetally from peripheral foci of retinal necrosis to posterior pole	Centrifugally with rapid confluence
Prognosis	Poor	Extremely poor

- Combined IV and intravitreal treatment with ganciclovir and foscarnet is the strategy of choice, as IV acyclovir does not treat PORN effectively.

- IV corticosteroids must be avoided in nearly all cases.

- Acetylsalicylic acid (100 mg per day) can be used to decrease platelet hyperaggregation that occurs in herpetic retinitis.

- Prophylactic argon laser retinopexy delimiting necrotic retinal areas can be applied in an effort to reduce the high risk of RRD, although studies are inconclusive about its advantages.

- Once RRD has occurred, vitrectomy with silicone oil tamponade is the management of choice. Some authors advocate performing early vitrectomy with intravitreal acyclovir lavage and laser demarcation to prevent RRD, although this has not led to an improvement in final visual acuity.

- Patients should be tested for comorbid conditions, such as AIDS. If HIV is found, highly active antiretroviral therapy (HAART) should be promptly instituted.

Prognosis

- Despite aggressive treatment, the prognosis is extremely poor. The final visual outcome

TABLE 9-4. Medical Treatment of PORN

Active Drug	Dose and Route of Administration	Toxicity
Ganciclovir	5 mg/kg IV b.i.d. for 3 weeks, then 5 mg/kg daily IVT injections: 1–2 mg/0.05 mL	Blood cells and liver
Foscarnet	180 mg/kg/day IV divided into 2–3 infusions for 3 weeks, then 90–120 mg/kg/day IVT injections: 1.2–2.4 mg/0.05 mL	Renal failure
Valgancyclovir	900 mg/day PO, after IV induction phase, as a maintenance regimen	Blood cells and liver
Valacyclovir	1 g PO t.i.d. as maintenance treatment	Renal failure

is no light perception in almost 60% of eyes, mainly related to total retinal necrosis and RRD.

- Ischemic optic neuropathy with further optic atrophy also precludes good visual restoration.

REFERENCES

Benz MS, Glaser JS, Davis JL. Progressive outer retinal necrosis in immunocompetent patients treated initially for optic neuropathy with systemic corticosteroids. *Am J Ophthalmol.* 2003;135(4):551–553.

Chau Tran TH, et al. Successful treatment with combination of systemic antiviral drugs and intravitreal ganciclovir injections in the management of severe necrotizing herpetic retinitis. *Ocul Immunol Inflamm.* 2003;11(2):141–144.

Engstrom RE, Jr., et al. The progressive outer retinal necrosis syndrome. A variant of necrotizing herpetic retinopathy in patients with AIDS. *Ophthalmology.* 1994;101(9):1488–1502.

Forster DJ, et al. Rapidly progressive outer retinal necrosis in the acquired immunodeficiency syndrome. *Am J Ophthalmol.* 1990;110(4):341–348.

Moorthy RS, et al. Management of varicella zoster virus retinitis in AIDS. *Br J Ophthalmol.* 1997;81(3):189–194.

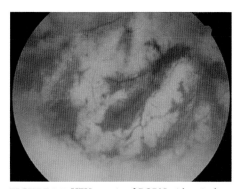

FIGURE 9-7. VZV-associated PORN with retinal necrosis and retinal hemorrhages in an AIDS patient.

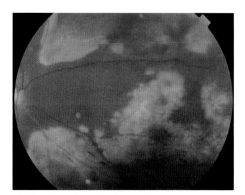

FIGURE 9-8. Multifocal areas of outer retinal necrosis in a patient with PORN.

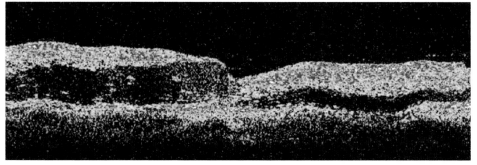

FIGURE 9-9. The OCT shows full thickness retinal involvement, most prominent in the outer retina. (Courtesy of Sunir J. Garg, MD, and Heather Shelsta, MD.)

CONGENITAL RUBELLA SYNDROME

P. Vijayalakshmi

Rubella is a mild systemic viral illness transmitted by respiratory droplets, and has an incubation period of 2 weeks. When a pregnant woman gets infected for the first time, the virus is transmitted transplacentally and it can lead to miscarriage, stillbirth, or to an infant with multiple systemic abnormalities. The range of congenital defects differs according to the gestational age of the child and the earlier in gestation that the infection occurs, the worse the damage; infection during the first 12 weeks usually results in cardiac and ocular involvement, while infection during the 12th to 28th weeks results in deafness and pulmonary artery stenosis. The consequences of rubella infection in utero are collectively termed *congenital rubella syndrome (CRS)*.

Etiology and Epidemiology

- Rubella is a single-stranded RNA virus and humans are the only host. The World Health Organization estimates that more than 100,000 children are born with CRS each year worldwide, most of them in developing countries.
- Vaccination tremendously reduces the occurrence of CRS.

Symptoms

- The symptoms depend on the organ systems involved and on the severity of damage. Parents often note leukocoria.

Signs (Figs. 9-10 to 9-16)

- Cardiac
  - Patent ductus arteriosus
  - Pulmonary artery stenosis
  - Atrial and ventricular septal defects

- Deafness
  - The most common finding is progressive sensorineural deafness, which occurs in 44% of cases.
  - Vestibular function is rarely impaired.
- Brain damage
  - Moderate to severe mental retardation
  - Spastic diplegia
  - Microcephaly
  - Schizophrenia-like clinical picture
  - Intrauterine growth retardation
  - Failure to thrive
  - Hepatosplenomegaly
  - Insulin-dependent diabetes mellitus
  - Meningoencephalitis
- Ocular signs
  - Cataract (usually bilateral, occasionally unilateral) occurs in the majority of patients.
  - Salt and pepper retinopathy: occurs in approximately 20% of patients. The appearance ranges from a fine stippling of the retinal pigment epithelium (RPE) to dark, patchy areas, and are most prominent in the posterior pole.
  - Congenital glaucoma (in 10% of cases)
  - Microphthalmos (occurs in 10% of cases)
  - Corneal edema in the absence of a raised IOP
  - Nystagmus
  - Strabismus
  - Optic atrophy
  - Dacryostenosis

Differential Diagnosis

- Other TORCH infections
  - *Toxoplasma gondii*
  - Others (syphilis, HIV, West Nile virus, varicella zoster, Epstein-Barr virus)

- **R**ubella
- **C**ytomegalovirus
- **H**erpes simplex virus

Diagnostic Evaluation

- The serum of an infant is tested for rubella-specific IgM. Older infants may need additional investigations such as IgG avidity test, RT-PCR for demonstration of virus in lens matter and other body fluids such as serum, throat secretions, and urine.

Treatment

- The treatment is directed to the affected organs and tissues. If a cataract is present, lens aspiration is performed in conjunction with primary posterior capsulorrhexis and anterior vitrectomy. Intraocular lenses (IOLs) are usually avoided in young children. A severe inflammatory response can follow cataract surgery and requires intensive therapy with topical steroids with or without systemic steroids. Glaucoma is initially managed medically followed by glaucoma surgery if needed.

Prognosis

- Poor when multiple systems are involved, and these children need a multidisciplinary team of a pediatrician, neurologist, ophthalmologist, otolaryngologist, and rehabilitation personnel.

REFERENCES

Vijayalakshmi P, Rajasundari TA, Prasad NM, et al. Prevalence of eye signs in congenital rubella syndrome in South India: a role for population screening. *Br J Ophthalmol.* 2007;91(11):1467–1470.

Vijayalakshmi P, Srivastava KK, Poornima B, et al. Visual outcome of cataract surgery in children with congenital rubella syndrome. *J AAPOS.* 2003;7(2):91–95.

Vijaylakshmi P, Muthukkaruppan VR, Rajasundari A, et al. Evaluation of a commercial rubella IgM assay for use on oral fluid samples for diagnosis and surveillance of congenital rubella syndrome and postnatal rubella. *J Clin Virol.* 2006;37(4):265–268.

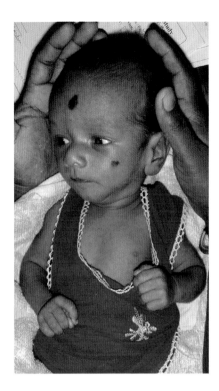

FIGURE 9-10. This child has congenital rubella syndrome. Although full term, the baby is small for his gestational age. There is leukocoria due to a cataract in the left eye.

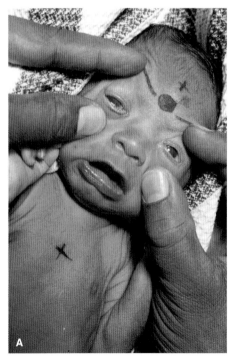

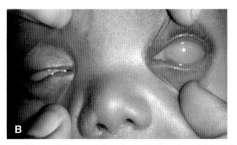

FIGURE 9-11. **A.** This child had bilateral cornea clouding and is small for gestational age. **B.** Another child with cloudy corneas.

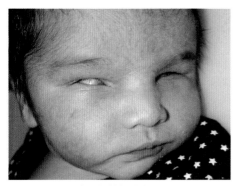

FIGURE 9-12. This child has bilateral microphthalmos.

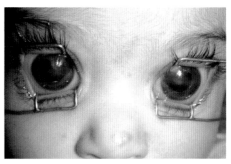

FIGURE 9-13. This child has corneal scarring and buphthalmos due to congenital glaucoma.

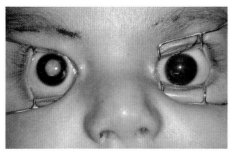

FIGURE 9-14. There is a mature cataract in the right eye and an early cataract in the left eye.

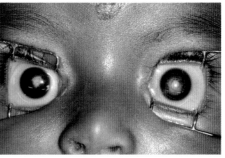

FIGURE 9-15. This child has a bilateral posterior capsular cataract.

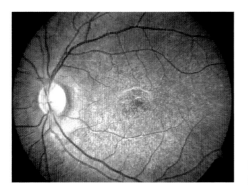

FIGURE 9-16. There is diffuse mottling of the RPE, giving a salt and pepper fundus in rubella retinopathy.

WEST NILE VIRUS

Sunir J. Garg and Moncef Khairallah

West Nile virus is a single-stranded RNA virus transmitted by mosquitoes. It causes a bilateral uveitis, with multifocal chorioretinal lesions that have a target-shaped and/or linear appearance.

Etiology and Epidemiology

- West Nile virus was first identified in Uganda, and is endemic to many parts of the world.

- Although birds are the natural host of the virus, the virus is transmitted by mosquitoes. West Nile virus is in the same virus family as yellow fever, dengue fever, and Japanese encephalitis.

- Patients older than 50 years and those with diabetes may be more susceptible to ocular manifestations.

Symptoms

- Only 20% of infected people have systemic symptoms such as fever, headache, nausea and vomiting, malaise, myalgias, joint pain, vertigo, confusion, aphasia and ataxia, lymphadenopathy, and skin rashes.

- Less than 1% of infected people develop severe CNS symptoms, including mental status changes, sensory and motor neuropathies, and encephalitis.

- Patients with ocular involvement get blurry vision, floaters, photophobia, and peripheral field loss.

Signs (Figs. 9-17 to 9-19)

- Patients have bilateral ocular involvement.

- The most characteristic finding is multiple, discrete, circular cream-colored lesions scattered throughout the mid-periphery, periphery, and posterior pole that become pigmented and "punched out" over time.

- In diabetic patients, these chorioretinal lesions are more prevalent in the posterior pole, and tend to be larger and more numerous.

- Linear clustering of chorioretinal lesions, following the course of the retinal nerve fiber layer, is a common finding.

- Retinal hemorrhages

- Bilateral vitritis

- Transient mild anterior chamber cells

- Retinal arteriolar narrowing and/or occlusion, vascular sheathing

- Optic disk edema and optic atrophy

- Patients may develop choroidal neovascular membranes late in the course of the disease

Differential Diagnosis

- Tuberculosis (TB)

- Syphilis

- Sarcoidosis

- Systemic lupus erythematosus

- Herpes virus

- Lyme disease

- Epstein-Barr virus

- Ocular histoplasmosis

- Multifocal choroiditis

- Vogt-Koyanagi-Harada disease

- Rift Valley fever

- Rubella

Diagnostic Evaluation

- Clinical exam is the most helpful.

- Fluorescein angiography (FA) can demonstrate the chorioretinal lesions. In early stages of infection, the angiogram can shows early blockage with late staining. Chronic lesions will show "target-shaped" focal areas of hypofluorescence surrounded by hyperfluorescence.

- Indocyanine green angiography (ICGA) shows more lesions in the form of hypofluorescent spots that those appreciated clinically or by fluorescein angiography.

- Visual field testing can show nonspecific field defects.

- MRI can demonstrate myelitis (a nonspecific sign).

- IgM and IgG can be elevated, both in the serum and in cerebrospinal fluid.

Treatment

- Supportive, as this is a self-limited disease

- Topical steroids can be used to treat anterior segment inflammation.

Prognosis

- Generally good, with most patients retaining good central acuity.

- Patients with more significant vascular occlusion can experience significant vision loss to the 20/400 range.

REFERENCES

Chan CK, Limstrom SA, Tarasewicz DG, et al. Ocular features of West Nile virus infection in North America: a study of 14 eyes. *Ophthalmology.* 2006;113:1539–1546.

Khairallah M, Ben Yahia S, Attia S, et al. Linear pattern of West Nile virus-associated chorioretinitis is related to retinal nerve fibres organization. *Eye (Lond).* 2007; 21(7):952–955.

Khairallah M, Ben Yahia S, Ladjimi A, et al. Chorioretinal involvement in patients in patients with West Nile virus infections. *Ophthalmology.* 2004;111(11): 2065–2070.

Khairallah M, Yahia SB, Letaief M, et al. A prospective evaluation of factors associated with chorioretinitis in patients with West Nile virus infection. *Ocul Immunol Inflamm.* 2007;15(6):435–439.

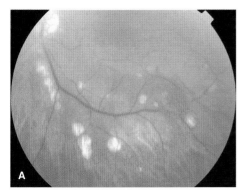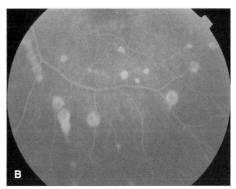

FIGURE 9-17. Fundus photograph (**A**) and fluorescein angiogram (**B**) of the left eye of a 64-year-old diabetic woman with serologically proven West Nile virus infection show numerous small and large atrophic chorioretinal lesions in the posterior pole and mid-periphery. There is also nonproliferative diabetic retinopathy.

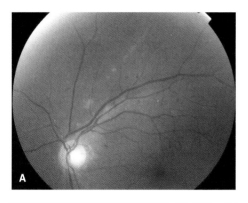

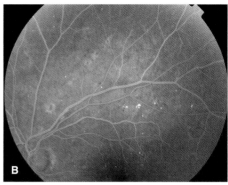

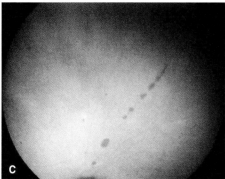

FIGURE 9-18. A. Red-free fundus photograph of the left eye of a diabetic man with serologically proven West Nile virus infection shows chorioretinal lesions extending superotemporally in a linear pattern from the optic disk. Note the presence of multifocal retinal arterial sheathing. There is also nonproliferative diabetic retinopathy. **B.** Fluorescein angiogram of the same eye shows central hypofluorescence and peripheral hyperfluorescence of the chorioretinal lesions. **C.** Late-phase ICGA of the same eye shows well-delineated hypocyanescent choroidal lesions, which are more numerous than those appreciated clinically or by FA.

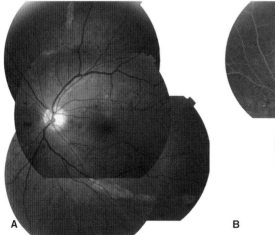

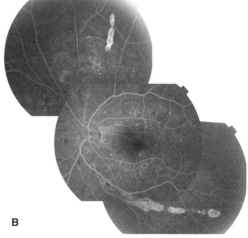

FIGURE 9-19. A. Fundus photograph of the left eye of a 58-year-old man with serologically proven West Nile virus infection shows multiple, inactive chorioretinal lesions of various sizes. Note the linear clustering of several chorioretinal lesions (curvilinear pattern in the vicinity of inferior major temporal vessels, and a radial pattern superiorly). There also are features of nonproliferate diabetic retinopathy. **B.** Fluorescein angiogram of the same eye shows more lesions than that observed clinically. Several lesions show the typical "target-like appearance" with central hypofluorescence and peripheral hyperfluorescence.

CHIKUNGUNYA

S. Lalitha Prajna and S. R. Rathinam

Chikungunya is a self-limited viral illness characterized by fever, fatigue, rash, arthralgias, and myalgias. However, more recent outbreaks have been associated with sight, as well as life-threatening complications.

Etiology and Epidemiology
- It is an arthropod-borne, single-stranded RNA alphavirus, belonging to the family Togaviridae and it is transmitted by the bite of the mosquito *Aedes aegyptei.*
- It is endemic in parts of Africa and Asia. Major epidemic outbreaks occurred in 2005.

Symptoms
- Systemic
  - Acute fever, chills, headache, fatigue, nausea, vomiting, myalgias, and a diffuse maculopapular rash.
  - Polyarticular and migratory joint pains
- Ocular
  - Photophobia, red eye, blurred vision, floaters, and retro-orbital pain
  - Loss of vision, color vision deficits, central or centrocecal scotoma, and peripheral field defects.

Signs (Figs. 9-20 to 9-22)
- Nodular episcleritis
- Mild granulomatous or nongranulomatous anterior uveitis
- Pigmented, diffuse keratic precipitates either over the central or the entire corneal endothelium, and stromal edema.
- Chikungunya retinitis. This can be differentiated from herpetic retinitis as Chikungunya retinitis has markedly less vitreous reaction and typically has posterior pole involvement, whereas herpetic retinitis in immunocompetent individuals has significant vitritis and multiple, focal lesions of retinitis in the retinal periphery.
- Optic neuritis, neuroretinitis, and retrobulbar neuritis.

Differential Diagnosis
- Toxoplasmosis
- Herpetic viral retinitis
- Syphilis
- Cat-scratch disease
- Dengue fever
- CMV retinitis

Diagnostic Evaluation
- Virus isolation and RT-PCR are useful during the initial viremic phase, whereas serologies (IgM antibody) are useful after 10 days of infection.

Treatment
- Systemic
  - Treatment is mainly supportive and includes rest, hydration, nonsteroidal anti-inflammatory agents, acetaminophen (paracetamol), and corticosteroids for refractory arthritis. Chloroquine has also been used to treat the joint pain.
- Ocular
  - Topical steroid eye drops for anterior uveitis.
  - IV/oral acyclovir and oral prednisone may be used to treat confluent retinitis. However, the efficacy of acyclovir against this virus has not yet been established.

Prognosis
- The visual prognosis is good in cases of anterior uveitis, but may be poor in cases of posterior segment involvement.

REFERENCES

Lalitha P, Rathinam S, Banushree K, et al. Ocular involvement associated with an epidemic outbreak of chikungunya virus infection. *Am J Ophthalmol.* 2007;144(4):552–556.

Mahendradas P, Ranganna SK, Shetty R, et al. Ocular manifestations associated with chikungunya. *Ophthalmology.* 2008;115(2):287–291.

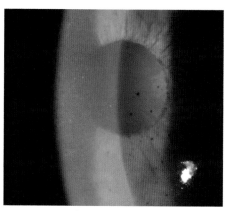

FIGURE 9-20. There are multiple, diffuse, pigmented keratic precipitates in chikungunya anterior uveitis.

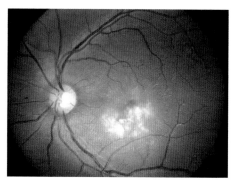

FIGURE 9-21. This patient has macular retinitis with areas of outer retinal whitening and hard exudates in the outer plexiform layer.

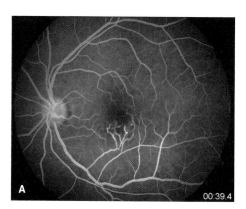

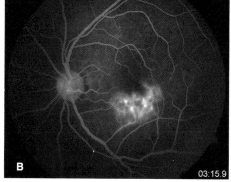

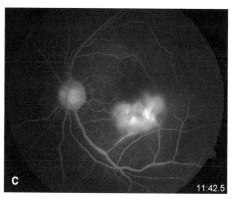

FIGURE 9-22. A. This frame of the late venous phase of the fluorescein angiogram shows irregular hypofluorescence in the inferior macula, with enlargement of foveal avascular zone. The hypofluorescence is due to reduced perfusion as a result of capillary closure and also due to blocked fluorescence secondary to the retinitis. **B.** Later frame of the angiogram demonstrates leakage from the vasculitis secondary to retinitis. **C.** Late phase shows continued leakage from an altered inner blood retinal barrier secondary to vasculitis and retinitis.

SPIROCHETES

SYPHILIS

*Julie Gueudry, Bahram Bodaghi,
and Phuc LeHoang*

Syphilis is a sexually transmitted disease. It has been called "the great masquerader" due to its ability, particularly in the tertiary stage, to mimic numerous types of uveitis. Ocular syphilis is an uncommon but diagnostically important manifestation of the disease and it can result in major complications without appropriate treatment.

Etiology and Epidemiology

- Syphilis is caused by the spirochete *Treponema pallidum*.
- It is transmitted almost exclusively by sexual contact.
- There have been recent syphilis outbreaks, especially in patients with AIDS. Patients with HIV are more likely to contract syphilis, and may have more rapid disease progression.
- Approximately 84% of cases occur in males.
- Ocular findings can occur in primary, secondary, latent, and tertiary syphilis.

Symptoms

- Pain, redness, photophobia
- Decreased vision, floaters
- Skin changes and mucous membrane lesions
- Fever, headache

Signs (Figs. 9-23 to 9-29)

- Ocular
  - Primary syphilis
    - Manifestations are limited to chancre of the eyelid and the conjunctiva.

  - Secondary syphilis (unilateral or bilateral)
    - Cutaneous rash of the eyelids and blepharitis are common, as is anterior uveitis.
    - Conjunctivitis mimicking trachoma has been reported.
    - Dacryocystitis and dacryoadenitis are less common.
    - Keratitis, episcleritis, and scleritis have been described.
    - Chorioretinitis, neuroretinitis, papillitis, exudative retinal detachment, vasculitis, and acute posterior placoid chorioretinopathy occur later during the secondary stage.

  - Tertiary syphilis (unilateral or bilateral)
    - In addition to the other signs seen in secondary disease, gummas of the eyelid, interstitial keratitis, pseudo-retinitis pigmentosa, optic atrophy, and Argyll Robertson pupil can be seen.
      - Argyll Robertson pupils are bilateral small pupils that do not constrict when exposed to light, but do constrict when the eye accommodates.

  - If the patient has HIV, the syphilis manifests itself differently. They can get yellow, placoid, subretinal lesions (acute syphilitic posterior placoid chorioretinopathy). They can also just have vitritis.

- Systemic
  - Primary syphilis occurs 2 weeks to 2 months after inoculation.
    - The chancre (a painless ulcer) begins at the inoculation site, and may have associated regional lymphadenopathy.
  - Secondary syphilis occurs 1 to 3 months after untreated primary syphilis.
    - A maculopapular or pustular cutaneous rash, often on the trunk, palms, and soles, commonly occurs.

▸ Mucous membrane lesions and generalized lymphadenopathy are also fairly common.

  ▸ Acute syphilitic meningitis is a less common finding.

▪ Latent syphilis

  ▸ No clinical manifestations

▪ Tertiary syphilis occurs months to years after untreated secondary syphilis.

  ▸ Benign tertiary syphilis with gummas of the skin and bone can occur.

  ▸ Cardiovascular involvement (aortitis, aortic valve insufficiency, and cardiovascular aneurysms) cause significant morbidity and mortality.

  ▸ Neurosyphilis occurs in 5% to 10% of patients, and includes meningitis, headaches, sensorimotor loss, cranial nerve palsies, and seizures.

● Congenital syphilis is rare and results from transplacental transmission. Only 60% of infected fetuses become newborns.

  ▪ Systemic manifestations include rhinitis within the first few months of birth, and a maculopapular rash. Late findings include notched incisors (Hutchinson's teeth), saddle-nose deformity, and sensorineural hearing loss.

  ▪ It can present with various ocular findings, including:

    ▸ Bilateral interstitial keratitis

    ▸ Acute or chronic uveitis

    ▸ Secondary cataract

    ▸ Salt and pepper chorioretinitis

Differential Diagnosis

● As syphilis can look like all forms of ocular inflammation, it should be considered in all kinds of uveitis.

Diagnostic Evaluation

● Laboratory tests should include both non-treponemal and treponemal tests.

  ▪ The nontreponemal tests, Venereal Disease Research Laboratory (VDRL) and rapid plasmin reagin (RPR) are non-specific for *Treponema pallidum,* so false-positive are possible. These tests are also used to assess treatment response.

  ▪ The main treponemal test is fluorescent *Treponema* antibody–absorption (FTA-Abs). It is specific for *Treponema pallidum,* so false-positive results are less common, but may still occur during pregnancy and in patients with autoimmune disorders. Once infected, patients will be positive for life.

  ▪ HIV serology should be obtained as coinfection is possible.

  ▪ Dark field microscopy, electron microscopy, and immunofluorescence can also be used.

● Lumbar puncture should be considered to exclude asymptomatic neurosyphilis.

  ▪ Patients with ocular syphilis should have CSF evaluation for VDRL titers, total protein, and cell counts.

Treatment

● Uveitis should be considered to be a manifestation of neurosyphilis and treated accordingly, even though this point remains controversial.

● The recommended treatment for neurosyphilis is penicillin G sodium (18 to 24 million units IV daily) or penicillin G procaine (2.4 million units IM daily) plus probenecid PO for 10 to 14 days.

● Ceftriaxone (2 g/day IV or IM for 10 to 14 days) may be considered in penicillin-allergic patients. However, cross-sensitivity exists and this agent has not been tested for the management of neurosyphilis. Some authors recommend penicillin desensitization for these patients prior to starting the cephalosporin.

● Cycloplegics and topical corticosteroids may be useful if anterior segment inflammation is present, but they should be considered solely an adjunct to antibiotic therapy.

● Patients should be monitored for a Jarisch-Herxheimer reaction, which occurs most often in secondary syphilis treated with penicillin (prophylaxis with corticosteroids may help in some cases).

● Patients should also be evaluated and treated for other sexually transmitted diseases, including HIV, gonorrhea, and chlamydia. In the United States, patients with sexually transmitted diseases should be reported to the local Board of Health.

Prognosis

● If patients receive prompt therapy, the prognosis is usually good with full visual recovery.

● Retinitis may resolve without scarring within a few days after initiation of specific antibiotics.

● If untreated, chronic progressive intraocular inflammation and complications may occur.

REFERENCES

Aldave AJ, King JA, Cunningham ET Jr. Ocular syphilis. *Curr Opin Ophthalmol.* 2001;12(6):433–441.

Chao JR, Khurana RN, Fawzi AA, et al. Syphilis: reemergence of an old adversary. *Ophthalmology.* 2006;113(11): 2074–2079.

Tran TH, Cassoux N, Bodaghi B, et al. Syphilitic uveitis in patients infected with human immunodeficiency virus. *Graefes Arch Clin Exp Ophthalmol.* 2005;243(9): 863–869.

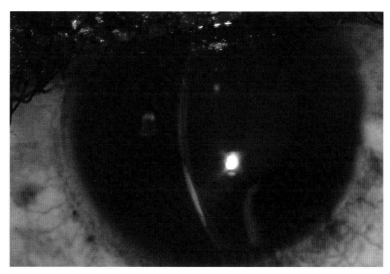

FIGURE 9-23. Slit-lamp photograph showing interstitial keratitis associated with congenital syphilis.

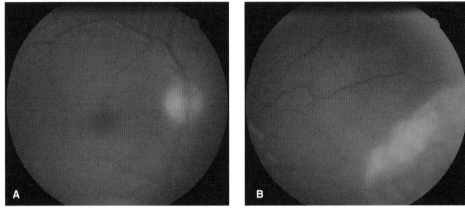

FIGURE 9-24. Fundus photographs of a patient with uveitis associated with syphilis. **A.** There is vitritis that is obscuring the posterior pole. **B.** A peripheral retinal infiltrate is present nasally.

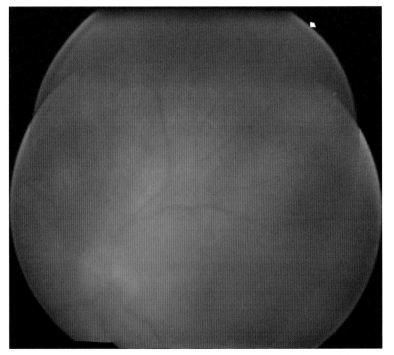

FIGURE 9-25. Fundus photograph of a patient with resolved uveitis due to syphilis reveals salt and pepper chorioretinitis.

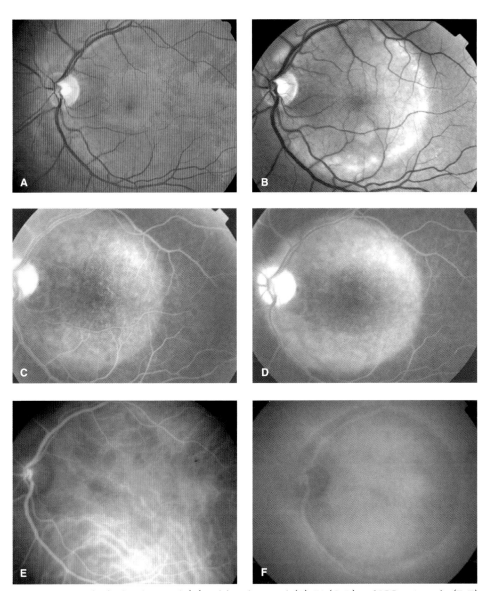

FIGURE 9-26. Color fundus photograph (**A**), red-free photograph (**B**), FA (**C, D**), and ICG angiography (**E, F**) of an acute syphilitic posterior placoid chorioretinitis, often seen in patients with HIV.

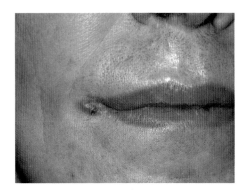

FIGURE 9-27. Perlèche (angular stomatitis) in a patient with syphilitic uveitis.

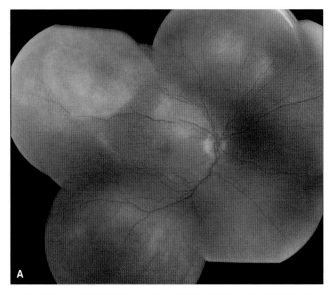

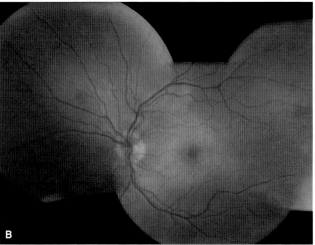

FIGURE 9-28. This 44-year-old man presented with bilateral decreased vision. He had a recent skin rash that was diagnosed as mononucleosis. His vision was 20/80 OD and 20/800 OS. **A.** Color fundus photo of the right eye shows large, patchy, multifocal yellow areas in the outer retina/choroid. **B.** The left eye has a similar, placoid lesion involving the macula.

(continued)

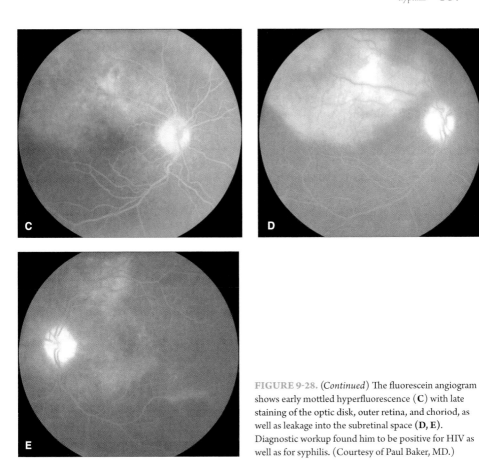

FIGURE 9-28. (*Continued*) The fluorescein angiogram shows early mottled hyperfluorescence (**C**) with late staining of the optic disk, outer retina, and choriod, as well as leakage into the subretinal space (**D, E**). Diagnostic workup found him to be positive for HIV as well as for syphilis. (Courtesy of Paul Baker, MD.)

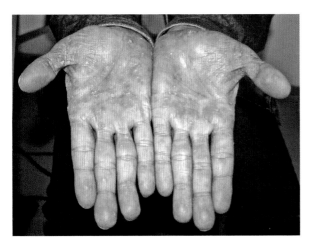

FIGURE 9-29. This patient with secondary syphilis has multiple, raised, erythematous lesions on the palms of the hands.

LYME DISEASE

Sunir J. Garg ▪

Lyme disease is a multisystem disease that can cause eye, skin, joint, heart, and neurologic problems.

Etiology and Epidemiology

● It is caused by a spirochete, *Borrelia burgdorferi,* which is transmitted by the *Ixodes* deer tick.

● In the United States, tick-endemic areas are along the Northeast Coast, the upper Midwest, and in northern California and Oregon.

● Lyme disease has also been reported in Europe, Australia, China, and Japan.

● Infected people will often have a history of camping or hiking.

Symptoms

● These patients can develop essentially all types of ocular inflammation, ranging from a mild conjunctivitis in the early stages, to retinal vasculitis and optic neuropathy. They can also develop cranial neuropathies.

● Early in the disease course, patients get flu-like symptoms, but they can develop significant arthritis, cardiac problems, headaches, and changes in mental status.

● Approximately 50% of patients will recall being bitten by a tick.

Signs (Figs. 9-30 to 9-33)

● Lyme disease is divided into three stages:

▪ Stage 1: Patients have flu-like symptoms, including fevers, myalgias, and arthralgias, often with regional lymphadenopathy. Three-fourths of patients will have erythema chronicum migrans. It starts as a red papule that enlarges to form a ring or target-shaped rash. If untreated, these lesions often grow to several centimeters to nearly a meter in size, and then fade over the course of 3 to 4 weeks. Although it occurs in up to two-thirds of patients, many people may not recall having this sign. Early eye findings include conjunctivitis and episcleritis. In Europe, patients are infected with *Borrelia afzelii,* which can cause a lymphocytoma (of the earlobe or areola) and acrodermatitis chronica atrophicans (a violaceous area of atrophy followed by fibrosis on the dorsal aspect of the hands and feet).

▪ Stage 2: This stage occurs 2 to 3 weeks to several years after infection. Patients may develop cardiac conduction defects (heart block), followed later by severe arthritis. Neurologically, they can get severe headaches, meningitis, and peripheral and cranial neuropathies, including a seventh nerve palsy. The ocular signs include conjunctivitis, keratitis, iridocyclitis, intermediate uveitis, vitritis, choroiditis, vasculitis, serous retinal detachments, and optic neuritis. They may also have diplopia from a third, fourth, fifth, or sixth nerve palsy, and may develop orbital myositis.

▪ Stage 3: These patients have prolonged arthritis and encephalitis. As a result, they can have chronic fatigue and can develop ataxia and dementia. Although they can develop any of the eye findings listed above, bilateral keratitis is the most common manifestation.

Differential Diagnosis

● Syphilis: If one cannot remember what Lyme does, it is a spirochete like syphilis, and has similar manifestations.

● Sarcoidosis

● TB

● Intermediate uveitis

● Vogt-Koyanagi-Harada syndrome

Diagnostic Evaluation

- Lab tests for Lyme disease are good, but they are most helpful when combined with a high clinical suspicion.

    - Antibodies to Lyme disease are present for several weeks after infection. ELISA testing (followed by a Western blot) is useful. False negatives are common, both in the early stage of the disease and after treatment with antibiotics. False positives also occur, especially if the patient has had syphilis. (Because Lyme disease and syphilis are both spirochetes, there is some cross-reactivity with the tests, so one should order both syphilis and Lyme titers).

    - In Lyme endemic areas, 10% to 15% of patients may be antibody positive. If so, positive serology along with erythema chronicum migrans or one of the classic manifestations of Lyme disease makes the diagnosis. If not an endemic area, the patient should have two or more of the classic symptoms before the diagnosis is made.

    - Cerebrospinal fluid may show pleocytosis, but it is frequently unremarkable.

Treatment

- Antibiotics: For very early stage disease, treatment with oral amoxicillin, doxycycline, or erythromycin may be considered. For later stages, consider IV penicillin or ceftriaxone, and patients may need long-term treatment. If the patient has a penicillin allergy, use doxycycline.

Prognosis

- Approximately one-fourth to one-third of patients with untreated erythema chronicum migrans will develop stage 2 disease. Less than 10% of these patients will develop chronic arthritis or neurologic disease. Once severe arthritis or neurologic symptoms occur, the symptoms persist despite antibiotic therapy.

REFERENCES

Mikkilä HO, Seppälä IJ, Viljanen MK, et al. The expanding clinical spectrum of ocular lyme borreliosis. *Ophthalmology.* 2000;107(3):581–587.

Stanek G, Strle F. Lyme borreliosis. *Lancet.* 2003;362: 1639–1647.

Stanek G, Strle F. Lyme borreliosis: a European perspective on diagnosis and clinical management. *Curr Opin Infect Dis.* 2009;22(5):450–454.

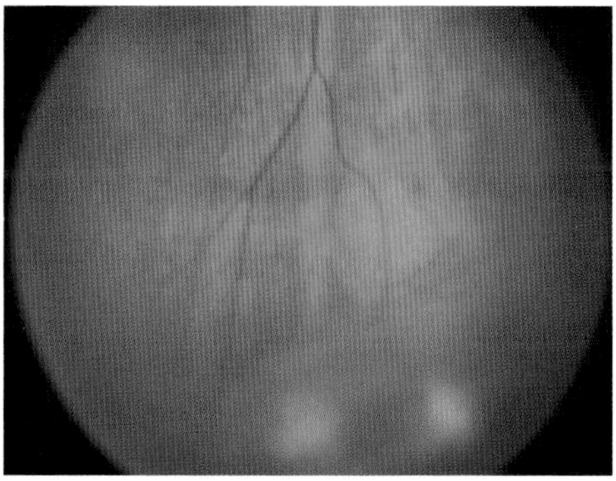

FIGURE 9-30. This patient had intermediate uveitis due to Lyme disease. There are snowballs present inferiorly.

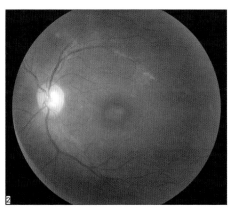

FIGURE 9-31. There is old vasculitis along the retinal venules in a patient with secondary Lyme disease.

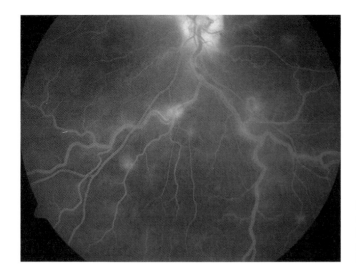

FIGURE 9-32. FA can demonstrate late staining of the retinal vessels and optic disk when retinal involvement is present.

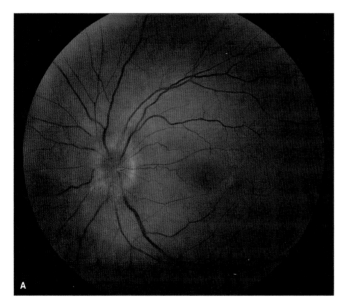

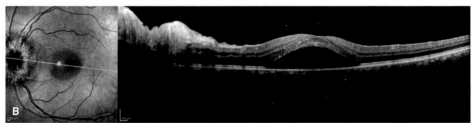

FIGURE 9-33. A. A 55-year-old man presented with sudden onset of decreased vision in the left eye. Optic disk edema was present. **B.** OCT confirmed peripapillary edema and also revealed subretinal fluid. (Courtesy Robert Sergott, MD, and Brandon Johnson, MD.)

LEPTOSPIROSIS

S. R. Rathinam

Leptospirosis is a re-emerging zoonotic disease. An anicteric fever occurs in the majority of cases, often with severe headache, nausea, vomiting, and severe muscle pain. Others develop an icteric, septicemic form called Weil's syndrome. Uveitis can occur 3 to 6 months after onset of systemic illness. The nonspecific and variable clinical presentation makes the diagnosis of both systemic and ocular leptospirosis difficult.

Etiology and Epidemiology

• Leptospirosis is a water-borne systemic illness caused by a spirochete. Infected animals pass the organism in their urine, and people in contact with animals, such as cattle farmers, butchers, and veterinarians are at higher risk. The leptospires enter human through intact mucosa or abraded skin.

• It occurs worldwide, and is endemic in tropical countries, especially those with heavy rainfall. People in these areas can contract the illness indirectly through contaminated soil and water, and outbreaks can occur after floods. It also occurs in overcrowded, poor areas where it likely transmitted by rodents.

Symptoms

• Pain, redness, photophobia, and decreased vision in one or both eyes.

Signs (Figs. 9-34 to 9-37)

• Infection with leptospirosis is usually divided into two phases. The initial, systemic phase is called the septicemic phase, and several months later, the immune phase occurs.

▪ Septicemic phase

▸ Conjunctival chemosis/congestion, subconjunctival hemorrhage

▸ Scleral icterus (jaundiced appearance) is diagnostic of Weil's disease.

▪ Immune phase

▸ Uveitis typically occurs 6 months after systemic onset, although it may occur soon after onset of systemic illness. The uveitis is usually either nongranulomatous, acute and mild, or posterior and severe.

▸ Acute anterior/panuveitis

▸ Hypopyon occurs in 12% of cases

▸ Cataract

▸ Membranous vitreous opacities, vitreous cells, snowballs as a "string of pearls"

▸ Disk hyperemia

▸ Retinal vasculitis occurs in 50% of eyes.

Differential Diagnosis

• HLA-B27–associated anterior uveitis

• Behçet's disease

• Sarcoidosis

• Toxoplasmosis

• Endogenous endophthalmitis

• Acute retinal necrosis

• Febrile illnesses: These range from milder forms of diseases such as influenza and malaria, to severe illnesses such as dengue and yellow fever, and septicemia.

Diagnostic Evaluation

• Microscopic agglutination test (MAT) is the gold standard. Seroconversion or a titer above 1:400 dilution is diagnostic for systemic leptospirosis. In chronic leptospirosis, a titer of 1:100 dilution is considered positive.

• Other tests available include dark field microscopy, ELISA, macroscopic agglutination, LEPTO dipstick, and lateral flow assays.

Treatment

- Leptospires are sensitive in vitro to most antimicrobial agents, including penicillin, amoxicillin, doxycycline, and ceftriaxone.

- Severe systemic leptospirosis is treated with IV penicillin G, 1.5 million units q6h for 1 week.

- For mild to moderate cases, doxycycline 100 mg b.i.d. for 1 week is effective. Topical/periocular/systemic steroids are added depending upon the disease severity. Cycloplegics are beneficial for severe anterior uveitis.

Prognosis

- As most people have mild disease, leptospiral uveitis generally carries a good prognosis.

REFERENCES

Priya CG, Rathinam SR, Muthukkaruppan V. Evidence for endotoxin as a causative factor for leptospiral uveitis in humans. *Invest Ophthalmol Vis Sci.* 2008;49(12): 5419–5424.

Shukla D, Rathinam SR, Cunningham ET Jr. Leptospiral uveitis in the developing world. *Int Ophthalmol Clin.* 2010;50(2):113–124.

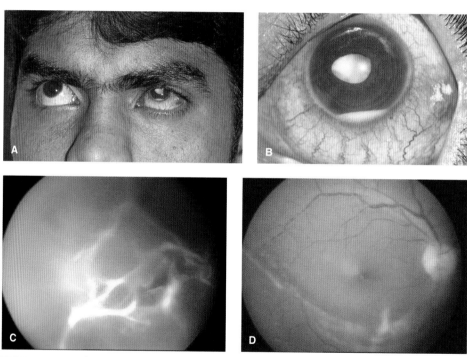

FIGURE 9-34. A. There is a unilateral hypopyon and cataract in a young male patient with leptospiral uveitis. **B.** There is diffuse conjunctival injection with ciliary flush, a hypopyon and a pearly white cataract in the left eye. **C.** There is 3+ vitreous haze with free-floating veil-like vitreous membranes, which are characteristic of leptospiral uveitis. There is disk hyperemia present as well. **D.** The right eye of the same patient has mild vitritis with a vitreous veil present inferiorly, disk hyperemia, and retinal vasculitis involving the superotemporal retinal vein.

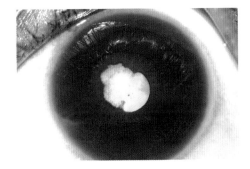

FIGURE 9-35. This patient has posterior synechiae and a partially absorbed cataract.

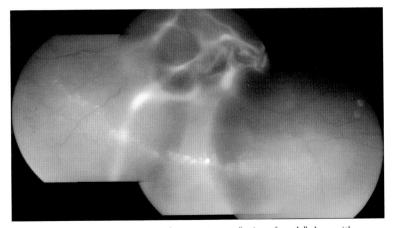

FIGURE 9-36. Fundus examination showing vitreous "string of pearls" along with significant vitritis.

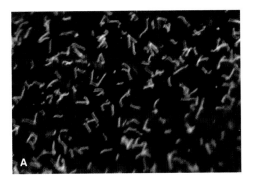
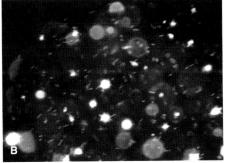

FIGURE 9-37. **A.** The bright spots are free moving leptospires in liquid medium seen under dark field microscopy. **B.** Microagglutination test. If one adds the serum of a patient with presumed leptospirosis to the MAT culture, and the person was indeed infected with *Leptospira*, one finds agglutinated leptospires in liquid medium under dark field microscopy. This is an example of a positive test.

MYCOBACTERIA

INTRAOCULAR TUBERCULOSIS

Vishali Gupta and Amod Gupta

Intraocular TB occurs secondary to hematogenous spread of *Mycobacterium tuberculosis* from the primary source (usually the lung) or from secondary lesions.

Epidemiology and Etiology

- Prevalence rates of TB as a cause of uveitis are highly variable, ranging from 0.5% in the United States to 9.6% in India. It is most prevalent in South and Southeast Asia, Russia, Peru, and central and southern Africa.

- Intraocular TB results when macrophages containing bacilli escape from the pulmonary granuloma(s) via the lymphatic and blood circulatory systems and reach the eye where they remain dormant.

- Reactivation of these dormant bacilli at some stage of life may produce active tubercular uveitis.

- Some of the ocular manifestations are likely due to an immune-mediated hypersensitivity response.

- Most patients with active ocular TB do not have a history of systemic or pulmonary TB.

Signs and Symptoms (Figs. 9-38 to 9-43)

- Granulomatous anterior uveitis, including mutton-fat keratic precipitates, iris nodules, and broad posterior synechiae

- Intermediate uveitis

- Posterior uveitis (the most common manifestation of TB uveitis)

  ▪ Choroidal tubercles are the most common manifestation and are the result of hematogenous seeding.

  ▪ Subretinal abscess or granulomas

▪ Serpiginous-like choroiditis: may present as: multifocal discrete lesions that become confluent and show wave-like progression; or diffuse, larger, yellowish white, plaque-like lesions.

▪ Retinal vasculitis, which is an obliterative vasculitis and can result in retinal neovascularization.

▪ Exudative retinal detachment

- Cystoid macular edema

- Neuroretinitis

- Atypical presentations: pigmented hypopyon, endophthalmitis.

Differential Diagnosis

- Sarcoidosis

- Syphilis

- Intraocular tumors (subretinal abscesses mimic tumors)

- Eales' disease

- Serpiginous choroiditis (Unlike TB, these patients tend to have: little to no vitritis, bilateral involvement, and a larger, more confluent lesion, which extends mainly from the disk and usually is confined to the posterior pole.)

Diagnostic Evaluation

- Tuberculin skin test/Mantoux skin test (PPD)

  ▪ Induration of less than 5 mm is a negative result.

  ▪ Induration of 5 to 10 mm is considered positive in patients with nodules on chest radiography, those with exposure to people with active TB, and in immunosuppressed patients, including HIV.

  ▪ Induration of 11 to 15 mm is considered positive in health care workers and people living in endemic areas.

  ▪ Greater than 15 mm of induration is considered positive in all people.

- Interferon-gamma assay tests including quantiferon-TB gold test (QFT-G) and T-SPOT TB test

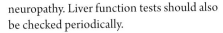

Both are more specific than the PPD test, as there are less false-positive results due to prior BCG vaccine.

In active TB, the T-SPOT test is more sensitive than the PPD test.

- Chest x-ray and chest CT scan. Chest CT may be more sensitive than chest x-ray.

- Histopathologic examination and culture from intraocular fluid

- PCR

- FA is useful to assess the amount of vasculitis, breakdown of the blood-retinal barrier, cystoid macular edema, disturbances of the retinal pigment epithelium, and to assess areas of retinal nonperfusion and neovascularization.

- ICGA helps to identify areas of choroidopathy, including active and atrophic lesions.

Treatment

- The treatment consists of a four-drug regimen, which includes isoniazid 5 mg/kg/day, rifampicin 10 mg/kg/day, ethambutol 15 mg/kg/day, and pyrazinamide 20 to 25 mg/kg/day. Ethambutol and pyrazinamide are stopped after 2 months and the rest of the drugs are continued for 4 to 16 months.

- It is important to give pyridoxine (vitamin B6) 10 mg along with the above agents, as it can prevent isoniazid-related peripheral neuropathy. Liver function tests should also be checked periodically.

- Patients also need concomitant corticosteroids to minimize the damage resulting from delayed-hypersensitivity response.

- Initiation of anti-TB treatment without concomitant corticosteroids may cause paradoxical worsening.

- Pan-retinal laser photocoagulation should be performed in cases of significant nonperfusion, or if neovascularization is present.

- Ethambutol can cause optic neuropathy.

Prognosis

- The prognosis is good if the disease is diagnosed in a timely fashion and if TB-specific therapy is initiated.

REFERENCES

Bansal R, Gupta A, Gupta V, et al. Role of anti-tubercular therapy in uveitis with latent/manifest tuberculosis. *Am J Ophthalmol.* 2008;146(5):772–779.

Gupta A, Bansal R, Gupta V, et al. Ocular signs predictive of tubercular uveitis. *Am J Ophthalmol.* 2010;149(4): 562–570.

Vasconcelos-Santos DV, Rao PK, Davies JB, et al. Clinical features of tuberculous serpiginouslike choroiditis in contrast to classic serpiginous choroiditis. *Arch Ophthalmol.* 2010;128(7):853–858.

Vasconcelos-Santos DV, Zierhut M, Rao NA. Strengths and weaknesses of diagnostic tools for tuberculous uveitis. *Ocul Immunol Inflamm.* 2009;17(5):351–355.

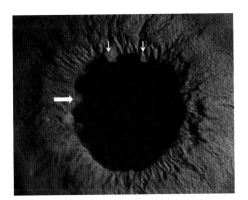

FIGURE 9-38. This patient had presumed tubercular granulomatous anterior uveitis with Koeppe nodules (thin arrows) and posterior synechiae (solid arrow).

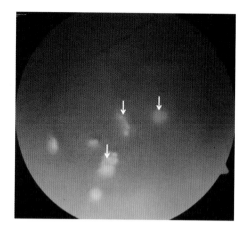

FIGURE 9-39. Fundus photograph of a patient with vitritis shows multiple snowballs inferiorly (arrows).

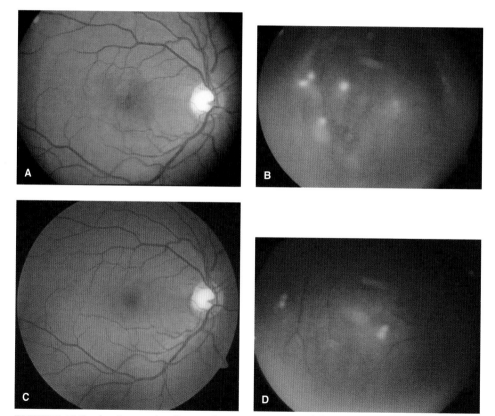

FIGURE 9-40. Fundus photographs of intermediate uveitis with CME (**A**) and vitritis with snowballs (**B**). The patient's Mantoux skin test showed induration greater than 10 mm, and the chest radiograph showed hilar lymphadenopathy. Fundus photographs taken 3 months after treatment show resolution of both the CME (**C**) as well as the snowballs (**D**). The visual acuity improved from 20/80 to 20/30.

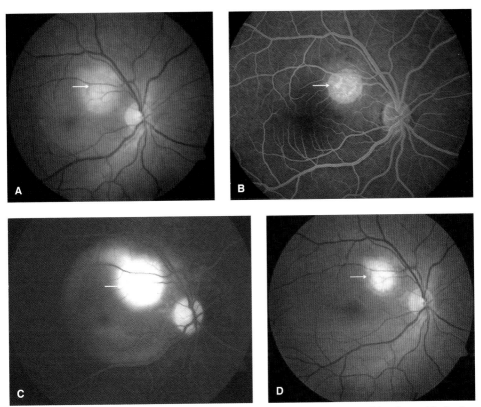

FIGURE 9-41. A. There is a choroidal tubercle (arrow) with an adjoining exudative retinal detachment. The fundus fluorescein angiograms show a well-demarcated choroidal tubercle early (**B**) and increasing hyperfluorescence with pooling of dye in the area of exudative detachment in the late phase (**C**). **D.** A few months after treatment, the tubercle has healed (arrow) with resolution of subretinal fluid. The patient's visual acuity improved to 20/20.

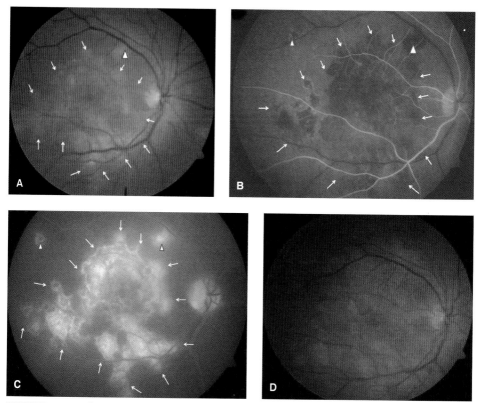

FIGURE 9-42. A. There is a diffuse, large patch of choroiditis involving the posterior pole (arrows). Additionally, this patient also has a few isolated patches of active choroiditis (arrowhead). This has an appearance similar to serpiginous chorioretinopathy. Fundus fluorescein angiograms show initial hypofluorescence (arrows; **B**) with late hyperfluorescence and diffusion of dye into adjacent retina (arrows; **C**). **D.** The active choroiditis resolved 3 months after starting anti-TB treatment.

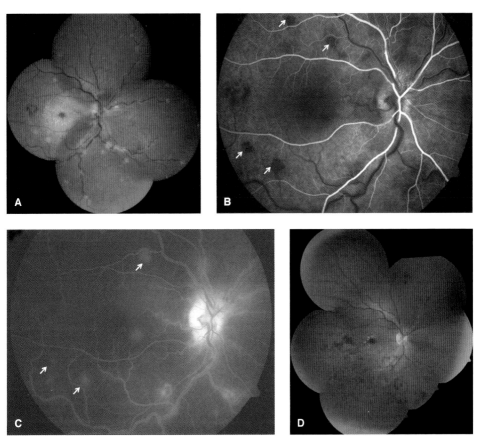

FIGURE 9-43. A. There is patchy retinal vasculitis choroiditis and optic disk edema along with hard exudates in the outer plexiform layer (neuroretinitis). **B.** The fluorescein angiogram of the right eye shows early hypofluorescence of the choroidal lesions (arrows). **C.** Later in the angiogram, the areas of choroiditis appear hyperfluorescent (arrows). Note the disk hyperfluorescence and patchy areas of leakage from the retinal vessels. **D.** The fundus photograph of the right eye 4 months after treatment shows resolution of disk edema, choroiditis patches, and vasculitis with partial resolution of the macular star. Retinal hemorrhages are still present.

HANSEN'S UVEITIS (LEPROSY)

S. R. Rathinam

Leprosy, also known as Hansen's disease, is a chronic communicable disease commonly seen in the tropics and subtropics. Leprosy is a systemic disease that has one of the highest rates of ocular complications.

Etiology and Epidemiology

- The causative agent is *Mycobacterium leprae,* an obligate intracellular acid-fast bacillus.

- It spreads via the nasal secretions of an infected person to another individual's oral or nasal mucosa through respiratory droplets. It is not usually spread through direct skin contact. It has a bimodal distribution, and affects children under 15 and adults over 30 years old.

- Most patients with leprosy live in countries where the disease is endemic, including Brazil, Nigeria, Madagascar, India, Myanmar, and Indonesia. Approximately 500,000 new cases occur annually. Ten to 12 million people are affected worldwide, with 3% to 7% having vision loss. Leprosy damages the Schwann cells of the peripheral nerves, which results in damage to the limbs, skin, nerves, and eyes.

Symptoms

- Pain, redness, defective vision
- Loss of sensation on the skin that can result in anesthesia.

Signs (Figs. 9-44 to 9-51)

- The spectrum of disease is decided by the host's immune response. Clinically, leprosy is classified in two forms. The tuberculoid (paucibacillary) form is milder, can cause wasting of the small muscles of the hands, has few skin lesions, and only causes ocular surface problems due to fifth and seventh nerve damage (which can result in corneal scarring from corneal anesthesia, trichiasis, trauma, etc.). The lepromatous (multibacillary) form is more contagious and severe. These patients have colored or hypopigmented papules and nodules, loss of temperature, touch, pain, and ultimately deep pressure sensations, neuropathic pain and anesthesia, and can have extensive ocular inflammation with:

  - Cataracts (the leading cause of blindness due to age, steroids, and inflammation)
  - Erythematous, tender nodules on face (lepromas)
  - Episcleritis, scleritis
  - Bilateral granulomatous uveitis
  - Iris pearls, iris atrophy
  - Loss of eyelashes and eyebrows (madarosis)

Differential Diagnosis

- TB
- Sarcoidosis

Diagnostic Evaluation

- Slit-skin smear test: Rod-shaped bacteria can be seen in a smear taken from the affected skin.

- Histologic study of full-thickness skin biopsy for host response (in hematoxylin and eosin stain) and for demonstration of acid-fast bacilli (in Fite-Faraco modification of the carbol fuchsin stain) is the gold standard test.

- No serologic tests are available, and it cannot be grown in culture. PCR may be useful.

Treatment

- Paucibacillary leprosy: Supervised monthly single dose of 600 mg of rifampicin and a daily unsupervised dose of 100 mg of dapsone for a total of 6 months.

- Multibacillary leprosy: Supervised monthly single dose of 600 mg of rifampicin with 300 mg of clofazimine in addition to an unsupervised daily dose of 100 mg dapsone with 50 mg clofazimine for 12 months. This is multidrug therapy that is safe and currently is provided free by World Health Organization.

- Depending upon the severity of inflammation, topical and systemic steroids are needed for ocular inflammation. Cataract surgery and treatment of lagophthalmos and refractive error are useful as needed.

Prognosis

- Early systemic treatment and adequate inflammatory control with steroids give a better prognosis.

REFERENCES

Chaudhry IA, Shamsi FA, Elzaridi E, et al. Initial diagnosis of leprosy in patients treated by an ophthalmologist and confirmation by conventional analysis and polymerase chain reaction. *Ophthalmology.* 2007;114(10): 1904–1911.

Hogewegand M, Keunen JEE. Prevention of blindness in leprosy and the role of the Vision 2020 Programme. *Eye.* 2005;19:1099–1105.

Rathinam SR. Leprosy uveitis in the developing world. *Int Ophthalmol Clin.* 2010;50(2):99–111.

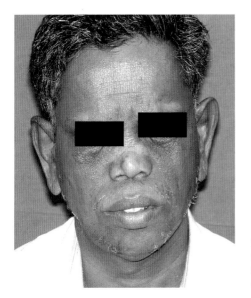

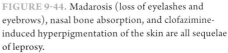

FIGURE 9-44. Madarosis (loss of eyelashes and eyebrows), nasal bone absorption, and clofazimine-induced hyperpigmentation of the skin are all sequelae of leprosy.

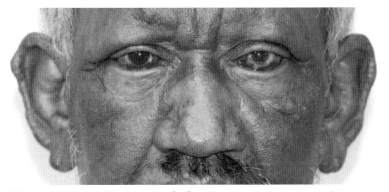

FIGURE 9-45. Deformity of the pinna (ear), madarosis, and scleritis occur in lepromatous leprosy.

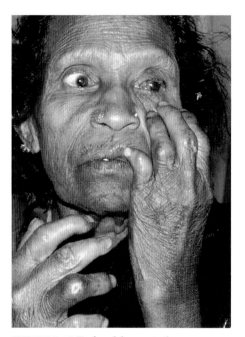

FIGURE 9-46. Profound damage to the nervous system can cause trophic ulcers and finger deformation.

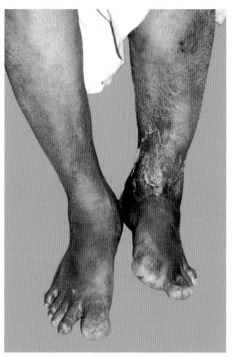

FIGURE 9-47. Extreme degree of tissue loss in lepromatous leprosy.

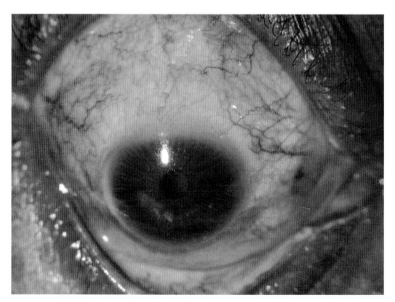

FIGURE 9-48. Diffuse scleritis can occur in leprosy.

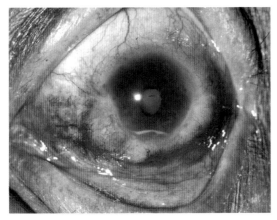

FIGURE 9-49. This patient developed conjunctival lepromas on the nasal aspects of the cornea.

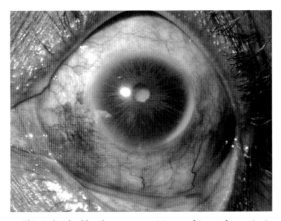

FIGURE 9-50. This individual has lepromatous iris atrophic patches, miosis, and scleritis.

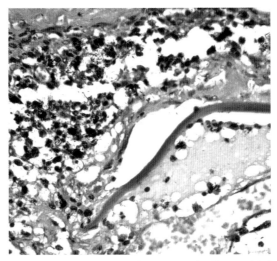

FIGURE 9-51. Biopsy of a conjunctival leproma showing Lepra bacilli in modified carbol fuchsin stain.

PARASITES, BACTERIA, FUNGI, AND NEMATODES

OCULAR TOXOPLASMOSIS

Chloe Gottlieb, Robert Nussenblatt,
and H. Nida Sen

Ocular toxoplasmosis, caused by the parasite *Toxoplasma gondii*, is the most common cause of posterior uveitis. Cats are the definitive host for the parasite; humans (intermediate host) acquire the infection via consumption of undercooked meat or unwashed vegetables, drinking oocyst-contaminated water, or through congenital transmission.

Etiology and Epidemiology

- It is the most common infectious chorioretinitis in the United States.

- Approximately 22% of the U.S. population is believed to be infected with *T. gondii*.

  - Prevalence in other parts of the world is significantly higher (i.e., Brazil).

  - Ocular toxoplasmosis may occur in 2% of those infected with *T. gondii*. The ocular disease can occur after either congenital or acquired disease.

  - Approximately 2000 to 7500 symptomatic ocular infections occur annually in the United States.

  - The risk of recurrent ocular disease is greatest in the first year following an episode of toxoplasmic retinochoroiditis.

Symptoms

- Blurred vision, floaters

- Scotomas

- Pain

This contribution to the work was done as part of the authors' official duties as NIH employees and is a work of the United States Government.

- Photophobia

- Patients may be asymptomatic (peripheral chorioretinal scars may be identified incidentally during a dilated exam).

Signs (**Figs. 9-52 to 9-55**)

- An active area of chorioretinitis at the border of a pigmented chorioretinal scar (this is the hallmark of ocular toxoplasmosis)

- Decreased visual acuity, visual field defects

- Normal or elevated intraocular pressure

- A white or cream-colored chorioretinal lesion

- Granulomatous panuveitis with a prominent vitritis; the classic description is a "headlight in the fog"

- Keratic precipitates, either granulomatous or stellate

- Retinal vasculitis (arteriolitis adjacent to the chorioretinitis)

- Branch retinal vein or artery occlusion

- Papillitis with or without an afferent pupillary defect

- Atypical and more severe presentations may occur in patients with HIV and other patients who are immunosuppressed. A brain abscess needs to be ruled out in immunocompromised patients with toxoplasmosis.

Diagnostic Evaluation

- Serologic testing for *T. gondii* is very helpful in classifying patients.

- Toxoplasmic chorioretinitis is a clinical diagnosis that is supported by a positive *Toxoplasma* serology.

  - A positive IgG, however, is not specific to the ocular disease. It only indicates prior infection, either ocular or systemic.

  - Elevated IgM confirms that the infection has been recently acquired.

  - In cases where multiple etiologies are being considered, a negative serology for

T. gondii is helpful to rule out toxoplasmosis as a cause.

▪ The presence of elevated *Toxoplasma*-specific intraocular antibody can be sought by testing the aqueous or vitreous (Goldmann-Witmer coefficient).

▪ PCR can be performed on a very small amount of aqueous or vitreous with high specificity.

▪ Western blot and immunoblotting of ocular fluids can also be performed in order to establish the diagnosis.

Treatment

● The chorioretinitis is usually self-limited; however, therapy should be considered under certain circumstances:

▪ A significant decrease in vision to below 20/40 or a two-line decrease in vision from baseline

▪ A lesion within the temporal arcade or in close proximity to the fovea, optic nerve, or a large retinal vessel

▪ Complications such as significant retinal or vitreous hemorrhage or retinal vascular occlusion

▪ Frequently recurring disease with a risk of vision loss

▪ Children when needed to prevent amblyopia

▪ Immunocompromised patients

▪ Patients who are functionally monocular

● There are a number of medications and a number of drug combinations that have been used with success. These include:

▪ Sulfadiazine (1 g q.i.d.), along with pyrimethamine (50 mg once, then 25 mg b.i.d., administered with folinic acid 3 mg, three to four times a week) and oral prednisone

▸ As pyrimethamine can cause thrombocytopenia, a platelet count should be performed at baseline, and weekly thereafter.

▪ Clindamycin, sulfadiazine, and prednisone

▸ Clindamycin has the advantage of being able to be injected intravitreally or subconjunctivally, but it can cause pseudomembranous colitis.

▪ Trimethoprim-sulfamethoxazole

▪ Atovaquone

● Prednisone should be started 12 to 24 hours after the antibiotics. For sulfa-allergic patients, clindamycin can be used instead of a sulfa drug. Spiramycin has been used in pregnant patients and is available in the United States with special approval as an orphan drug. Patients on the above medications should be monitored with laboratory studies.

Prognosis

● Usually good, especially if chorioretinal lesions are peripheral and the patient is otherwise healthy.

▪ Patients usually have a complete resolution of symptoms with full visual recovery.

● If the macula or optic nerve is affected, vision loss and a scotoma may result.

● Recurrences are possible and most commonly occur in the first year after an episode. Patients should be warned that a new area of chorioretinitis might develop at the border of an inactive scar. Continued trimethoprim/sulfamethoxazole has been shown to reduce recurrences in people at high risk.

● Severe inflammation can lead to vitreous changes/condensation, which can lead to a retinal detachment.

● Choroidal scarring and atrophy may lead to choroidal neovascularization with further vision loss.

● In immunocompromised patients: *T. gondii* has a predilection for encysting within ocular, muscle, and brain tissue, therefore patients who are immunocompromised should be referred to an infectious disease specialist for evaluation of a possible CNS infection.

REFERENCES

Holland GN. Ocular toxoplasmosis: a global reassessment. Part I: epidemiology and course of disease. *Am J Ophthalmol.* 2003;136(6):973–988. PubMed PMID:14644206.

Jones JL, Holland GN. Annual burden of ocular toxoplasmosis in the US. *Am J Trop Med Hyg.* 2010;82(3):464–465.

Nussenblatt RB, Whitcup SM. *Uveitis: Fundamentals and Clinical Practice.* 3rd ed. Philadelphia: Mosby;227.

Silveira C, Belfort R Jr, Muccioli C, et al. The effect of long-term intermittent trimethoprim/sulfamethoxazole treatment on recurrences of toxoplasmic retinochoroiditis. *Am J Ophthalmol.* 2002;134(1):41–46.

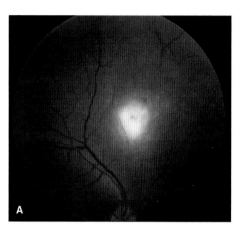

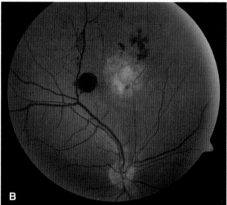

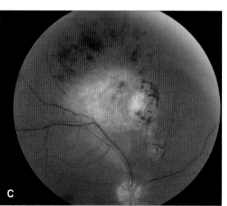

FIGURE 9-52. An immunocompromised patient with acquired toxoplasmosis (note the lack of vitreous haze due to immune compromise) who had several recurrences over 5 years. The initial episode of retinochoroiditis occurred with vasculitis (**A**). A branch retinal vein occlusion (BRVO) has occurred during resolution of the initial lesion (**B**) and during a recurrence (**C**).

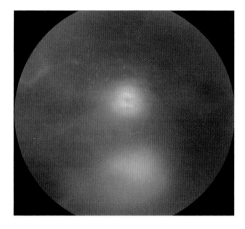

FIGURE 9-53. Recurrence of toxoplasmosis. Dense vitritis and two active lesions adjacent to a pigmented chorioretinal scar, giving the appearance of a "headlight in the fog."

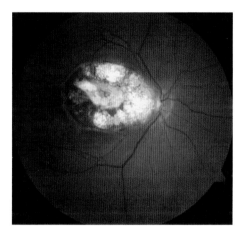

FIGURE 9-54. Congenital toxoplasmosis. An excavated, pigmented chorioretinal scar involving the central macula and the optic nerve.

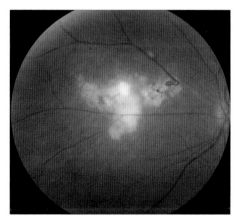

FIGURE 9-55. An active area of resolving chorioretinitis adjacent to a scar. There is vascular sheathing of a vessel leading to the optic nerve and a chorioretinal anastomosis in the old scar. Early Kyrieleis plaques are seen lining the arterioles around the lesion.

OCULAR TOXOCARIASIS

Uwe Pleyer

Toxocariasis is an infectious disease caused by *Toxocara canis* or *Toxocara cati*. It occurs when a person (usually a child) ingests food or soil contaminated by the feces of an infected animal.

Epidemiology and Etiology

- Human seroprevalence for *Toxocara* antibodies is between 2% and 80%, and varies with factors such as geographic location, socioeconomic status, and dietary habits.

- Most patients have exposure to puppies or kittens.

- *Toxocara* larvae have been found in both rural and metropolitan areas.

- The highest prevalence is in the southeastern United States, Japan, and Argentina.

- The risk for developing ocular toxoplasmosis in seropositive individuals is low: 0.1% to 1%. However, the prevalence likely is under-reported as it occurs mainly in children.

- The average age for developing ocular toxoplasmosis is 7 years.

- Following ingestion, second-stage larvae migrate through the intestine and enter the blood stream. The larvae are encysted by a focal granulomatous reaction most commonly in the brain, eyes, lung, and liver, where they remain alive for months.

Symptoms

- *Toxocara* typically causes unilateral, often asymptomatic, intraocular inflammation.

- Patients may have blurred vision, pain, photophobia, and floaters.

- Strabismus or leukocoria are common.

- However, in young children, it may go undetected despite severe visual impairment.

Signs (Figs. 9-56 to 9-59)

- There are two forms: ocular and systemic (visceral larva migrans, VLM) and they rarely coexist.

- Ocular

  - Clinical manifestations are almost exclusively *uni*lateral. In order of frequency, clinical manifestations appear at/as:

    ▶ Peripheral retina/vitreous (the most common presentation)

      – One or more focal, whitish granuloma(s)

      – Vitritis with traction bands and membranes

      – Retinal detachment

      – Usually in people aged 6 to 40 years

    ▶ Posterior pole (this has the best prognosis)

      – Whitish-grey granuloma variable in size

      – Macular heterotopia (from traction)

      – Epiretinal membrane

      – Retinal detachment

      – Secondary atrophy or hyperplasia of RPE

      – Retinochoroidal vascular anastomoses may occur.

      – This is most common in people aged 6 to 14.

    ▶ Chronic endophthalmitis

      – Mainly caused by host immune response against parasitic antigens

      – Relatively asymptomatic (painless), dense vitreous reaction

      – Leukocoria

      – Secondary complications

        □ Retinal detachment

        □ Neovascular glaucoma

        □ Phthisis bulbi

- Usually occurs in children aged 2 to 9 years
  - ▶ Optic nerve involvement
    - Rarely optic neuritis can occur
  - ▶ Anterior segment involvement
    - Rarely will patients develop anterior uveitis or scleritis
  - ▶ Patients may develop cystoid macular edema (CME) at any stage.
- Systemic (VLM)
  - VLM tends to affect the youngest children (3 and under), and presents as:
    - ▶ Pneumonitis
    - ▶ Hepatomegaly
    - ▶ Pneumonia
    - ▶ Myocarditis

Differential Diagnosis

- Endogenous bacterial endophthalmitis
- Retinoblastoma (presents in younger children, calcium is usually present)
- Coats' disease (exudative retinal detachment, primary retinal telangiectasis)
- Retinopathy of prematurity (bilateral, microvascular disease)
- Persistent hyperplastic primary vitreous (PHPV) (congenital condition, often with microphthalmia, cataract)
- Familial exudative vitreoretinopathy (FEVR) (autosomal dominant, family history, bilateral, microvascular changes)

Diagnostic Evaluation

- Diagnosis is based on clinical presentation and correlation with lab findings.
- ELISA testing for toxocara antibodies and eosinophilia in serum is more helpful in VLM than for ocular disease; for ocular toxoplasmosis, an aqueous humor or vitreous specimen is better. Stool samples are usually negative.

- B-scan ultrasonography may demonstrate:
  - A solid, highly reflective mass
  - Vitreous membranes at the posterior pole
  - Vitreous traction and secondary retinal detachment
- CT scan: Presence of intraocular calcification may allow differentiation from retinoblastoma

Treatment

- During active vitritis, either systemic or periocular steroids may be considered.
- Antihelminthic agents have been suggested; however, no large, controlled data are available, but albendazole 10 mg/kg/day for 2 weeks might be helpful in controlling, but not eradicating, the disease.
- Vitrectomy should be considered in order to:
  - Remove traction caused by vitreous bands
  - Remove epiretinal membranes
  - Repair retinal detachments
  - Relieve traction if macular heterotopia occurs

Prognosis

- It is variable, but can be poor depending upon location and secondary complications.

REFERENCES

Althcheh J, Nallar M, Conca M, et al. Toxocariasis: aspectos clinicos y de laboratorio en 54 pacientes. *Ann Pediatr.* 2003;58:425–431.

Stewart JM, Cubillan LDP, Cunningham ET. Prevalence, clinical features, and causes of vision loss among patients with ocular toxocariasis. *Retina.* 2005;25:1005–1013.

Torun N, Liekfeld A, Hartmann C, et al. Ocular toxoplasmosis antibodies in aqueous humor and serum. *Ophthalmologe.* 2002;99(2):109–112.

Yokoi K, Goto H, Sakai J, et al. Clinical features of ocular toxocariasis in Japan. *Ocul Immunol Inflamm.* 2003;11: 269–275.

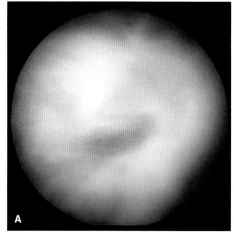
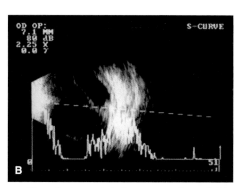

FIGURE 9-56. **A.** A fundus photograph of a 34-year-old man with ocular toxocariasis demonstrates dense vitritis. This is the typical appearance of a patient with "pseudo" endophthalmitis. **(B)** Combined A- and B-scan ultrasonography reveals a funnel-shaped retinal detachment and a hyperechoic subretinal granuloma in the same patient.

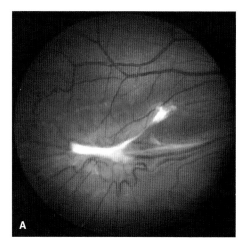
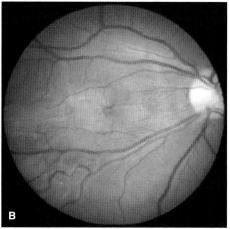

FIGURE 9-57. **A.** A fundus photograph demonstrates an epiretinal membrane in a 17-year-old boy. **B.** Fundus photograph 3 months after vitrectomy with removal of epiretinal membrane was performed. A vitreous sample was obtained and revealed high IgG production against *Toxocara canis* in the vitreous (GWC >80). The visual acuity did not improve after vitrectomy.

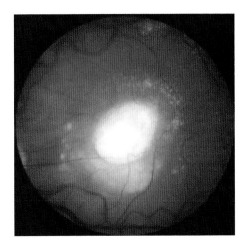

FIGURE 9-58. This 17-year-old girl had a subretinal granuloma with central scar formation. Her vision was 20/400. She had a high serum IgG titer for *Toxocara canis*.

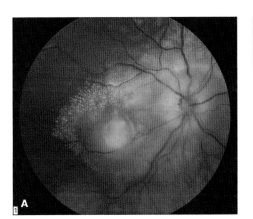

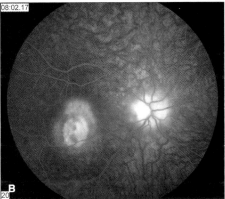

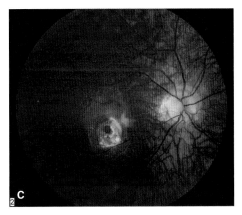

FIGURE 9-59. **A.** This 8-year-old girl had progressive vision loss down to count fingers. She described an overall "darkness" to her vision. She had a submacular lesion with optic neuritis. **B.** The fluorescein angiogram reveals late staining of the granuloma with disk hyperfluorescence. **C.** She did not receive treatment. Five months later, her vision had improved to 20/60 with involution of the lesion. There is a subretinal fibrosis with alteration of the retinal pigment epithelium. (Courtesy of Sunir J. Garg, MD.)

CAT-SCRATCH DISEASE

Julie Gueudry and Bahram Bodaghi

Cat-scratch disease (CSD), or ocular *Bartonella* infection, is a bacterial infection that causes two major types of ocular involvement: conjunctivitis and neuroretinitis. Generally occurring in children, adolescents, and young adults, the diagnosis is based on a typical clinical presentation and a specific serology. Most cases are benign and are self-limited. Prevention remains important in order to reduce the incidence of the disease and its potential complications. More severe cases require antibiotics.

Etiology and Epidemiology

- It is caused by *Bartonella henselae,* a small gram-negative rod that is prevalent worldwide.
- The domestic cat or kitten is the principal animal vector.
- Most patients will have a recent history of cat bites, cat scratches, and/or cat flea bites. It can also be transmitted if cat saliva or the feces of the cat flea comes into contact with the conjunctiva or with an exposed wound.
- Kittens have a higher rate of infection than adult cats.
- It occurs in immunocompetent individuals of all ages but is more frequent in children and young adults.

Symptoms

- Unilateral eye redness, foreign body sensation, and epiphora
- Blurred vision
- Patients may develop a fever, nausea, vomiting, and sore throat, which occurs within 2 weeks of onset of ocular symptoms. Patients may then develop regional lymphadenopathy.

Signs (Figs. 9-60 to 9-62)

- Usually, but not exclusively, unilateral
- Conjunctivitis is seen with parinaud oculoglandular syndrome, which is characterized by:
  - Palpebral swelling
  - Granulomatous nodule on the conjunctiva
  - Discharge is often present and tends to be serous
  - Preauricular, submandibular, or cervical lymphadenopathy is the classic feature of this disease.
  - Mild systemic symptoms of malaise, fatigue, and nausea may occur in 10% to 30% of patients
- Neuroretinitis
  - Possible cause of Leber idiopathic stellate neuroretinitis
  - May be unilateral or bilateral
  - Optic nerve swelling with peripapillary hemorrhages may occur. The classic stellate macular hard exudates may follow a few weeks later.
  - Vitreous cells
  - Granulomatous anterior uveitis may occur without optic neuritis
  - Neuroretinitis is not a complication of CSD-related conjunctivitis
  - Focal retinochoroiditis with white infiltrates and retinal necrosis may also occur. It usually is associated with vitreous and/or anterior chamber cells, and optic disk swelling may be present.

Differential Diagnosis

- Parinaud oculoglandular conjunctivitis:
  - Tularemia
  - TB
  - Syphilis
  - Sarcoidosis

- Lymphogranuloma venereum due to *Chlamydia trachomatis*
- Ocular sporotrichosis
- Other causes of optic disk edema associated with a macular star that should be considered:
  - Malignant hypertension
  - Pseudotumor cerebri with a macular hemi-star
  - Sarcoidosis
  - Syphilis
  - TB
  - Toxoplasmosis
  - Toxocariasis
  - Lyme disease
  - Leptospirosis

Diagnostic Evaluation

- *Bartonella henselae* serology with indirect immunofluorescent assays or ELISA testing. These have a moderate false-negative rate.
- Warthin-Starry silver impregnation stain
- Direct identification through tissue culture is challenging.
- PCR for the detection of *B. henselae* 16S ribosomal DNA in ocular fluids can be considered.

Treatment

- The disease is usually self-limited and the ideal treatment has not been defined.
- Parinaud oculoglandular conjunctivitis: azithromycin 500 mg by mouth the first day then 250 mg daily for 4 more days.
- Severe intraocular infection: doxycycline (100 mg given PO b.i.d.) or trimethoprim-sulfamethoxazole can be used, occasionally

in conjunction with rifampin (300 mg PO b.i.d.).

- Doxycycline and rifampin appear to shorten the course of disease and hasten visual recovery.
- Doxycycline is not used in children below 12 years of age, as tooth discoloration is a concern.
- Duration of treatment is usually 4 weeks in immunocompetent patients and 4 months in immunocompromised patients.
- Prevention is paramount; currently, there is no vaccine available and any cat bite or scratch must be immediately washed and disinfected.

Prognosis

- Long-term prognosis is excellent in most cases and most patients will recover their vision within 1 to 4 weeks.
- The macular star may take 6 to 12 months to fully resolve.
- Some individuals may develop a mild or severe visual loss due to optic neuropathy or macular atrophy.

REFERENCES

Cunningham ET, JE Koehler. Ocular bartonellosis. *Am J Ophthalmol.* 2000;130:340–349.

Curi AL, Machado D, Heringer G, et al. Cat-scratch disease: ocular manifestations and visual outcome. *Int Ophthalmol.* 2010;30(5):553–558.

Drancourt M, Berger P, Terrada C, et al. High prevalence of fastidious bacteria in 1520 cases of uveitis of unknown etiology. *Medicine (Baltimore).* 2008;87:167–176.

Jones DB. Cat-scratch disease. In: Pepose JS, Holland GN, Wilhelmus KR, editors. *Ocular infection and immunity.* St. Louis: Mosby Year Book; 1996:1389–1397.

Solley WA, Martin DF, Newman NJ, et al. Cat scratch disease: posterior segment manifestations. *Ophthalmology.* 1999;106(8):1546–1553.

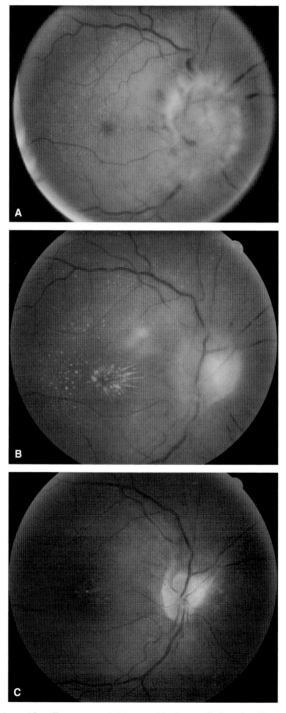

FIGURE 9-60. A. Patient with stellate neuroretinitis caused by *Bartonella henselae*. The vision at presentation was hand motion. **B.** There was progressive improvement several weeks after antibiotic therapy. **C.** One year later, the final vision was 20/200 due to optic and macular atrophy.

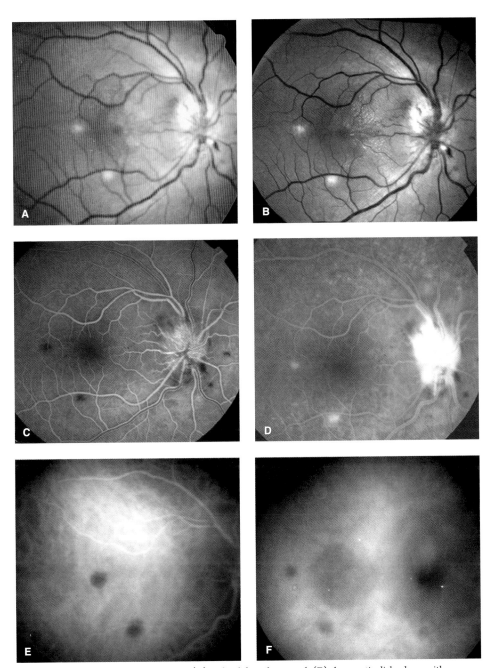

FIGURE 9-61. Color fundus photograph (**A**) and red-free photograph (**B**) show optic disk edema with a macular star. There are some intraretinal hemorrhages and two small areas of chorioretinitis temporal to the fovea. **C, D.** FA shows staining of the optic disk and chorioretinal lesions in the late frames. **E, F.** ICG angiography shows hypocyanescence in the areas of chorioretinitis. There are also larger areas of hypocyanescence around the disk and under the macula.

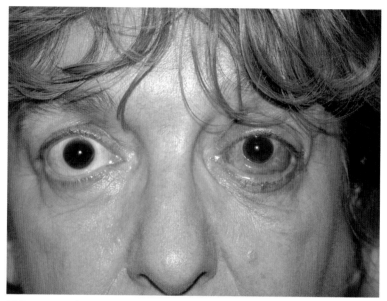

FIGURE 9-62. This patient has Parinaud's oculoglandular syndrome. The left eye has conjunctival injection with epiphora. The left preauricular node is enlarged.

WHIPPLE'S DISEASE

Valérie Touitou and Bahram Bodaghi

Whipple's disease is a systemic infectious disease caused by *Tropheryma whipplei*. Ocular involvement remains rare but the diagnosis should be considered in patients with uveitis or neuro-ophthalmologic manifestations who also have chronic diarrhea and weight loss and who do not improve, and may even worsen, despite use of corticosteroids.

Epidemiology

- The incidence is approximately 18 and 30 cases of systemic disease per 100,000 people annually. This incidence is likely an underestimate.
- Ocular disease occurs in approximately 3% of cases of systemic Whipple's disease.
- The mean age at onset of the disease is 50 years.
- Three-fourths of infected patients are men.

Etiology

- Whipple disease is caused by the bacteria *Tropheryma whipplei,* but it took nearly 50 years to isolate the organism.
  - 1952: First patient cured by antibiotics (chloramphenicol) suggesting a bacterial origin of the disease
  - 1992: First identification of the bacillus
  - 2000: First culture of *Tropheryma whipplei* achieved

Signs and Symptoms (**Figs. 9-63 and 9-64**)

- Systemic
  - Usually precedes ocular involvement and includes:
    - Chronic weight loss is the most common symptom. Patients may also have nonspecific fevers.
    - Chronic diarrhea, abdominal pain, steatorrhea
    - Arthralgias (usually more peripheral than axial, and is polyarticular rather than monoarticular). The arthralgias are often migratory.
    - Chronic lymphadenopathy (which is often mediastinal)
    - Ascites and pleuritis
    - Cutaneous hyperpigmentation, thrombopenic purpura
    - Heart murmurs, endocarditis, myocarditis, arrhythmia
    - Central motor deficit, dementia, hypothalamopituitary involvement, epilepsy, poly- or mono-neuritis
- Ocular
  - Findings may occur in the absence of any systemic symptoms.
    - Keratitis
    - Patients may develop a chronic, bilateral, posterior, or panuveitis. It is usually granulomatous with a few keratic precipitates and limited posterior synechiae.
    - Choroiditis
    - Scleritis
    - Ophthalmoplegia, supranuclear gaze palsy
    - Oculomasticatory myorhythmia (pendular nystagmus associated with tongue or mandibular myoclonus)
    - Papilledema, retrobulbar neuritis, optic nerve atrophy

Differential Diagnosis

- Sarcoidosis
- TB
- Behçet's disease
- Ulcerative colitis
- Histoplasmosis

- Multifocal choroiditis
- Intraocular and systemic lymphoma
- Amyloidosis
- *Mycobacterium avium intracellulare* infection
- Ankylosing spondylitis

Diagnostic Evaluation

- Most patients have the diagnosis made late in the disease course due to the nonspecific signs and symptoms. Tissue is required to establish the diagnosis. The most common tests are:

  - Immunohistochemistry: PAS-positive "foamy" macrophages are seen in tissue biopsies (duodenal, vitreous, lymph node)

  - PCR: PCR of saliva and stool specimens are useful as screening tests. PCR of duodenal biopsies, lymph node biopsies, aqueous humor, vitreous, or CSF specimens can be used to identify the 16S-rRNA gene.

Treatment

- Antibiotics must cross the blood–brain barrier and be administered for a prolonged period of time in order to reduce the risk of relapses.
- Cerebral Whipple's disease:
  - Induction (2 weeks)
    - Either penicillin 1.2 million units or ceftriaxone IV 2 g b.i.d. in addition to streptomycin 1 g/day for 2 weeks, *or*

    - IV trimethoprim (800 mg)-sulfamethoxazole (160 mg) (TMP-SMX) b.i.d. or t.i.d. for 1 to 2 weeks
  - Follow-up treatment (1 year)
    - TMP-SMX (960 mg b.i.d.), *or*
    - Oral cefixime (400 mg once daily). Usually TMP-SMX is preferred for long-term treatment.

  - Due to Whipple's effect on gastrointestinal absorption, patients should also receive folic acid supplementation.

- Ocular Whipple's disease: There is no consensus on treatment. Prolonged antibiotic therapy for at least 1 year is required in to order to avoid relapses.

Prognosis

- The prognosis is variable as most patients are diagnosed late in the disease course, when significant CNS or cardiac changes may have occurred.

REFERENCES

Chan RY, Yannuzzi LA, Foster CS. Ocular Whipple's disease: earlier definitive diagnosis. *Ophthalmology.* 2001;108(12):2225–2231.

Drancourt M, Raoult D, Lépidi H, et al. Culture of Tropheryma whipplei from the vitreous fluid of a patient presenting with unilateral uveitis. *Ann Intern Med.* 2003;16;139(12):1046–1047.

Lagier JC, Lepidi H, Raoult D, et al. Systemic Tropheryma whipplei: clinical presentation of 142 patients with infections diagnosed or confirmed in a reference center. *Medicine (Baltimore).* 2010;89(5):337–345.

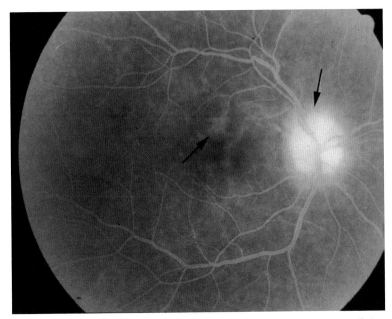

FIGURE 9-63. Chronic posterior uveitis with papillitis and vascular leakage at the posterior pole in a patient with Whipple's disease.

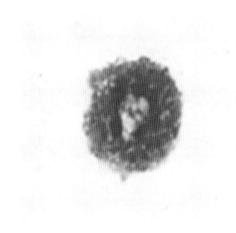

FIGURE 9-64. Periodic acid-Schiff positive macrophage inclusions in the vitreous specimen of a patient with chronic uveitis who was diagnosed with Whipple's disease.

DIFFUSE UNILATERAL SUBACUTE NEURORETINITIS

Carlos Alexandre de Amorim Garcia

Diffuse unilateral subacute neuroretinitis (DUSN) is a unilateral ocular infectious disease caused by nematodes capable of infiltrating the subretinal space. It can cause a diffuse chorioretinitis, or "wipe-out" of the RPE.

Etiology and Epidemiology

• DUSN usually occurs in healthy children and young adults with no significant past ocular history.

• It most commonly occurs in people in tropical climates and is the second leading cause of unilateral blindness in northeast Brazil. It is also found in the United States, India, and some Asian and European countries.

• Several species of nematodes of various sizes may cause DUSN, including: *Toxocara canis, A. caninum, Strongyloides stercoralis, Ascaris lumbricoides,* and *B. procyonis.*

• Identification of the organism is based on a combination of careful measurement of the parasite's dimensions, serologic testing (limited role), and epidemiologic studies.

Symptoms

• The clinical course is characterized by periods of activity and remission.

• Less commonly, patients may have pain, photophobia, and redness.

• Decreased visual acuity and central or paracentral scotomas that can be severe in the late stages of the disease.

Signs (Figs. 9-65 to 9-68)

• Early stage

  ▪ Mild to moderate vitritis, mild optic disk edema, and recurrent crops of evanescent, multifocal, white-yellowish lesions at the level of the outer retina, RPE and choroid which are clustered in only one region of the retina.

  ▪ Less frequent signs include: iridocyclitis, perivenous exudation, subretinal hemorrhages, and serous retinal detachment.

  ▪ The worm can be seen during any stage of the disease. When present, they are typically in the vicinity of the active white-yellowish lesions. A live nematode is seen as a white, mobile, often glistening worm that is gently tapered at both ends and varies in length from 400 to 2,000 μm.

• Late stage

  ▪ Most patients in whom DUSN is suspected clinically are in the chronic phase. These patients have severe vision loss, with the vast majority of patients having less than 20/200 vision.

  ▪ Eyes often have diffuse depigmentation of the RPE, most prominent in the peripapillary and peripheral retina.

  ▪ The diffuse RPE loss leads to optic nerve atrophy and severe retinal arteriole narrowing.

  ▪ There is an increased retinal inner limiting membrane reflex.

  ▪ Occasionally, recurrent crops of evanescent, multifocal, white-yellowish lesions at the level of the outer retina and choroid occur.

  ▪ Evidence of white-yellowish subretinal tunnels or tracks, which are suggestive of larva migration in the subretinal space

Differential Diagnosis

• Early stage

  ▪ Multifocal choroiditis

  ▪ Acute posterior multifocal placoid pigment epitheliopathy

- Multiple evanescent white dot syndrome
  - Birdshot chorioretinitis
  - Sympathetic ophthalmia
  - Nonspecific optic neuritis and papillitis
- Late stage
  - Posttraumatic chorioretinopathy
  - Retinitis pigmentosa
  - Occlusive vascular disease
  - Sarcoidosis
  - Toxic retinopathy

Diagnostic Evaluation

- The main test is biomicroscopy using the three-mirror Goldman lens or 78-diopter lens.
- Blood serologies, blood smears and stool samples are not helpful. Occasionally eosinophilia is found.
- FA in the early stage of the disease demonstrates hypofluorescence of the focal white yellowish lesions of active retinitis followed by late staining. In the advanced states, there is an irregular increase in background choroidal fluorescence.
- ICGA shows hypofluorescent dark spots.
- Electroretinogram: DUSN is characterized by a diffuse retinal inflammation that causes significant electrophysiologic alterations to both the a- and b-waves.
- Goldman perimetry is useful for evaluating the visual field before and after treatment.

Treatment

- When a live worm is found, laser treatment to kill the nematode is useful at any disease stage. Successful treatment can improve visual acuity and reduce inflammatory ocular signs.
- Oral treatment: Albendazole 400 mg/day for 30 days can be used when a live worm is not found.

Prognosis

- Good if larva is visualized in the early stage.
- Poor if the diagnosis is delayed.

REFERENCES

Cortez R, Denny JP, Mendoza RM, et al. Diffuse unilateral subacute neuroretinitis in Venezuela. *Ophthalmology.* 2005;112:2110–2114.

Garcia CA, Gomes AH, Garcia Filho CA, et al. Early-stage diffuse unilateral subacute neuroretinitis: improvement of vision after photocoagulation of the worm. *Eye.* 2004;18:624–627.

Garcia CA, Gomes AH, Vianna RN, et al. Late-stage diffuse unilateral subacute neuroretinitis: photocoagulation of the worm does not improve the visual acuity of affected patients. *Int Ophthalmol.* 2005;26:39–42.

Gass JD, Braunstein RA. Further observations concerning the diffuse unilateral subacute neuroretinitis syndrome. *Arch Ophthalmol.* 1983;101:1689–1697.

Gass JDM. Diffuse unilateral subacute neuroretinitis. In: Gass JDM, ed. *Stereoscopic Atlas of Macular Disease: Diagnosis and Treatment.* 4th ed. St. Louis: Mosby-Year Book Inc.; 1997:622–628.

Souza EC, Casella AMB, Nakashima Y, et al. Clinical features and outcomes of patients with diffuse unilateral subacute neuroretinitis treated with oral albendazole. *Am J Ophthalmol.* 2005;140:437.

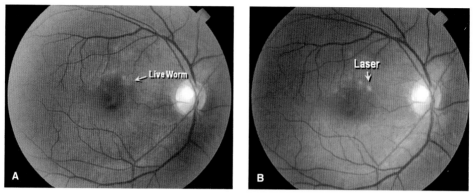

FIGURE 9-65. Note the active white-yellowish evanescent lesions in the early stage with a small live worm (**A**) and after focal laser photocoagulation (**B**).

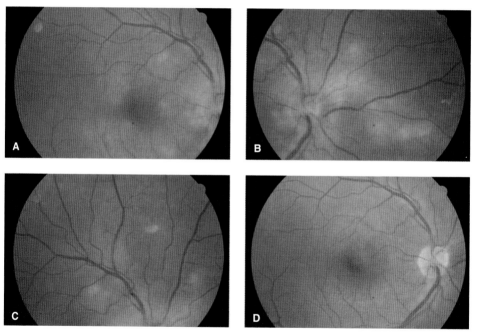

FIGURE 9-66. A–C. Note the active white-yellowish evanescent lesions in the early stage of a patient in whom no live worm could be found. **D.** The same patient 60 days after albendazole treatment.

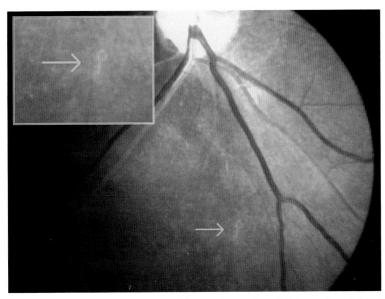

FIGURE 9-67. Note the optic atrophy, narrowing of the retinal arterioles and widespread mottled depigmentation of the retinal pigment epithelium. The subretinal worm was located (and highlighted in the inset).

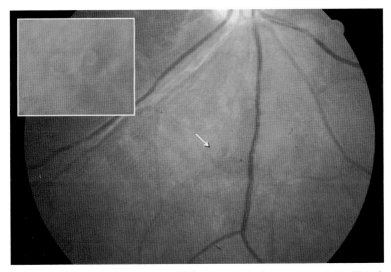

FIGURE 9-68. Fundus findings in the late stages of diffuse unilateral subacute neuroretinitis. Note the optic atrophy and arteriolar attenuation with presence of a live worm (enlarged in the inset).

ONCHOCERCIASIS

Jason F. Okulicz

Onchocerciasis (river blindness) is a chronic infection caused by the nematode *Onchocerca volvulus* and primarily affects the skin and eye.

Etiology and Epidemiology

- Onchocerciasis is endemic in Africa, where approximately 95% of all infected people live. It also occurs in Latin America and Yemen. Infection reduces life expectancy by an average of 10 years.

- Onchocerciasis is a major cause of blindness, with approximately two million people having blindness or severe visual impairment.

- The nematode *Onchocerca* volvulus is transmitted from person to person by the bite of a black fly (genus *Simulium*), which breeds near freely flowing waterways, thus the name "river blindness."

- Microfilariae enter the skin and mature into adults, forming nodules in the subdermal connective tissue, often at bony prominences.

- Microfilariae released from the adult worms migrate to various sites, most commonly to the subepidermal lymphatics and the eye.

- Ocular penetration by microfilariae begins through the bulbar conjunctiva at the limbus, then they invade the cornea, anterior chamber, and iris.

- The microfilariae enter the posterior segment via hematogenous spread or via the ciliary nerves.

- When the microfilariae die, the host incites an immune response, which is responsible for most of the ocular and dermatologic complications.

Symptoms

- Early symptoms include fever, arthralgias, and transient urticaria of the face and trunk.

- Pruritus is common; however, some patients have no pruritus, while other have severe, continuous itching.

- Conjunctivitis or photophobia may occur early, with blindness becoming increasingly common as time goes on.

Signs (Figs. 9-69 to 9-75)

- Onchocercoma, which are subcutaneous nodules, can be found anywhere.

- A maculopapular rash is common, while skin lichenification, hypopigmentation, or hyperpigmentation can also occur. More severe disease is characterized by skin ulcerations, epidermal atrophy, hanging groin (due to atrophic inguinal skin), femoral and inguinal lymphadenitis, and generalized corporal atrophy.

- Microfilariae may be seen within the cornea or migrating freely in the anterior chamber and vitreous humor.

- Corneal infiltration of microfilariae causes punctate keratitis that over time can cause sclerosing keratitis.

- Corneal opacification and neovascularization secondary to inflammation induced by dead microfilariae occur as lymphocytes and eosinophils infiltrate the peripheral cornea and lead to a sclerosing keratitis.

- Anterior uveitis

  - Nongranulomatous or granulomatous inflammation occurs early and may result from invasion of the iris and ciliary body by the microfilariae or as a response to dead microfilariae.

  - Iritis occurs in about 10% to 20% of cases with ocular involvement.

This contribution to the work was done as part of the author's official duties as an NIH employee and is a work of the United States Government.

▦ A pseudo-hypopyon composed of microfilariae can occur.

▦ Posterior synechiae may cause inferior pupil distortion giving the classic pear-shaped iris, and may lead to pupillae occlusio et seclusio, iris bombe, iris atrophy, inflammatory or angle closure glaucoma, and cataract.

● Chorioretinitis is present in 10% to 25% of patients with ocular involvement, and diffuse RPE mottling with subretinal fibrosis can occur.

● The macula is generally spared, with central visual acuity maintained until late in the disease.

● Optic atrophy can be found in 25% of cases with ocular involvement

Differential Diagnosis

● Syphilis

● Yaws

● Scleroderma

● Uveitic glaucoma or chronic angle closure glaucoma

● HSV infection

● Anterior ischemic optic neuropathy

● Sarcoidosis

● Trachoma

● TB

● Interstitial keratitis

● Atopic keratoconjunctivitis

● Neurotrophic keratopathy

Diagnostic Evaluation

● Traditionally, the diagnosis is based on a "skin snip," which entails obtaining a 3- to 5-mg skin snip from an affected area and examining the tissue for direct visualization of microfilariae.

▦ Most sensitive and specific test overall

▦ Less sensitive for early or mild infections

▦ Becoming increasingly unacceptable to local populations due to invasiveness

● PCR tests can be used to amplify parasite DNA sequences from skin snips and increase sensitivity.

● Direct visualization of microfilariae by slit-lamp examination of the cornea and anterior chamber of the eye.

● Other tests

▦ Rapid-format antibody cards

▸ Utilize serum specimens to detect antibodies, such as IgG4 antibodies to recombinant *Onchocerca volvulus* antigen Ov16

▦ Dipstick assays

▸ Detect oncho-C27 antigen in urine or tears, and have high sensitivity and specificity

Treatment

● Ivermectin is the drug of choice given its high efficacy and low toxicity.

▦ Prevents ocular disease and eliminates skin disease

▦ A single 150 mcg/kg dose clears microfilariae from skin for several months.

▦ Does not affect adult worms

▦ Adverse reactions are similar to the systemic responses of dying microfilariae

▸ Fever, edema, pruritus, lymphadenitis, and body aches

▦ Frequency of administration is controversial

▸ Up to 33% of patients in nonendemic areas cured with a single dose

▸ Most patients require additional therapy given the lifespan of adult worms is 12 to 15 years.

▸ Annual ivermectin appears to reduce intraocular inflammation.

- Doxycycline

  - Targets symbiotic *Wolbachia* bacteria essential for worm fertility

  - Usual course is doxycycline 100 mg PO b.i.d. for 6 weeks in addition to ivermectin

  - Combination ivermectin and doxycycline therapy has been shown to reduce microfilarial load, which may affect transmission and may reduce or prevent blindness.

Prognosis

- Generally is good in patients who receive proper therapy before irreversible ocular lesions develop.

- Ivermectin treats skin manifestations and thereby reduces morbidity and improves quality of life.

REFERENCES

CDI Study Group. Community-directed interventions for priority health problems in Africa: results of a multi-country study. *Bull World Health Organ.* 2010;88(7):509–518.

Enk CD. Onchocerciasis—river blindness. *Clin Dermatol.* 2006;24:176–180.

Hopkins AD. Ivermectin and onchocerciasis: is it all solved? *Eye.* 2005;19:1057–1066.

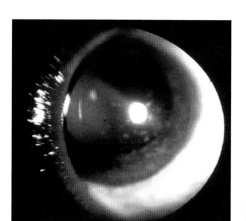

FIGURE 9-69. Photograph demonstrating punctate keratitis that results from infiltration of microfilariae.

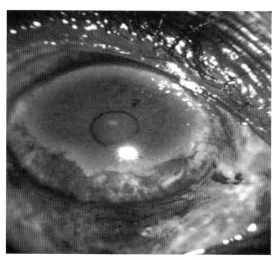

FIGURE 9-70. Photograph showing sclerosing keratitis.

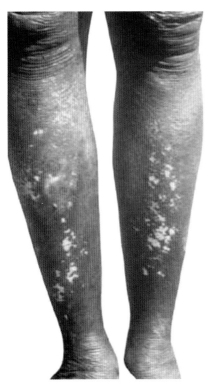

FIGURE 9-71. The "leopard-spot" pattern of skin depigmentation.

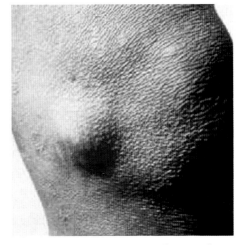

FIGURE 9-72. An onchocercoma adjacent to the knee.

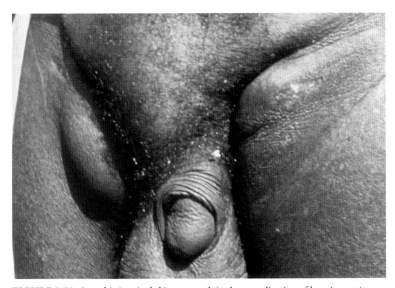

FIGURE 9-73. Atrophic inguinal skin can result in the complication of hanging groin.

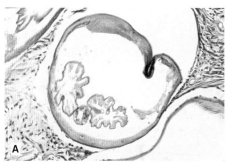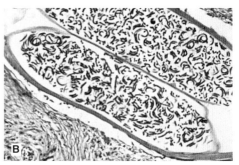

FIGURE 9-74. A. Photomicrograph of a skin biopsy specimen demonstrating an adult worm in cross-section (hematoxylin and eosin stain). **B.** Photomicrograph of a gravid adult female worm from skin biopsy specimen (hematoxylin and eosin stain).

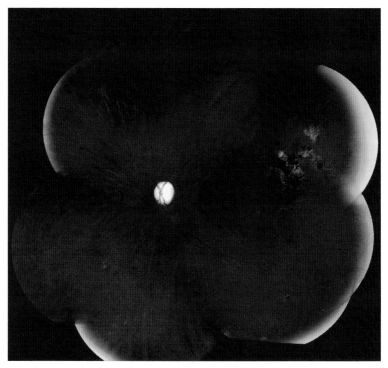

FIGURE 9-75. This patient has diffuse chorioretinal scarring due to onchocerciasis. (Courtesy of Nida Sen, MD, and Robert Nussenblatt, MD.)

LOIASIS

Rajeev Jain and Dinesh Selva

Loiasis, also known as Loa loa filariasis, African eye worm, Calabar swellings, and fugitive swellings, is due to a subcutaneous nematode (roundworm), *Loa loa,* which causes both cutaneous and ocular disease. Infected patients may have pruritus, subcutaneous swelling, migrating lesions, and marked eosinophilia. Adult worms are 25 to 70 mm long.

Etiology and Epidemiology

- Loiasis is endemic in the rainforest areas of western and central Africa. Sporadic cases occur in migrants to and travelers from these areas. It is a chronic infection, infecting millions of people.

- Transmission occurs through the bite of an infected female fly from the genus *Chrysops,* which is also known as the mango fly, deerfly, or horsefly. These blood-sucking flies introduce filarial larvae into the skin, where they develop into adults. The adults migrate subcutaneously and may be seen moving underneath the conjunctiva. Humans are the only known reservoir, and the nematode can live for several years in the subcutaneous tissue.

Signs and Symptoms (**Figs. 9-76 to 9-78**)

- Although the majority of infections are asymptomatic, skin and eye involvement may manifest clinically.
- Systemic
  - Calabar swellings are localized, inflammatory, nonerythematous subcutaneous swellings that are 15 to 20 mm in size. They occur in the extremities often adjacent to the joints, and last for a few days to a few weeks. They are areas of localized angioedema secondary to an immune response and can be associated with urticaria and pruritus.
  - Patients may have migratory myalgias, arthralgias, and pitting edema of the extremities.
  - Other hypersensitivity reactions include glomerulonephritis, motor and sensory deficits, asthma, endomyocardial fibrosis, and eosinophilia.
- Ocular
  - The worm can migrate under the conjunctiva. Patients may present with a red and painful eye with conjunctival injection, chemosis, or subconjunctival hemorrhage. However, patients may be asymptomatic or note only mild ocular irritation or a sensation of movement across the ocular surface.
  - The adult worm may be seen moving underneath the conjunctiva or as an immobile, coiled translucent structure. Painful eyelid swelling has also been reported. Less commonly, the worm may be visible in the anterior chamber.

Diagnostic Evaluation

- Direct isolation of Loa loa worm from the calabar swellings or subconjunctival tissue provides the most definitive diagnosis.
- The diagnosis may also be made by demonstration of microfilariae in the blood. Blood collection should be performed during the daytime, between 10 am and 2 pm, when microfilarial density is highest. However, microfilariae may be absent in bloodstream in cases of unisexual infection and undetectable in up to 30% of patients who have bisexual infections.
- Significant eosinophilia is often present. Patients may also have elevated IgE.
- Although antigen detection using immunoassay for circulating antigens is possible, a high level of antigenic cross reactivity between different helminthic antigens has limited its use.

Treatment

- Drugs

  ▪ The drug of choice remains diethylcarbamazine citrate (DEC) 6 mg/kg/day divided t.i.d. and taken for at least 2 weeks. It is effective against microfilariae and less effective against adult worms, so repeated treatments may be required for complete cure. However, this should be used with caution, as DEC may precipitate encephalopathy if there is high microfilarial load.

  ▪ If DEC is not tolerated or there is high risk of precipitating encephalopathy, albendazole 200 mg taken b.i.d. for 3 weeks should be considered. Repeated courses may be necessary.

  ▪ Ivermectin may also be given in a single dose of 200 to 400 μg/kg. However, there is a higher risk of precipitating encephalopathy, especially in areas that also are endemic for *Onchocerca*.

  ▪ Antihistamines and oral corticosteroids may also be required to treat allergic reactions that may develop as a consequence of dying microfilariae.

- Surgery

  ▪ Surgical extraction from the subconjunctival space or excision biopsy of calabar swelling can also be performed prior to institution of drug therapy. When the worm is visualized, subconjunctival or topical lidocaine can be used to anesthetize the eye. The visible worm can then be removed through a small conjunctival peritomy.

REFERENCES

Barua P, Barua N, Hazarika NK, et al. Loa loa in the anterior chamber of the eye: a case report. *Indian J Med Microbiol.* 2005;23:59–60.

Boussinesq M. Loiasis. *Annals of Tropical Medicine & Parasitology.* 2006:100(8):715–731.

Jain R, Chen JY, Butcher AR, et al. Subconjunctival Loa loa worm. *Int J Infect Dis.* 2008;12(6):e133–135.

Khetan VD. Subconjunctival Loa loa with Calabar swelling. *Indian J Ophthalmol.* 2007;55:165–166.

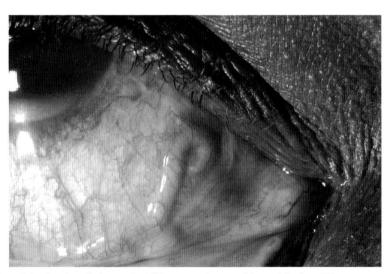

FIGURE 9-76. A subconjunctival worm is visible as a translucent, white, mobile thread-like structure under the inferior bulbar conjunctiva. (Reproduced from Jain R, Chen JY, Butcher AR, et al. Subconjunctival Loa loa worm. *Int J Infect Dis.* 2008;12(6):e133–135.)

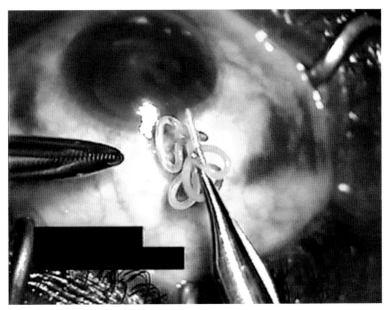

FIGURE 9-77. The female Loa loa worm is seen following surgical extraction through a conjunctival peritomy. (Reproduced from Jain R, Chen JY, Butcher AR, et al. Subconjunctival Loa loa worm. *Int J Infect Dis.* 2008;12(6):e133–135.)

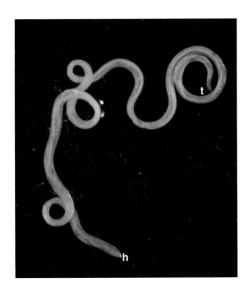

FIGURE 9-78. The adult female Loa loa excised from the patient in Figure 9-77. The length from the head (h) and tail (t) was 57.7 mm. It is approximately 0.5 mm wide. (Reproduced from Jain R, Chen JY, Butcher AR, et al. Subconjunctival Loa loa worm. *Int J Infect Dis.* 2008;12(6):e133–135.)

OCULAR CYSTICERCOSIS

Kim Ramasamy

Cysticercosis is a systemic illness caused by dissemination of the larval form of the pork tapeworm, *Taenia solium*. When humans ingest contaminated soil, water, or undercooked pork that contains *T. solium* cysticerci, the individual becomes the definitive host and carries an intestinal adult tapeworm (taeniasis). A person with tapeworm sheds eggs and tapeworms in their feces. When humans ingest eggs of *T. solium,* they develop cysticercosis within organs (similar to what happens in pigs), and are an accidental intermediate host. It is this type of ingestion that can lead to the ocular findings.

Etiology and Epidemiology

• Infection with eggs results from ingestion of the larvae through infected food handlers, ingestion of fruit and vegetables contaminated with human waste, or by feces-contaminated water supplies in endemic areas. The eggs become larvae that cross the intestinal wall, enter the blood or lymphatic circulation, and then go to the eye, muscles, and neural tissue. Cysticercosis affects an estimated 50 million people worldwide. It is found in areas with poor sanitation, and endemic areas include Latin America including Mexico, sub-Saharan Africa, India, and East Asia.

• Ocular and orbital cysticercosis most commonly occurs in children and young adults.

Symptoms

• Blurry vision and floaters. In cases of ruptured cysticercosis, patients may be much more symptomatic from the ensuing inflammatory reaction. Patients may have diplopia or strabismus.

• Patients with neurocysticercosis can develop epilepsy.

Signs (Figs. 9-79 to 9-83)

• Translucent cyst with or without characteristic undulating movements may be present in the subretinal space, vitreous cavity, conjunctiva, anterior segment, extraocular muscles, eyelid, or orbit. Occasionally, the worm crosses the macula causing significant vision loss. If the cyst ruptures, the patient may develop profound vitritis, proliferative vitreoretinopathy, uveitis, rhegmatogenous or exudative retinal detachment, retinal hemorrhages, disk edema, cyclitic membrane formation, and phthisis. Orbital cysticercosis is characterized by proptosis, globe displacement, strabismus, and restricted motility.

Differential Diagnosis

• Toxocara

• Masquerade syndromes

• Endogenous endophthalmitis

• Severe toxoplasmosis

Diagnostic Evaluation

• The organism is often visible via slit-lamp exam and indirect ophthalmoscopy.

• If a hazy media is present, B-scan ultrasonography can be used to visualize the cyst.

• CT scan of the brain is used to diagnose neurocysticercosis, and whole-body CT can be used for systemic screening.

• The parasite can be found in stool samples, and antibodies can be detected from the blood or stool.

Treatment

• Medical: Niclosamide and praziquantel are used to treat adult worms and praziquantel and metrifonate can be used for cysticercosis. These medications should be administered with concomitant steroids as death of the worm can result in significant intraocular inflammation.

• Surgical removal of the parasites is useful. If the cyst is present in anterior chamber, a paracentesis may be attempted. Pars plana vitrectomy with removal of cyst is useful for intraocular cysticercosis.

Prognosis

- The prognosis is poor in cases of ruptured cysticercosis with severe inflammation.

REFERENCES

Madigubba S, Vishwanath K, Reddy G, et al. Changing trends in ocular cysticercosis over two decades: an analysis of 118 surgically excised cysts. *Indian J Med Microbiol.* 2007;25(3):214–219.

Rath S, Honavar SG, Naik M, et al. Orbital cysticercosis: clinical manifestations, diagnosis, management, and outcome. *Ophthalmology.* 2010;117(3):600–605, 605.e1. Epub 2010 Jan 8.

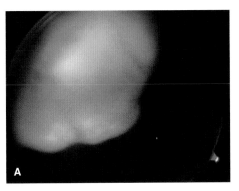

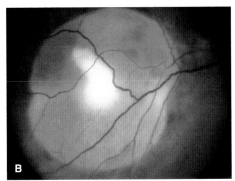

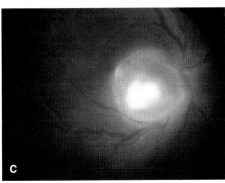

FIGURE 9-79. **A.** Translucent cyst with characteristic undulating movements that appears like a "living mobile pearl." **B.** The scolex (the "head" of the worm) protruding out of the cyst. **C.** The cyst is in the subretinal space.

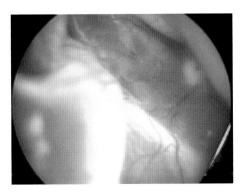

FIGURE 9-80. The subretinal cysticercosis has caused a exudative retinal detachment.

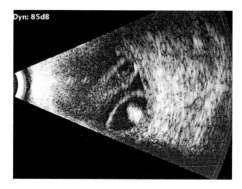

FIGURE 9-81. The B-scan ultrasonogram demonstrates the subretinal cysticercosis and the scolex.

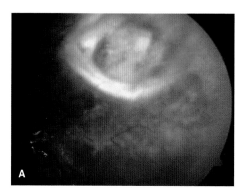

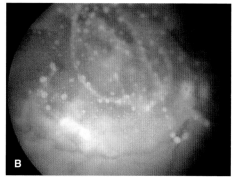

FIGURE 9-82. **A.** The cyst bored a hole from the subretinal space, through the retina and entered the vitreous cavity. This passage incited inflammation, leaving behind a chorioretinal scar. **B.** The ruptured cysticercosis caused intense vitreous reaction.

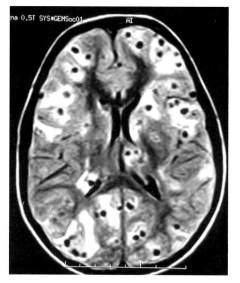

FIGURE 9-83. Intracranial cysticercosis shown in FLAIR MRI image in which fluid appears dark. The CSF in the ventricles appears dark as do the numerous round black "holes" which are fluid-filled cysts. The bright signal around the cysts is edema in the adjacent brain parenchyma. The degree of disease is extensive, with cortical, subcortical, and deep brain lesions. (Interpretation courtesy of Michael Dutka, MD.)

RHINOSPORIDOSIS

S. R. Rathinam

Rhinosporidiosis is a chronic granulomatous disease that affects the mucosa of the nose, conjunctiva, lacrimal sac, or urethral meatus. The lesion presents as a discrete, friable, painless, slow-growing, polypoidal, pedunculated, or sessile mass.

Etiology and Epidemiology

- The causative agent, *Rhinosporidium seeberi,* is an endosporulating microorganism. Spores are transmitted from dust and contaminated water; bathing in stagnant water in endemic areas is considered a major risk factor. The presumed mode of infection is from its natural aquatic habitat through the mucosa or traumatized epithelium. It is endemic in India, Sri Lanka, South America, Malawi, Kenya, Uganda, and the Congo.

Symptoms

- Rhinitis, epistaxis, and nasal obstruction
- Foreign body sensation
- Red eye
- Dark-colored swelling on the eye

Signs (**Figs. 9-84 to 9-87**)

- The most common involvement is the nasal and nasopharyngeal mucosa, followed by the eye.
- The polyps are a red, fleshy, conjunctival lesion with small yellow-white dots on its surface representing the sporangia.
- When the infection is in the bulbar conjunctiva, there is no space for the oculosporidium to grow out as a polyp as the affected area is compressed by the lids. Hence, these lesions are usually sessile and spread along the bulbar conjunctiva and grow deep toward the sclera. It has been postulated that some enzymatic substance produced by the organism corrodes the sclera, resulting in thinning and staphyloma formation. Patients may develop dacryocystitis.

Differential Diagnosis

- Episcleritis
- Scleritis
- Staphyloma
- Giant papillary conjunctivitis

Diagnostic Evaluation

- Histopathology is critical to confirm the diagnosis, as it very hard to culture. Staining the histopathology of the conjunctival scrapings with hematoxylin and eosin shows sporangia of different sizes containing spores.

Treatment

- Simple excision of the polyp with cryotherapy can work for smaller, circumscribed lesions.
- If there is lacrimal sac rhinosporidiosis, complete excision of the sac may be necessary.
- If a staphyloma occurs, cauterization of the base of staphyloma and homologous sclera graft can be performed.
- Oral dapsone 100 mg once or twice a day for 3 to 6 months may treat the infection.

Prognosis

- Recurrence, chronicity, spread to anatomically close sites and secondary bacterial infections are the most frequent complications.

REFERENCES

Arseculeratne SN. Recent advances in rhinosporidiosis and *Rhinosporidium seeberi*. *Indian J Med Microbiol.* 2002;20(3):119–131.

Capoor M, Khanna G, Rajni, et al. Rhinosporidiosis in Delhi, North India: Case Series from a Non-endemic Area and Mini-review. *Mycopathologia.* 2009;168: 89–94.

Fredricks DN, Jolley JA, Lepp PW, et al. *Rhinosporidium seeberi*: a human pathogen from a novel group of aquatic protistan parasites. *Emerg Infect Dis.* 2000;6(3):273–282.

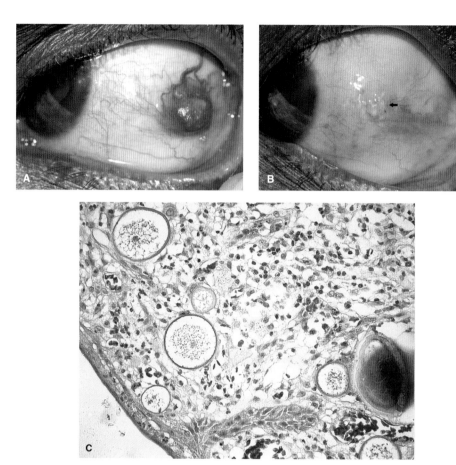

FIGURE 9-84. A. Conjunctival rhinosporidiosis approximately 5 mm in diameter with characteristic pale, yellow-white spots scattered on the surface. **B.** The patient underwent excision of the growth, and a postexcision photograph shows intact scleral tissues (arrow). **C.** Histopathologic sections with hematoxylin and eosin stain shows the sporangia in various stages of maturity enclosed in a thick chitinous wall with infiltration of chronic inflammatory cells. (H and E, × 400.)

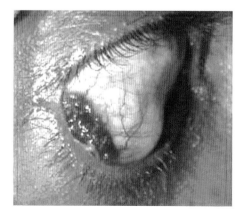

FIGURE 9-85. This is an advanced conjunctival polyp with the characteristic pale yellow-white spots with associated early scleral ectasia/staphyloma.

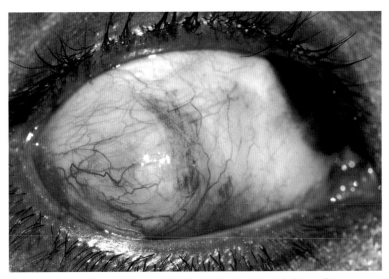

FIGURE 9-86. This person has more significant scleral ectasia with the uveal tissue apparent as the dark blue color.

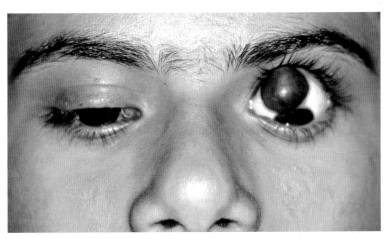

FIGURE 9-87. This person has complete scleral thinning superior to the cornea in the left eye with uveal prolapse.

CHAPTER 1

Endophthalmitis

POSTOPERATIVE ENDOPHTHALMITIS

Stephen G. Schwartz, Harry W. Flynn, Jr.,
and Roy D. Brod

ACUTE-ONSET POSTOPERATIVE ENDOPHTHALMITIS

Endophthalmitis is characterized by marked inflammation of intraocular tissues and fluids. In a patient with endophthalmitis, the etiology and most likely infecting organisms may be predicted by the clinical setting. The largest category is acute-onset postoperative endophthalmitis, generally defined as presenting within 6 weeks of intraocular surgery.

Etiology and Epidemiology

• Presents within 6 weeks of intraocular surgery

• Reported incidence rates are variable. In a recent large single-center series, reported rates were 0.025% overall, 0.028% following cataract surgery, 0.2% following secondary intraocular lens (IOL) implantation, 0.108% following penetrating keratoplasty, and 0.011% following 20-gauge pars plana vitrectomy (PPV).

• The Endophthalmitis Vitrectomy Study (EVS) recruited patients with acute-onset postoperative endophthalmitis following cataract surgery or secondary IOL implantation. In the EVS, 69% of patients had positive vitreous cultures. Of these, the most common etiologic organisms were coagulase-negative staphylococci.

• Preoperative risk factors include immune compromise (including diabetes mellitus), active systemic infection, active blepharitis or conjunctivitis, and disease of the lacrimal drainage system.

• Intraoperative risk factors include prolonged or complicated surgery, secondary IOL implantation, posterior capsular rupture, vitreous loss, iris prolapse, contaminated irrigating solutions or IOLs, and inferotemporal placement of clear corneal incisions. Some authors have suggested that a clear corneal, sutureless incision for cataract surgery is a risk factor for endophthalmitis.

- Postoperative risk factors include wound leak, vitreous incarceration in the wound, and contaminated eye drops.

Symptoms

- Rapid onset of visual loss, redness, and pain

Signs (Figs. 10-1 and 10-2)

- Marked intraocular (anterior chamber and vitreous) inflammation with anterior chamber fibrin and hypopyon
- Eyelid edema, conjunctival congestion, corneal edema, and retinal periphlebitis may occur to a variable degree.

Differential Diagnosis

- Toxic anterior segment syndrome (TASS) generally occurs earlier (within 1 or 2 days) and may be associated with little or no pain, as well as little or no posterior segment inflammation.
- Retained lens material
- Flare-up of pre-existing uveitis
- Triamcinolone acetonide particles
- Long-standing (dehemoglobinized) vitreous hemorrhage

Diagnostic Evaluation

- Acute-onset postoperative endophthalmitis is a clinical diagnosis, followed by laboratory confirmation.
- If the posterior segment cannot be visualized, B-scan ultrasonography may be helpful to rule out retinal detachment, suprachoroidal hemorrhage, or retained lens fragment.
- Aqueous and vitreous cultures. Vitreous samples are more likely to yield a positive culture than aqueous samples. Vitreous cultures may be obtained either with a needle (tap) or with PPV instrumentation.
- Commonly used culture media include 5% blood agar (most common organisms), chocolate agar (fastidious organisms, such as *N. gonorrhoeae* and *H. influenzae*), Sabouraud agar (fungi), thioglycollate broth (anaerobes), and anaerobic blood agar (anaerobes).
- Blood culture bottles may also be used and are helpful in after-hours cases.

Treatment

- The EVS reported that for patients with acute-onset postoperative endophthalmitis following cataract surgery or secondary IOL implantation and presenting visual acuity of light perception, PPV was associated with improved visual outcomes when compared to vitreous tap. For patients with hand motion vision or better, the results of intravitreal tap with injection of antibiotics were similar to PPV. In diabetic patients with presenting visual acuity of hand motions or better, there was a trend toward better visual outcomes in patients treated with PPV, but this was not statistically significant.
- The EVS treated all patients with intravitreal vancomycin (1 mg in 0.1 mL) and amikacin (0.4 mg in 0.1 mL). However, to reduce the risk of aminoglycoside toxicity, either ceftazidime (2.25 mg in 0.1 mL) or ceftriaxone (2 mg in 0.1 mL) may be considered.
- The EVS reported no additional visual benefit associated with the adjunctive use of systemic amikacin and ceftazidime. However, fourth-generation systemic fluoroquinolones such as moxifloxacin achieve intraocular penetration and may be considered for adjunctive use, although supporting evidence of efficacy is lacking.
- In patients with acute-onset postoperative endophthalmitis with suspected bacterial etiology, intravitreal dexamethasone (0.4 mg in 0.1 mL) may be considered.
- The EVS treated all patients with subconjunctival vancomycin (25 mg in 0.5 mL), ceftazidime (100 mg in 0.5 mL), and dexamethasone (6 mg in 0.25 mL). However, subsequent clinical trials have demonstrated that there may be no additional benefit associated with subconjunctival antibiotics.

- The EVS treated all patients with systemic prednisone (30 mg b.i.d. for 5 to 10 days). However, systemic corticosteroids should be used with caution in certain at-risk patients, including diabetics and the elderly.

- The EVS treated all patients with fortified topical vancomycin (50 mg/cc) and fortified topical amikacin (20 mg/cc), up to every hour. As a substitute, commercially available topical antibiotics (such as fourth-generation fluoroquinolones) may be considered. In addition, the EVS treated all patients with topical corticosteroids and cycloplegics.

- If the clinical status appears to be worsening at 48 to 72 hours, consideration should be given to reculturing and reinjection of antibiotics based on the initial culture results. If the initial culture was a needle tap, PPV can be considered for the subsequent procedure.

Prognosis

- The strongest predictor of final visual outcome in the EVS was presenting visual acuity. Therefore, prompt initiation of treatment is more important than any other factor, including vitreous tap versus PPV.

- Other predictors of less favorable outcomes in the EVS included older age, diabetes mellitus, corneal infiltrate, abnormal intraocular pressure, anterior segment neovascularization, absent red reflex, and open posterior capsule.

REFERENCES

Endophthalmitis Vitrectomy Study Group. Results of the Endophthalmitis Vitrectomy Study: a randomized trial of immediate vitrectomy and of intravenous antibiotics for the treatment of postoperative bacterial endophthalmitis. *Arch Ophthalmol.* 1995;113:1479–1496.

Lalwani GA, Flynn HW Jr, Scott IU, et al. Acute-onset endophthalmitis after clear corneal cataract surgery (1996–2005). Clinical features, causative organisms, and visual acuity outcomes. *Ophthalmology.* 2008;115: 473–476.

Schwartz SG, Flynn HW Jr, Scott IU. Endophthalmitis: classification and current management. *Exp Rev Ophthalmol.* 2007;2:385–396.

Wykoff CC, Parrott MB, Flynn HW Jr., et al. Nosocomial acute-onset postoperative endophthalmitis at a university teaching hospital (2002–2009). *Am J Ophthalmol.* 2010 Jul 7 [Epub ahead of print].

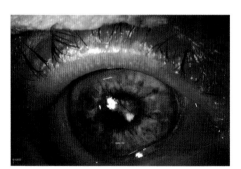

FIGURE 10-1. This person has conjunctival chemosis, injection, hypopyon, and fibrin in the anterior chamber, all indicative of acute-onset postoperative endophthalmitis.

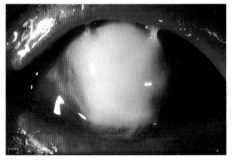

FIGURE 10-2. The patient has acute postoperative endophthalmitis. In this case, there is a profuse amount of purulent material with an opaque cornea, suggestive of an organism such as *Pseudomonas aeruginosa*.

DELAYED-ONSET (CHRONIC) POSTOPERATIVE ENDOPHTHALMITIS

Endophthalmitis is characterized by marked inflammation of intraocular tissues and fluids. Delayed-onset (chronic) postoperative endophthalmitis is defined as endophthalmitis presenting more than 6 weeks after intraocular surgery.

Etiology and Epidemiology

- Presents more than 6 weeks following intraocular surgery

- In one single-center series, the reported rate of delayed-onset postoperative endophthalmitis following cataract surgery was 0.017%.

- Common causative organisms in cases of chronic postoperative endophthalmitis include *P. acnes,* fungi, and various less virulent gram-positive and gram-negative organisms.

Symptoms

- Insidious onset of visual loss, redness, photophobia, and pain. Symptoms are typically less severe than in patients with acute-onset postoperative endophthalmitis.

Signs (Fig. 10-3)

- Slowly progressive intraocular inflammation with variable occurrence of hypopyon and keratic precipitates. A white intracapsular plaque may be present and may be indicative of *P. acnes* infection. Signs are typically less severe than in patients with acute-onset postoperative endophthalmitis.

- Eyelid edema, conjunctival congestion, corneal edema, and aqueous and vitreous inflammation may occur, but generally to a lesser degree than in acute-onset postoperative endophthalmitis.

Differential Diagnosis

- Noninfectious uveitis
- Retained lens material
- Triamcinolone acetonide particles
- Longstanding (dehemoglobinized) vitreous hemorrhage

Diagnostic Evaluation

- Delayed-onset (chronic) postoperative endophthalmitis is a clinical diagnosis, confirmed with laboratory testing.

- If the posterior segment cannot be visualized, B-scan ultrasonography may be helpful to rule out retinal detachment, suprachoroidal hemorrhage, and retained lens fragment.

- Cultures: Vitreous samples are more likely to yield a positive culture than are aqueous samples.

- Vitreous cultures may be obtained either with a needle (tap) or with PPV instrumentation.

- Commonly used culture media include 5% blood agar (most common organisms), chocolate agar (fastidious organisms, such as *N. gonorrhoeae* and *H. influenzae*), Sabouraud agar (fungi), thioglycollate broth (anaerobes), and anaerobic blood agar (anaerobes). If delayed-onset (chronic) postoperative endophthalmitis is suspected, the laboratory should be instructed to hold the cultures for at least 2 weeks to allow isolation of fastidious organisms.

- Blood culture bottles may also be used.

Treatment

- Many authors recommend initial PPV with capsulectomy in cases of chronic postoperative endophthalmitis. Alternatively, one may consider initial tap and inject, followed by more invasive surgery if the clinical examination does not improve. The Endophthalmitis Vitrectomy Study (EVS) did not enroll patients with delayed-onset (chronic) postoperative endophthalmitis, so its findings regarding vitreous tap versus PPV are not necessarily applicable to these patients. If PPV with capsulotomy or capsulectomy is not successful, explantation of the IOL and removal of the capsular bag may be necessary.

- Similar to acute-onset postoperative endophthalmitis, a reasonable initial treatment would include intravitreal vancomycin (1 mg in 0.1 mL) and amikacin (0.4 mg in 0.1 mL). However, to reduce the risk of aminoglycoside toxicity, either ceftazidime (2.25 mg in 0.1 mL) or ceftriaxone (2 mg in 0.1 mL) may be considered.

- If fungal endophthalmitis is suspected, either intravitreal amphotericin B (0.005 mg in 0.1 mL) or intravitreal voriconazole (0.1 mg in 0.1 mL) may be used. Adjunctive systemic antifungals may be used, typically in consultation with an internist or infectious disease specialist.

- In patients with suspected bacterial etiology, intravitreal dexamethasone (0.4 mg in 0.1 mL) may be considered. However, fungal infections are relatively more common in patients with delayed-onset (chronic) postoperative endophthalmitis, so intravitreal dexamethasone should be used with caution in these patients.

- Similar to acute-onset postoperative endophthalmitis, subconjunctival vancomycin (25 mg in 0.5 mL), ceftazidime (100 mg in 0.5 mL), and dexamethasone (6 mg in 0.25 mL) can be given.

- Similar to acute-onset postoperative endophthalmitis, systemic corticosteroids should be used with caution in certain at-risk patients, including diabetics and the elderly. In addition, fungal infections are relatively more common in these patients, so systemic corticosteroids should be used with caution if fungal infection is suspected.

- Fortified topical vancomycin (50 mg/cc) and fortified topical amikacin (20 mg/cc) may be beneficial. However, fortified topical antibiotics may require access to a compounding pharmacy, which may not be available in all locations. As a substitute, commercially available topical antibiotics (such as fourth-generation fluoroquinolones) may be considered. In addition, topical corticosteroids and cycloplegics are suggested.

Prognosis

- Because delayed-onset (chronic) postoperative endophthalmitis is frequently caused by indolent organisms, the prognosis may be slightly more favorable than for patients with acute-onset postoperative endophthalmitis caused by more virulent species.

REFERENCES

Al-Mezaine HS, Al-Assiri A, Al-Rajhi AA. Incidence, clinical features, causative organisms, and visual outcomes of delayed-onset pseudophakic endophthalmitis. *Eur J Ophthalmol.* 2009;19:804–811.

Clark WL, Kaiser PK, Flynn HW Jr, et al. Treatment strategies and visual acuity outcomes in chronic postoperative *Propionibacterium acnes* endophthalmitis. *Ophthalmology.* 1999;106:1665–1670.

Doshi RR, Arevalo JF, Flynn HW Jr, et al. Evaluating exaggerated, prolonged, or delayed postoperative intraocular inflammation. *Am J Ophthalmol.* 2010 July 12 [Epub ahead of print].

Schwartz SG, Flynn HW Jr, Scott IU. Endophthalmitis: classification and current management. *Exp Rev Ophthalmol.* 2007;2:385–396.

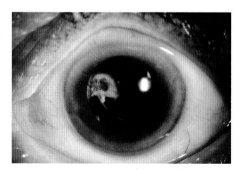

FIGURE 10-3. This eye had delayed-onset postoperative endophthalmitis. Externally, the eye is not injected, and no anterior chamber keratic precipitates or hypopyon is noted. The white plaque within the capsular bag is suggestive of *P. acnes,* which was the organism eventually isolated on cultures.

FILTERING BLEB-ASSOCIATED ENDOPHTHALMITIS

Endophthalmitis is characterized by marked inflammation of intraocular tissues and fluids. In a patient with endophthalmitis, the etiology and most likely infecting organisms may be predicted by the clinical setting. Endophthalmitis associated with filtering blebs has certain unique and important characteristics.

Etiology and Epidemiology

- It may present months to years following trabeculectomy.

- Reported incidence rates are variable. In a large single-center series, the reported rate was 0.2%.

- Preoperative risk factors include active blepharitis or conjunctivitis, contaminated eye drops, contact lens wear, and lacrimal drainage system abnormalities.

- Intraoperative risk factors include an inferior filtering bleb and use of antimetabolites.

- Postoperative risk factors include bleb leak, thin-walled blebs, bleb manipulations, or blebitis.

Symptoms

- Vision loss, redness, and pain. After the onset of initial symptoms, progression may be either rapid or insidious.

Signs (Figs. 10-4 and 10-5)

- Purulent (white) bleb
- Marked intraocular inflammation with anterior chamber fibrin and hypopyon
- Eyelid edema, conjunctival congestion, corneal edema, vitritis, and retinal periphlebitis may occur.

Differential Diagnosis

- Blebitis: Generally associated with less inflammation, less pain, and little or no vitreous inflammation

- Noninfectious uveitis
- Triamcinolone acetonide particles
- Longstanding (dehemoglobinized) vitreous hemorrhage

Diagnostic Evaluation

- Filtering bleb-associated endophthalmitis is a clinical diagnosis, followed by laboratory confirmation.

- If the posterior segment cannot be visualized, B-scan echography may be helpful to rule out retinal detachment or suprachoroidal hemorrhage.

- Ocular cultures: Vitreous samples are more likely to yield a positive culture than aqueous samples.

- Vitreous cultures may be obtained either with a needle (tap) or with PPV instrumentation.

- Commonly used culture media include 5% blood agar (most common organisms), chocolate agar (fastidious organisms, such as *N. gonorrhoeae* and *H. influenzae*), Sabouraud agar (fungi), thioglycollate broth (anaerobes), and anaerobic blood agar (anaerobes).

- Blood culture bottles may also be used and are helpful in after-hours cases.

Treatment

- Some authors recommend initial PPV in cases of filtering bleb-associated endophthalmitis. Alternatively, one may consider initial tap and inject, followed by more invasive surgery if the clinical examination does not improve. The EVS did not enroll patients with filtering bleb-associated endophthalmitis, so its findings regarding vitreous tap versus PPV are not necessarily applicable to these patients.

- Similar to acute-onset postoperative endophthalmitis, initial treatment includes intravitreal vancomycin (1 mg in 0.1 mL) and amikacin (0.4 mg in 0.1 mL). However, to reduce the risk of aminoglycoside toxicity, either ceftazidime (2.25 mg in 0.1 mL) or ceftriaxone (2 mg in 0.1 mL) may be considered.

• In patients with filtering bleb-associated endophthalmitis, intravitreal dexamethasone (0.4 mg in 0.1 mL) may be considered.

• Similar to acute-onset postoperative endophthalmitis, subconjunctival vancomycin (25 mg in 0.5 mL), ceftazidime (100 mg in 0.5 mL), and dexamethasone (6 mg in 0.25 mL) can be used.

• Similar to acute-onset postoperative endophthalmitis, systemic corticosteroids should be used with caution in certain at-risk patients, including diabetics and the elderly.

• Fortified topical vancomycin (50 mg/mL) and fortified topical amikacin (20 mg/mL) may be beneficial. However, fortified topical antibiotics may require access to a compounding pharmacy, which may not be available in all locations. As a substitute, commercially available topical antibiotics (such as fourth-generation fluoroquinolones) may be considered. In addition, topical corticosteroids and cycloplegics are suggested.

Prognosis

• Pre-existing visual loss (e.g., end-stage glaucoma) may limit visual recovery in these patients.

• Because streptococcal and gram-negative organisms are more frequent in this category, the visual outcomes may be worse than in cases of acute-onset postoperative endophthalmitis.

• Similar to acute-onset postoperative endophthalmitis, the strongest predictor of final visual outcome is presenting visual acuity. Therefore, prompt initiation of treatment is more important than any other factor, including vitreous tap versus PPV.

REFERENCES

Busbee BG, Recchia FM, Kaiser R, et al. Bleb-associated endophthalmitis: clinical characteristics and visual outcomes. *Ophthalmology.* 2004;111:1495–1503.

Endophthalmitis Vitrectomy Study Group. Results of the Endophthalmitis Vitrectomy Study: a randomized trial of immediate vitrectomy and of intravenous antibiotics for the treatment of postoperative bacterial endophthalmitis. *Arch Ophthalmol.* 1995;113:1479–1496.

Schwartz SG, Flynn HW Jr, Scott IU. Endophthalmitis: classification and current management. *Expert Review Ophthalmol.* 2007;2:385–396.

Sharan S, Trope GE, Chipman M, et al. Late-onset bleb infections: prevalence and risk factors. *Can J Ophthalmol.* 2009;44:279–283.

Smiddy WE, Smiddy RJ, Ba-Arth B, et al. Subconjunctival antibiotics in the treatment of endophthalmitis managed without vitrectomy. *Retina.* 2005;25:751–758.

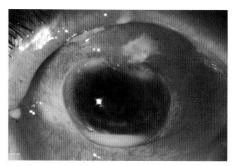

FIGURE 10-4. The superotemporal filtering bleb is ischemic centrally, and is surrounded by injection of the bleb and conjunctiva. There is corneal edema, hypopyon, and fibrin in the anterior chamber.

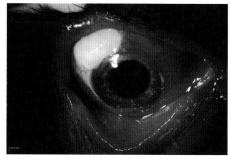

FIGURE 10-5. The infected superotemporal bleb is white, surrounded by an injected, red background, the typical appearance of bleb-associated endophthalmitis. There is mild corneal edema with a small hypopyon.

ENDOGENOUS ENDOPHTHALMITIS

*Manohar Babu Balasundaram
and S. R. Rathinam*

Endogenous endophthalmitis (EE) occurs due to hematogenous dissemination of bacteria or fungi to the eye. While many patients will have other evidence of systemic infection, such as endocarditis, urinary tract injection, pneumonia, skin infections, or meningitis, a number of patients may appear to be healthy. A good history and high clinical suspicion is very important in these cases.

Etiology and Epidemiology

- Compromised host defense and septic focus anywhere in the body

- Those with a history of IV drug abuse, indwelling catheters, diabetes, hepatobiliary infections, alcoholism, immunosuppressive disorders, and abdominal surgery are at higher risk.

- A number of organisms can cause EE, including: gram-positive organisms such as *Streptococcus* species, *Staphylococcus aureus*, and *Bacillus cereus;* gram-negative organisms such as *Klebsiella pneumonia, Escherichia coli,* and *Pseudomonas aeruginosa,* and fungi such as *Candida albicans* and *Aspergillus* species. Gram-positive organisms are predominantly responsible for EE in Western countries while gram-negative organisms and fungi are responsible for EE in Eastern countries.

Symptoms

- Systemic symptoms are nonspecific and depend on the primary source of systemic sepsis, and can include fever, chills, myalgias, and pain in the specific organ system involved.

- Ocular symptoms can include pain, blurry vision, photophobia, floaters. The disease is usually unilateral, but can be bilateral in up to 25% of cases.

Signs (Figs. 10-6 to 10-11)

- Anterior focal: Discrete foci of infection, seen as iris nodules or microabscesses, with injection, and anterior chamber cell

- Anterior diffuse: Severe inflammation, with lid edema, chemosis, corneal edema, and/or hypopyon

- Posterior focal: Whitish nodules or plaques, usually in the choroid, that rapidly involve the retina, with or without Roth spots, cotton wool spots, retinal vasculitis, vitritis, and/or vitreous snowballs

- Posterior diffuse: With intense vitreous inflammation

Differential Diagnosis

- Severe panuveitis
- Toxoplasmosis
- Leptospirosis
- Masquerade syndromes
- Postoperative endophthalmitis

Diagnostic Evaluation

- Cultures: Throat, nasal, blood, urine, indwelling catheters, and cerebrospinal fluid (CSF) and any other clinically evident septic foci should be considered for culture before initiation of antibiotic therapy. Often multiple sites are cultured at once.

- Abdominal ultrasound can be helpful to look for abscess formation, especially in the hepatobiliary system.

- Chest imaging can be used to identify abscess formation or pneumonia.

- Intraocular cultures from aqueous and vitreous can be helpful if there is no other positive specimen.

- Transthoracic and transesophageal echocardiograms can be useful to evaluate patients for endocarditis.

- Testing for immunocompromised states, including HIV should be considered.

Treatment

- Treatment is tailored to the organism and organ system involved, and mainly depends on identification of the causative agent.

- Systemic broad-spectrum IV antibiotics, such as vancomycin and an aminoglycoside/ or third-generation cephalosporin treats not only the systemic infection, but has reasonable intraocular penetration due to breakdown of the blood–eye barrier.

- Intravitreal antibiotics such as vancomycin 1 mg in 0.1 mL and amikacin 0.4 mg in 0.1 mL or ceftazidime 2.25 mg in 0.1 mL with or without PPV may be needed.

- In cases of proven or suspected fungal infection, a combination of oral or IV drug (amphotericin B 20 mg/day, fluconazole 400 mg/day, itraconazole 200 mg/day, voriconazole 400 mg b.i.d. × 1 day, then 200 mg b.i.d., or caspofungin), and intravitreal agents such as amphotericin B 5 µg/0.1 mL or voriconazole 100 µg/0.1 mL with or without

PPV are needed. Cases with more significant vitritis tend to do better with vitrectomy plus antifungal agents.

- Topical steroids and cycloplegics are used to control anterior segment inflammation.

Prognosis

- Poor prognosis is associated with virulent organisms, compromised systemic health and delay in diagnosis. Treatment of the primary focus of infection improves the prognosis.

REFERENCES

Arevalo JF, Jap A, Chee SP, et al. Endogenous endophthalmitis in the developing world. *Int Ophthalmol Clin.* 2010 Spring;50(2):173–187.

Jackson TL, Eykyn SJ, Graham EM, et al. Endogenous bacterial endophthalmitis: a 17-year prospective series and review of 267 reported cases. *Surv Ophthalmol.* 2003;48:403–423.

Smith SR, Kroll AJ, Lou PL, et al. Endogenous bacterial and fungal endophthalmitis. *Int Ophthalmol Clin.* 2007 Spring;47(2):173–183.

Wong JS, Chan TK, Lee HM, et al. Endogenous bacterial endophthalmitis. An East Asian experience and a reappraisal of a severe ocular affliction. *Ophthalmology.* 2000; 107:1483–1491.

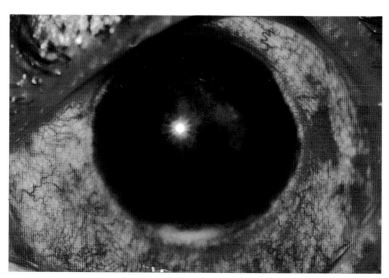

FIGURE 10-6. This person developed anterior diffuse EE with severe conjunctival injection, corneal edema, hypopyon, and posterior synechiae after IV fluid therapy for dehydration.

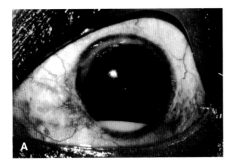

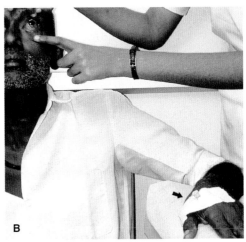

FIGURE 10-7. **A.** An HIV-positive patient developed EE with a hypopyon after experiencing sepsis secondary to an IV catheter. **B.** The patient developed sepsis due to an IV catheter from which *Pseudomonas* was cultured.

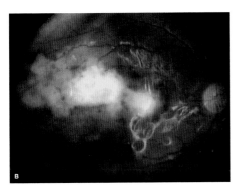

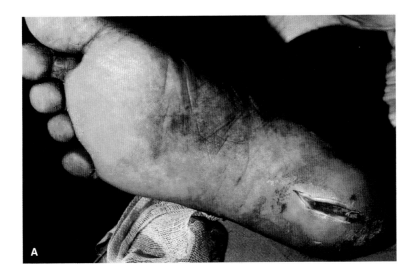

FIGURE 10-8. **A.** EE occurred as a result of an infected foot wound of a diabetic patient. **B.** There was a posterior focal subretinal abscess with hemorrhagic borders in this patient.

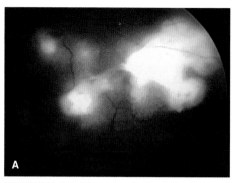 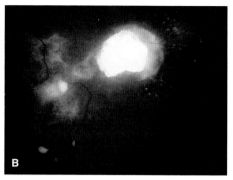

FIGURE 10-9. **A.** This patient had multifocal posterior endogenous endophthalmitis. The choroid shows purulent material with some breakthrough into the vitreous cavity before antibiotic therapy. **B.** The same patient after antibiotic treatment shows involution of the lesions with clearer media.

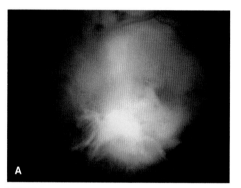 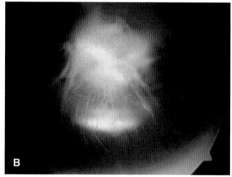

FIGURE 10-10. **A.** Posterior diffuse EE is characterized by intense vitreous inflammation. Prior to starting antibiotic therapy, the patient had diffuse vitritis, subretinal infiltrates, and hemorrhage. **B.** After treatment, the vitreous inflammation is less intense and the vitritis appears to be "firming up."

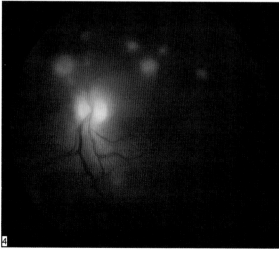

FIGURE 10-11. This person has candidemia, and developed vitreous "snowballs," which are often seen with endogenous candida endophthalmitis.

ENDOGENOUS FUNGAL ENDOPHTHALMITIS

Bahram Bodaghi and Phuc LeHoang

Endogenous fungal endophthalmitis usually occurs secondary to hematogenous dissemination of fungi in patients who have certain well-identified risk factors. Early diagnosis is important in order to avoid subsequent complications and a poor visual outcome.

Epidemiology

- Endogenous fungal endophthalmitis is uncommon.

- Patients of all ages, from neonates to the elderly, can develop it.

- It is important to identify risk factors such as IV hyperalimentation, catheter infection, immunosuppression, long-term systemic use of antibiotics, diabetes mellitus, cancer surgery, abdominal surgery, abortion, or IV drug abuse. These can facilitate early diagnosis, as well as help guide treatment.

- Approximately one-third of patients with candidemia will develop chorioretinitis or endogenous endophthalmitis.

- Ocular involvement should be considered a marker for a disseminated infection.

Etiology and Pathogenesis

- *Aspergillus* species, *Candida* species, *Cryptococcus neoformans,* and *Histoplasma capsulatum* are the major causes of endogenous fungal endophthalmitis.

- Endogenous fungal endophthalmitis develops slowly when compared to endogenous bacterial endophthalmitis.

- Lesions start at the level of the choroid, and subsequently break through into the vitreous, especially with *Candida* species.

- *Candida* species involve the vitreous as the prominent focus of infection, whereas *Aspergillus* species are predominantly at the level of retina, subretinal space, subretinal pigment epithelial space, and choroid.

Symptoms

- Patients may be asymptomatic, and patients who are seriously ill may not be able to voice any visual changes.

- In other cases, symptoms are due to chorioretinal and vitreous involvement and may include:

  - Floaters, blurred vision

  - Scotomata and photophobia

  - A red and painful eye

  - Visual loss due to macular involvement or dense vitritis

Signs (**Figs. 10-12 to 10-17**)

- Lesions are initially located at the level of the choroid and/or retina, and spread into the vitreous cavity in the late phase.

- The anterior segment initially may be normal. Over time, patients may develop anterior uveitis with ciliary injection, nongranulomatous keratic precipitates, posterior synechiae, flare cells, and in severe cases, a hypopyon.

- Early on, funduscopy shows small creamy-white lesions that may become difficult to see at the late stage due to vitreous involvement.

- Retinal hemorrhages may surround small necrotic lesions and appear similar to Roth spots.

- Vitreous abscess often have a "string-of-pearls" appearance.

- Periorbital and eyelid edema can rarely occur.

- Orbital abscess, orbital apex syndrome, and an optic neuropathy may be associated with *Aspergillus* ethmoid sinusitis.

Differential Diagnosis

- The early stage of the disease may mimic other types of intraocular inflammation, including:

    - The white dot syndromes, specifically multifocal choroiditis

    - Primary intraocular lymphoma or other masquerade syndromes

    - Acute retinal necrosis syndrome

    - Infectious chorioretinitis such as toxoplasmosis

    - Syphilis

Diagnostic Evaluation

- Cultures should be obtained from sources such as blood, urine, and IV lines in order to identify the organism and a possible underlying source. Chest imaging can also be considered as indicated by history.

- Identification of the fungus from an aqueous, vitreous, or retinal specimen can be obtained in select circumstances, but is not routinely needed.

- PCR applied to ocular fluids is a promising diagnostic tool but is not yet routinely used.

- Performed at an early stage, fluorescein angiography can help to confirm the presence of chorioretinitis.

- B-scan ocular ultrasonography should be used to assess the retina and vitreous in cases with severe media opacity.

Treatment

- When evaluating patients with ocular inflammation, looking for a treatable infection remains paramount. Systemic evaluation looking for an underlying source is critical.

- Early diagnosis of fungal endophthalmitis enables earlier treatment and a better final visual outcome.

- Spontaneous resolution remains extremely rare.

- IV and intravitreal administration of antifungal agents is the main therapeutic strategy.

- Patients with *Candida* endophthalmitis

    - Oral fluconazole and voriconazole are first-line agents.

    - In severe or imminently vision threatening cases, intravitreal amphotericin B, voriconazole, or caspofungin can be administered.

- Patients with *Aspergillus* endophthalmitis

    - Oral voriconazole is effective.

    - Intravitreal amphotericin B, voriconazole, or caspofungin can be used for more vision threatening cases.

- PPV with intravitreal antifungal injection should be performed in cases with significant vitreous involvement, for both diagnostic and therapeutic effect.

- The use of intravitreal corticosteroids remains controversial.

Prognosis

- There is a wide range of visual outcomes in cases of fungal endophthalmitis, depending on how soon the treatment is started, the stage of the disease, and the organism involved.

- The interaction between the host immune response and the burden of the infectious agent play a major role in affecting visual outcome.

- Despite aggressive treatment, the visual prognosis is often poor because of frequent macular involvement.

- Systemic fungal infection is a life-threatening condition.

REFERENCES

Cassoux N, Bodaghi B, Lehoang P, et al. Presumed ocular candidiasis in drug misusers after intravenous use of oral high dose buprenorphine (Subutex). *Br J Ophthalmol.* 2002;86:940–941.

Khan FA, Slain D, Khakoo RA. Candida endophthalmitis: focus on current and future antifungal treatment options. *Pharmacotherapy.* 2007;27:1711–1721.

Rao NA, Hidayat AA. Endogenous mycotic endophthalmitis: variations in clinical and histopathologic changes in candidiasis compared with aspergillosis. *Am J Ophthalmol.* 2001;132:244–251.

Shen X, Xu G. Vitrectomy for endogenous fungal endophthalmitis. *Ocul Immunol Inflamm.* 2009;17: 148–152.

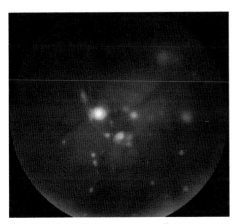

FIGURE 10-12. There are many small vitreous abscesses in a case of fungal endophthalmitis due to *Candida albicans.* (Courtesy of MidAtlantic Retina, the Retina Service of Wills Eye Institute.)

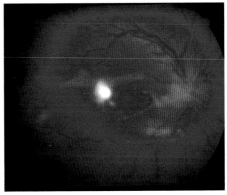

FIGURE 10-13. This patient had *Candida albicans*–associated chorioretinitis with a prominent white abscess temporal to the macula.

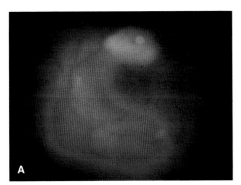

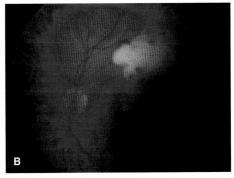

FIGURE 10-14. *Aspergillus fumigatus*–associated EE before **(A)** and after **(B)** vitrectomy shows a large area of chorioretinitis along the superotemporal arcade.

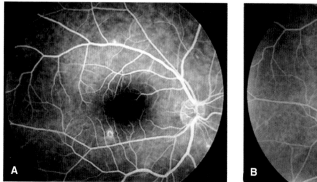
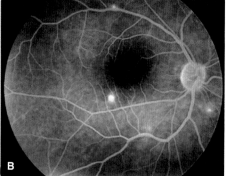

FIGURE 10-15. FA (early phase [**A**] and mid-phase [**B**]) showing the typical pattern of chorioretinitis (blocks early and stains late) in a case of *Candida albicans*–associated endophthalmitis.

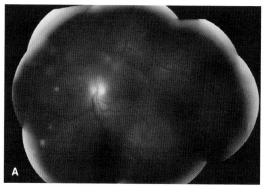
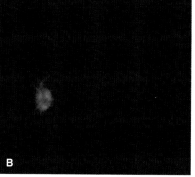

FIGURE 10-16. A. The color photograph shows multiple focal, round, white vitreous abscesses suggestive of candida. **B.** FA demonstrates nonspecific staining of the optic disk and vessels, as well as some blocking due to the vitreous inflammation.

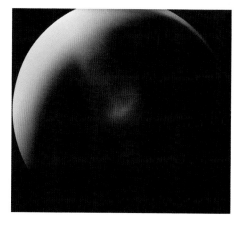

FIGURE 10-17. There is moderate vitritis as well as a yellow-white subretinal abscess with associated subretinal hemorrhage in this patient with *Aspergillus*. (Courtesy of Arunan Sivalingam, MD, and Eliza Hoskins, MD.)

AIDS-Related Eye Disease

Annal D. Meleth and Allison Dublin

As of 2007, over one million people in the United States, and over 33 million people worldwide are infected with the HIV virus. Men make up 75% of affected patients, and men who have sex with men and racial minorities are disproportionally affected. The HIV virus itself can cause retinopathy. Many of the more serious ocular manifestations of AIDS are due to opportunistic infections.

HIV RETINOPATHY

Human immunodeficiency virus (HIV) retinopathy is the most common ocular manifestation of HIV.

Epidemiology and Etiology

- It is uncommon if the CD4 is above 200, but it occurs in approximately 50% of patients with a CD4 less than 50.
- On histopathology, loss of pericytes, narrowing of the capillary lumen, and thickening of the basement membrane are the earliest manifestations of the disease.

Symptoms

- Patients are typically asymptomatic, but they may describe alterations of color vision, visual field changes, and reduced contrast sensitivity.

Signs

- Cotton wool spots (Fig. 11-1)
- Intraretinal hemorrhages
- Capillary microaneurysms, nonperfusion, and telangiectasis

Differential Diagnosis

- Diabetic retinopathy
- Hypertensive retinopathy
- Radiation retinopathy
- Venous occlusive disease
- Collagen vascular disease (lupus)

Prognosis

- The prognosis is almost uniformly good.

Treatment

- No specific treatment is required, and it usually regresses with highly active antiretroviral therapy (HAART).

REFERENCES

Holland GN. AIDS and ophthalmology: the first quarter century. *Am J Ophthalmol.* 2008;145(3):397–408.

Jabs DA. Ocular manifestations of HIV infection. *Trans Am Ophthalmol Soc.* 1995;93:623–683.

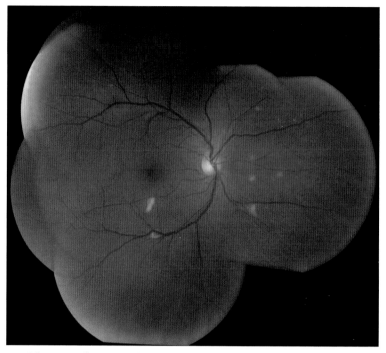

FIGURE 11-1. A few scattered cotton wool spots in a patient with HIV.

CYTOMEGALOVIRUS RETINITIS

Cytomegalovirus (CMV) retinitis is the most common ocular opportunistic infection in AIDS, and is characterized by yellow-white retinal necrosis and perivascular inflammation.

Epidemiology and Etiology

- The primary risk factor is the degree of immune compromise. Patients with a CD4 count below 50 cells/μL have more than a fourfold higher risk of developing CMV retinitis compared to patients with CD4 greater than 100 cells/μL.

- CMV retinitis is the most common ocular opportunistic infection in patients with AIDS, and is itself an AIDS-defining illness.

- In the pre-HAART era, it occurred in up to 40% of patients with AIDS and most patients died within 1 to 2 years after diagnosis. Fortunately, there has been a dramatic decrease in incidence in HAART era.

- Rhegmatogenous retinal detachments (RRDs) are also an important cause of vision loss in patients with CMV retinitis, developing in approximately 20% of patients.

Symptoms

- Painless vision loss
- Floaters
- Photopsias

Signs (Figs. 11-2 to 11-7)

- Perivascular inflammation with irregular patches of fluffy white retinitis and necrosis with associated scattered hemorrhages. It usually starts as a single lesion and then spreads outward as granular dots from that focus.

- Patients often have a granular lesion with multiple dots around the edge (representing advancing lesions) with central clearing that leads to a stippled retinal pigment epithelium.

- Additional features include:
  - Frosted branch angiitis
  - Chronic vitritis
  - Cystoid macular edema

- Progression typically occurs via expansion of previous retinal lesions, which can advance at a rate of up to 250 microns per week.
  - It typically advances faster anteriorly than posteriorly.

- Vision loss occurs via macular or optic nerve involvement from primary retinitis or secondarily with macular edema associated with paramacular involvement or due to retinal detachment.

Differential Diagnosis

- Acute retinal necrosis (ARN) starts as multiple lesions in the mid-peripheral that rapidly progress and is associated with substantial vitritis.

- Progressive outer retinal necrosis (PORN)
- Syphilis
- Toxoplasmosis

Diagnostic Evaluation

- Fundus photos can be used to follow disease progression.

- Fluorescein angiography (FA) demonstrates mottled hyperfluorescence of the expanding borders. There can be late staining of the retinal vessels near the area of infection.

- Autofluorescence: Advancing border often displays hyperautofluorescence.

- AC tap or vitreous tap with polymerase chain reaction (PCR) may be considered.

Treatment

- HAART with immune recovery arrests CMV retinitis progression.

■ Without HAART, 50% of patients experience CMV reactivation at maintenance dose of anti-CMV therapy.

● The clinician must consider concurrent CMV disease in other organ systems.

● Systemic therapy

■ Gancyclovir (5 mg/kg IV b.i.d.) for an induction period of 2 weeks followed by long-term maintenance (5 mg/kg IV q.d.)

■ Foscarnet (90 mg/kg IV b.i.d. or 60 mg/kg IV t.i.d.) for an induction period of 2 weeks followed by maintenance (90 mg/kg q.d.)

■ Cidofovir (5 mg/kg every week) for an induction period of 2 weeks followed by long-term maintenance (3 to 5 mg/kg IV q2wk)

■ Valgancyclovir (900 mg PO b.i.d.) is an orally administered prodrug of gancyclovir, which has an induction period of 2 weeks followed by maintenance (900 mg PO q.d.)

● Intravitreal therapy can be useful as systemic therapy can cause bone marrow suppression (gancyclovir and valgancyclovir) and renal toxicity (foscarnet and cidofovir). However, intravitreal injections need to be performed frequently. If a patient needs long-term therapy and systemic treatment cannot be continued, a gancyclovir implant (see below) should be considered.

■ Gancyclovir (2 mg/0.05 mL)

■ Foscarnet (1.2 mg/0.05 mL)

■ Fomivirsen (330 g intravitreal every week); withdrawn from the market

■ Combination

● Surgical therapy

▶ Gancyclovir implant (Vitrasert, Bausch and Lomb) is surgically placed in the pars plana and delivers gancyclovir for 6 to 8 months at +4 concentration of IV injection.

▶ May be a good option in patients with resistance and unilateral disease.

■ Retinal detachments in these cases are often complex with multiple retinal holes and often require vitrectomy with silicone oil tamponade.

● Resistance

■ Phenotypic and genotypic resistance can occur to gancyclovir, foscarnet, and cidofovir.

■ Gancyclovir resistance often secondary to mutations in the UL97 gene.

■ Rate of resistance has declined in HAART era (from 28% in pre-HAART to approximately 9% in HAART era).

■ Reports exist of gancyclovir-resistant CMV in serum with susceptible CMV in aqueous and vitreous samples.

Prognosis

● Dependent on extent of retina involved, but has dramatically improved in HAART era.

REFERENCES

Jabs DA, van Natta ML, Thorne JE, et al. Course of cytomegalovirus retinitis in the era of highly active antiretroviral therapy: Second eye involvement and retinal detachment. *Ophthalmology.* 2004;111:2232–2239.

Musch DC, Martin DF, Gordon JF, et al. Treatment of cytomegalovirus retinitis with a sustained-release ganciclovir implant. The Ganciclovir Implant Study Group. *N Engl J Med.* 1997;337(2):83–90.

Studies of Ocular Complications of AIDS Research Group, in collaboration with the AIDS Clinical Trials Group. Mortality in patients with the acquired immunodeficiency syndrome treated with either foscarnet or ganciclovir for cytomegalovirus retinitis. *N Engl J Med.* 1992;326(4):213–220.

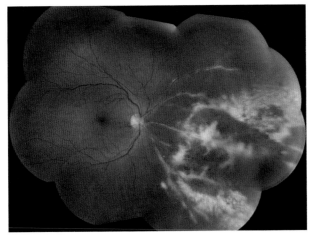

FIGURE 11-2. Active CMV retinitis in a patient who underwent bone marrow transplantation.

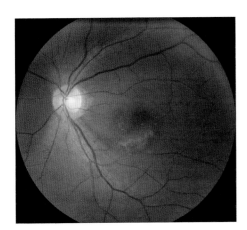

FIGURE 11-3. CMV retinitis in this case is limited to perimacular area with necrotizing retinitis along the inferior arcade, intraretinal hemorrhage, and granularity surrounding fovea.

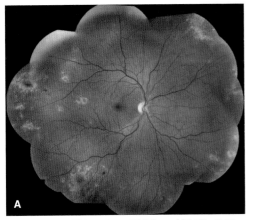

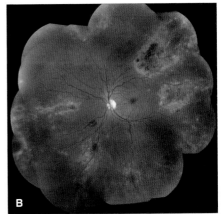

FIGURE 11-4. This patient with bilateral CMV retinitis confirmed with PCR has extensive white areas of retinitis in the mid-periphery with scattered hemorrhages in both eyes.

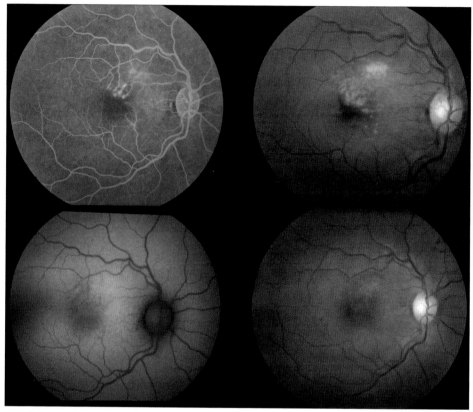

FIGURE 11-5. Note the area of CMV retinitis superior to fovea (upper right) and vascular staining and leakage on FA (upper left). Fundus autofluorescence shows hyperautofluorescence in the corresponding area (lower left). Lower right frame shows resolution of retinitis following ganciclovir implant.

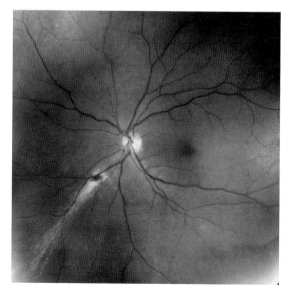

FIGURE 11-6. CMV retinitis with "brush-fire" appearance along the inferonasal quadrant in a patient with HIV.

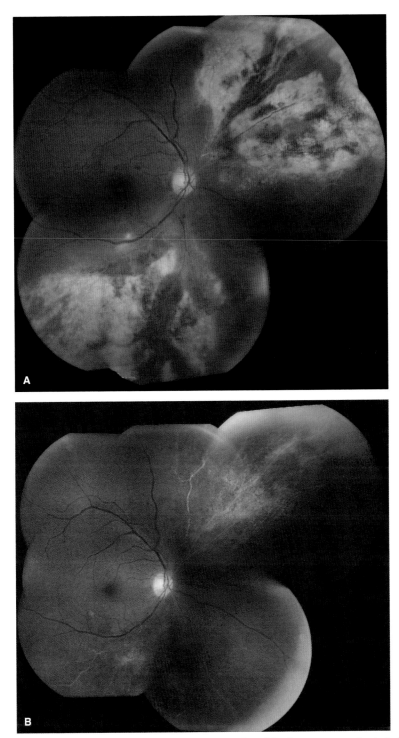

FIGURE 11-7. A. This patient had CMV retinitis with the classic "pizza" fundus appearance of retinal whitening with scattering retinal hemorrhages. **B.** Within 1 month of starting HAART therapy and oral valgancyclovir, there was marked improvement. (Courtesy of Paul Baker, MD.)

IMMUNE RECOVERY UVEITIS

Immune recovery uveitis (IRU) represents a response to antigens and it occurs in patients who have immune-reconstitution after having had retinitis. Although it most commonly occurs in patients with CMV retinitis, it can also occur following infection with tuberculosis or toxoplasmosis.

Epidemiology and Etiology

- It typically occurs in patients who have had prior CMV retinitis.
- The risk increases with the extent of retinal involvement.
- Incidence estimates vary widely, but typically occurs in approximately 10% of patients with immune recovery.

Symptoms

- Vision loss
- Floaters
- Photopsias

Signs

- Posterior synechiae
- Cataract
- Vitritis
- Optic disk edema
- Cystoid macular edema
- Epiretinal membrane
- Proliferative vitreoretinopathy
- Vitreous hemorrhage

Differential Diagnosis

- CMV retinitis
- ARN
- Toxoplasmosis

Diagnostic Evaluation

- IL-12 is typically elevated in vitreous (vs. CMV retinitis).
- The CMV PCR from an anterior chamber or vitreous tap may be negative.

Treatment

- Both periocular and intravitreal triamcinolone, as well as low-dose oral steroids, can be administered depending on immune status. The efficacy of these treatments is variable.
- Generally, the CMV does not reactivate with steroid treatment, but patients should be followed for this.

Prognosis

- The outcome is variable and depends upon the degree of inflammation and presence of posterior segment complications. Patients may have some long-term vision loss as a result of IRU.

REFERENCES

Kempen JH, Min YI, Freeman WR, et al. Risk of immune recovery uveitis in patients with AIDS and cytomegalovirus retinitis. *Ophthalmology*. 2006;113:684–694.

Morrison VL, Kozak I, LaBree LD, et al. Intravitreal triamcinolone acetonide for the treatment of immune recovery uveitis macular edema. *Ophthalmology*. 2007;114:334–339.

ACUTE RETINAL NECROSIS

Acute retinal necrosis (ARN) is rare and consists of a full-thickness retinal necrosis associated with vitritis and occlusive vasculopathy. It is caused by the herpes simplex virus (HSV) and typically occurs in immunocompetent patients.

Epidemiology and Etiology

- The herpes viruses, including varicella zoster virus (VZV), HSV-1, HSV-2, EBV, and CMV all have caused ARN.
- The mean age of onset is age 50, but it can occur at any age.
- ARN is typically unilateral at onset. ARN is bilateral (BARN) in 10% to 36%, and the second eye becomes involved usually within 6 weeks of the first, although several years of separation are possible.

Symptoms

- Mild to moderate eye pain
- Vision loss
- Floaters
- Photopsias

Signs (Fig. 11-8)

- American Uveitis Society diagnostic criteria
  - One or more foci of retinal necrosis with discrete borders in the peripheral retina
  - Rapid circumferential progression of necrosis in the absence of treatment
  - Evidence of occlusive vasculitis with arteriolar involvement
  - Prominent inflammation in the anterior and posterior chambers
- Other manifestations
  - Optic neuritis
  - Scleritis, episcleritis

- Neovascularization and vitreous hemorrhage related to occlusive disease

Differential Diagnosis

- PORN
- CMV retinitis
- Toxoplasmosis
- Syphilis
- Sarcoidosis
- Tuberculosis

Diagnostic Evaluation

- PCR of aqueous or vitreous with demonstration of virus
- Color fundus photography can be used to document disease progression.
- FA demonstrates hypofluorescence in the areas of occlusive vasculopathy, late hyperfluorescence in the areas of activity, and hyperfluorescence of neovascularization (if present).

Treatment

- IV acyclovir, along with systemic corticosteroids with or without intravitreal antiviral therapy, has been the standard therapy for a number of years.
  - In addition to treating the affected eye, it reduces risk of bilateral involvement and extension of disease.
- Treatment does not reduce the risk of RRD.
- Recent reports suggest that treatment with oral valacyclovir, the prodrug of acyclovir, achieves similar bioavailability and treatment success and avoids inpatient admission.
- RRDs usually need to be treated with vitrectomy and long-acting gas/silicone oil tamponade.
- Some investigators recommend prophylactic laser retinopexy in order to reduce the rate

of retinal detachment; however, the efficacy of this approach is variable.

Prognosis

- The final visual outcome is usually poor. Fifty percent of patients are 20/200 or worse 3 months after disease onset, and this increases to 75% by 3 years. The prognosis is related to initial visual acuity. RRD occurs in 50% of patients and portends a poor visual outcome.

- The newer antiviral agents do not appear to offer a better final visual outcome.

REFERENCES

Aizman A, Johnson MW, Elner SG. Treatment of acute retinal necrosis syndrome with oral antiviral medications. *Ophthalmology.* 2007;114(2):307–312. Epub 2006 Nov 21.

Tibbetts MD, Shah CP, Young LH, et al. Treatment of acute retinal necrosis. *Ophthalmology.* 2010;117(4):818–824. Epub 2010 Jan 15.

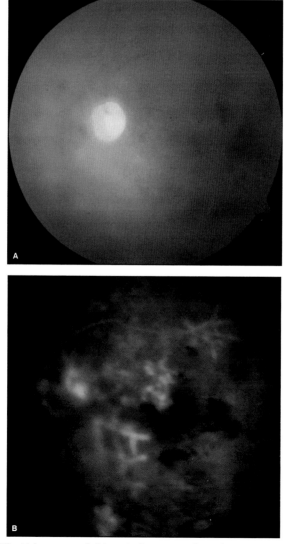

FIGURE 11-8. **A.** ARN with large areas of white retinal necrosis with overlying vitritis. **B.** FA demonstrates significant occlusive vasculopathy and neovascularization.

PROGRESSIVE OUTER RETINAL NECROSIS

Progressive outer retinal necrosis (PORN) is characterized by outer retinal necrosis. Like ARN, it is associated with herpes virus, but unlike ARN, it occurs in immunocompromised patients. The visual outcome is poor.

Epidemiology and Etiology

- It occurs in severely immunocompromised patients, most commonly in those with AIDS.
  - In the pre-HAART era it occurred in up to 2% of patients, but is less common now.
- Typically, it is caused by varicella zoster and herpes simplex viruses.
- It is bilateral in over two-thirds of cases.
- Two-thirds of patients have a history of cutaneous herpes zoster.

Symptoms

- Painless vision loss
- "Curtain" visual field defect

Signs (Fig. 11-9)

- Presenting vision ranges from near-normal to NLP.
- Patchy, multifocal outer retinal whitening, typically outside of the posterior pole with macular involvement in one-third at the time of presentation.
- Extremely rapid progression (hours to days) to full-thickness retinal necrosis
- Minimal to no vitritis
- No vasculitis
- Afferent pupillary defect

Differential Diagnosis

- ARN involves the entire retina, while PORN is outer retinal. ARN has moderate to severe vitritis and vasculitis, and uncommonly involves the posterior pole.
- CMV retinitis
- Syphilis
- Tuberculosis

Diagnostic Evaluation

- Patients should be tested for HIV if an underlying diagnosis is unknown.
- PCR to detect the virus in the vitreous
- FA: Demonstrates outer retinal defect that blocks early and stains late. Unlike ARN, there is a lack of vasculitis.
- Fundus autofluorescence: Early hypofluorescence followed by a stippled autofluorescence pattern.

Treatment

- Combination intravitreal and intravenous antiviral therapy with long-term maintenance therapy in patients who are persistently immunocompromised should be considered, but the visual outcome remains poor.
- The underlying cause of immunosuppression should be treated.
- Aggressive management of RRDs with vitrectomy and silicone oil tamponade.

Prognosis

- Despite aggressive treatment, the visual outcome is poor with 67% of patients progressing to NLP in one series.
- Two-thirds of patients may also develop a retinal detachment.

REFERENCES

Engstrom RE Jr, Holland GN, Margolis TP, et al. The progressive outer retinal necrosis syndrome. A variant of necrotizing herpetic retinopathy in patients with AIDS. *Ophthalmology.* 1994;101(9):1488–1502.

Kim SJ, Equi R, Belair ML, et al. Long-term preservation of vision in progressive outer retinal necrosis treated with combination antiviral drugs and highly active antiretroviral therapy. *Ocul Immunol Inflamm.* 2007; 15(6):425–427.

Spaide RF, Martin DF, Teich SA, et al. Successful treatment of progressive outer retinal necrosis syndrome. *Retina.* 1996;16(6):479–487.

Yin PD, Kurup SK, Fischer SH, et al. Progressive outer retinal necrosis in the era of highly active antiretroviral therapy: successful management with intravitreal injections and monitoring with quantitative PCR. *J Clin Virol.* 2007;38(3):254–259. Epub 2007 Feb 5.

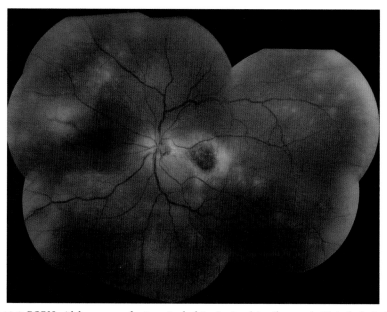

FIGURE 11-9. PORN with large areas of outer retinal whitening involving the macula. Note the lack of vitritis and vasculitis.

FUNGAL RETINITIS

Fungal retinitis is a rare cause of visual compromise in patients with AIDS, and it is typically associated with systemic fungemia (Fig. 11-10).

Cryptococcus neoformans

- It is a yeast that causes infection through inhalation.

- Historically, this was a common cause of meningitis in AIDS patients.

- It affects the eye either through hematogenous spread or through extension from the optic nerve.

  - The most common ocular manifestations are optic neuropathy and choroiditis, but it can also cause optic atrophy, endophthalmitis, vitreoretinal abscesses, and extraocular muscle palsies (usually the sixth nerve).

- Treatment with intravenous amphotericin B plus intravitreal amphotericin B with or without vitrectomy should be considered.

Paracoccidiomycosis

- This fungal infection is more common in Central and South America. It is the most common cause of systemic mycosis in Brazil. It is rarely seen in AIDS patients.

- Typical manifestations include parinaud oculoglandular syndrome.

  - It can also cause choroidal granuloma, vitritis, and endophthalmitis.

- Treatment with intravenous amphotericin B plus intravitreal amphotericin B with or without vitrectomy should be considered.

Candida

- *Candida* endophthalmitis is uncommon among AIDS patients.

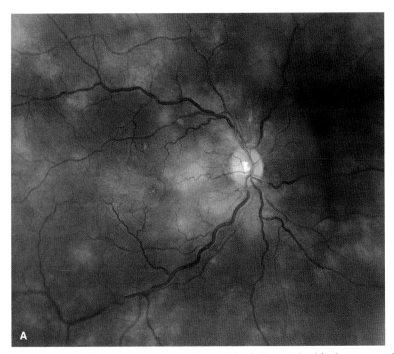

FIGURE 11-10. This patient with AIDS presented with fever and a headache. **A.** Dilated fundus exam revealed multiple, deep, yellow plaques scattered throughout the posterior pole is typical of *Cryptococcus neoformans*.

(continued)

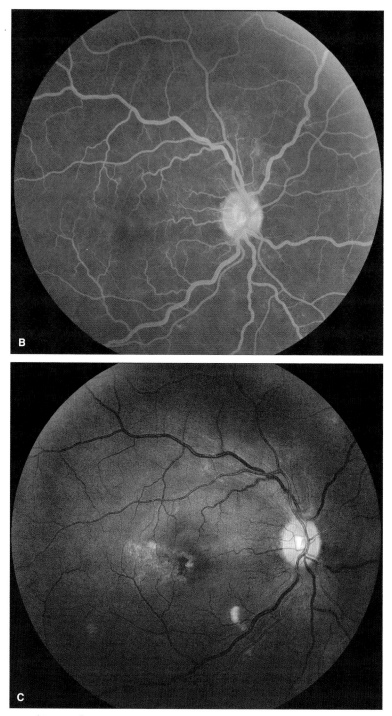

FIGURE 11-10. (*Continued*) **B.** FA revealed nonspecific late staining of the choroidal lesions. **C.** One month after starting amphotericin, there was resolution of the yellow lesions. Diffuse mottling of the retinal pigment epithelium is present, most notably in the macula. (Courtesy of Paul Baker, MD.)

PNEUMOCYSTIS CARINII (JIROVECII) CHOROIDITIS

*P*neumocystis carinii (PC) choroiditis is a rare cause of choroidopathy in patients with AIDS and often serves as a marker of disseminated systemic disease.

Epidemiology and Etiology

- It is rare.
- PC causes pneumonitis. For a number of years, the prophylaxis for PC pneumonitis was aerosolized pentamidine. However, this did not provide prophylaxis to the eyes. There has been a dramatic decrease in ocular PC since the use of systemic prophylaxis.
- The majority of patients (three-fourths) have bilateral disease.

Symptoms

- As the lesions cause a choroiditis and usually have no associated inflammation, patients are typically asymptomatic.

Signs

- Affected patient usually exhibit deep, multifocal cream-orange plaques that range in size from 300 to 3,000 microns and are located in the midperipheral and posterior choroid.

Differential Diagnosis

- Tuberculosis
- Intraocular lymphoma
- Sarcoidosis
- Metastatic disease
- Syphilis
- *Cryptococcus*

Diagnostic Evaluation

- FA demonstrates early hypofluorescence of the lesions with late staining.

Treatment

- Double-strength trimethoprim-sulfamethoxazole IV or oral for 21 days, followed by long-term prophylaxis is very effective.

Prognosis

- PC typically resolves with treatment.

REFERENCES

Gupta A, Hustler A, Herieka E, et al. Pneumocystis choroiditis. *Eye (Lond).* 2010;24(1):178.

Morinelli EN, Dugel PU, Riffenburg R, et al. Infectious multifocal choroiditis in patients with acquired immune deficiency syndrome. *Ophthalmology.* 1993;100:1014–1021.

KAPOSI'S SARCOMA

K aposi's sarcoma (KS) is a common tumor related to human herpes virus-8 infection. It typically occurs in patients with AIDS and affects the eyelids or the adnexal skin.

Epidemiology and Etiology

- Oculocutaneous KS may precede, follow, or occur concomitantly with systemic disease.

- Associated with HHV-8

- It is most commonly seen in patients with AIDS, but can also occur in persons of Mediterranean or African descent, as well as in organ transplant patients.

Symptoms

- Ocular irritation secondary to tear film abnormalities

Signs (Figs. 11-11 and 11-12)

- Patients usually have a violaceous tumor that affects the conjunctiva, lid margin, or eyelid skin.

  - Conjunctival lesions usually appear as an elevated subconjunctival reddish mass, and are more common in the inferior for-nix and on the tarsal conjunctiva.

  - Eyelid lesions usually present as a firm subcutaneous purplish nodule.

- One staging system defines KS as:

  - Stage 1: A patch that is less than 3 mm in height and present for less than 4 months

  - Stage 2: A larger plaque that is flat, which is also less than 3 mm in height and present for less than 4 months

  - Stage 3: A nodule greater than 3 mm in height and present for more than 4 months

Differential Diagnosis

- Subconjunctival hemorrhage

- Conjunctival melanosis
- Pyogenic granuloma
- Squamous cell carcinoma
- Conjunctival lymphoma
- Lymphangioma

Diagnostic Evaluation

- Histopathology demonstrates spindle-shaped cells with inflammatory cells and extravasated red blood cells.

  - Stage 1: Flat dilated vascular channels

  - Stage 2: Plump fusiform endothelial cells lining dilated vascular channels, with a few foci of immature spindle cells

  - Stage 3: Densely packed spindle cells with hyperchromatic nuclei and mitotic figures

- Systemic evaluation should be performed to identify any extraocular tumors.

Treatment

- The most effective treatment is immune reconstitution.

- Intralesional injection of α-interferon, vinblastine, and triamcinolone have all been used.

- External beam radiation can be effective.

Prognosis

- Typically, most patients have an indolent course. Tumor recurrence is fairly common.

REFERENCES

Chang Y, Cesarman E, Pessin MS, et al. Identification of herpesvirus-like DNA sequences in AIDS-associated Kaposi's sarcoma. *Science.* 1994;266:1865–1869.

Dugel PU, Gill PS, Frangieh GT, et al. Treatment of ocular adnexal Kaposi's sarcoma in acquired immune deficiency syndrome. *Ophthalmology.* 1992;99:1127–1132.

International Collaboration on HIV and Cancer. Highly active antiretroviral therapy and incidence of cancer in human immunodeficiency virus-infected adults. *J Natl Cancer Inst.* 2000;92:1823–1830.

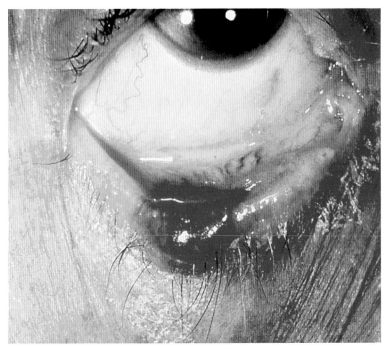

FIGURE 11-11. Kaposi's sarcoma appears as an elevated red tumor on the lid margin in a patient with AIDS. (Courtesy of Robert Penne, MD.)

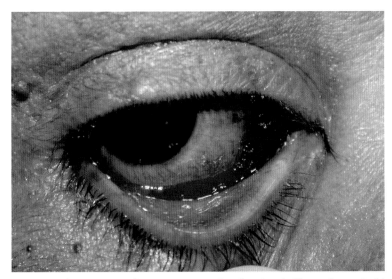

FIGURE 11-12. Kaposi's sarcoma can often appear as a pseudo-subconjunctival hemorrhage as in this patient with AIDS. (Courtesy of Ajay Manchandia, MD.)

Drug-Induced Uveitis

Nehali V. Saraiya and Debra A. Goldstein ▪

Uveitis is usually due to immune or infectious causes; however, certain systemic or local drugs may also precipitate intraocular inflammation. In general, the pathogenesis of drug-induced inflammation is not well understood. It is hypothesized that direct and/or indirect mechanisms are involved. Direct mechanisms are thought to play a role with topically or intracamerally instilled drugs and usually are observed soon after medication use. Indirect mechanisms result from immune complex deposition in uveal tissues, immune reactions to antigens liberated from antibiotic-induced death of a microorganism, or drug-induced alteration of melanin's ability to scavenge free radicals. These mechanisms may result in intraocular inflammation weeks to months after initial use of the drug.

The most common medications implicated in drug-induced uveitis are discussed in the following pages.

RIFABUTIN

Rifabutin is prescribed for the treatment and prophylaxis of *Mycobacterium avium* complex (MAC) infection in HIV-positive patients. Symptoms of acute uveitis may present 2 weeks to more than 7 months following initiation of therapy. Uveitis has been reported to occur with rifabutin alone as well as in combination with other antimicrobial agents such as azithromycin, erythromycin, clarithromycin, ethambutol, and fluconazole. It has been reported with doses as low as 300 mg per day. It recurs with re-challenge and increases in severity with dose escalation.

Symptoms
- Unilateral or bilateral
- Pain
- Redness
- Photophobia
- Blurred vision

Signs

- Conjunctival injection
- Keratic precipitates
- Anterior chamber cell/flare with or without hypopyon
- Vitreous cell
- Perivascular retinal infiltrates

Treatment

- Discontinue rifabutin.
- Treat inflammation with topical steroids and cycloplegic agents.

Prognosis

- In most cases, uveitis resolves within 1 to 2 months of discontinuation of rifabutin and administration of topical corticosteroids, with favorable outcomes (complete resolution of symptoms and normalization of vision in many cases).

REFERENCES

Jacobs DS, Piliero PJ, Kuperwaser MG, et al. Acute uveitis associated with rifabutin use in patients with human immunodeficiency virus infection. *Am J Ophthalmol.* 1994;118(6):716–722.

Moorthy RS, Valluri S, Jampol LM. Drug induced uveitis. *Surv Ophthalmol.* 1998;42(6):557–570.

CIDOFOVIR

Cidofovir has been used intravenously and intravitreally for the treatment of cytomegalovirus (CMV) retinitis. Anterior uveitis has been reported to occur in 26% to 59% of patients receiving IV cidofovir after a median of 4 to 11 doses. Hypotony and uveitis have also been reported following IV cidofovir in a patient with nonocular CMV infection (encephalitis) and an otherwise normal fundus exam, suggesting a direct effect of the drug on the ciliary body. Anterior uveitis also occurs with intravitreal cidofovir for treatment of CMV retinitis. One cases series reported anterior uveitis in 26% of patients after a single intravitreal cidofovir injection. Concomitant use of systemic probenecid decreased the frequency of inflammation. Because of its association with immune recovery uveitis, cidofovir should not be used if immune recovery is expected.

Signs and Symptoms

- Pain, redness, photophobia, tearing, and decreased vision

- Unilateral or bilateral nongranulomatous anterior uveitis with or without keratic precipitates, posterior synechiae, hypopyon, and anterior vitreous cell

- The uveitis may be severe and fibrinous, and accompanied by hypotony.

Treatment and Prognosis

- Aggressive topical steroid and cycloplegic agents

- Cessation of cidofovir is usually required.

- Outcome is variable with potential for permanent structural complications such as posterior synechiae and hypotony.

REFERENCES

Ambati JK, Wynne KB, Angerame MC, et al. Anterior uveitis associated with intravenous cidofovir use in patients with cytomegalovirus retinitis. Br J Ophthalmol. 1999;83(10):1153–1158.

Kempen JH, Min YI, Freeman WR, et al. Studies of Ocular Complications of AIDS Research Group. Risk of immune recovery uveitis in patients with AIDS and cytomegalovirus retinitis. Ophthalmol. 2006;113(4): 684–694.

Moorthy RS, Valluri S, Jampol LM. Drug induced uveitis. Surv Ophthalmol. 1998;42(6):557–570.

BISPHOSPHONATES

Bisphosphonates are used to inhibit bone resorption in patients with osteoporosis and to manage hypercalcemia associated with osteolytic bone cancer, metastatic disease to bone, and Paget's disease of bone. Ocular inflammation has been reported most commonly with pamidronate disodium, but is also seen with other agents in this class including zoledronic acid, alendronate sodium, risedronate sodium, and etidronate disodium. Onset has been reported anywhere from 24 hours to weeks after initiation of therapy.

Symptoms

- Unilateral or bilateral
- Redness
- Pain
- Photophobia
- Blurred vision

Signs

- Conjunctivitis
- Episcleritis
- Scleritis (Fig. 12-1)
- Iritis: Anterior chamber reaction with cell/flare

Treatment

- Nonspecific conjunctivitis seldom requires treatment; NSAID eye drops may provide symptomatic relief. In these cases, the bisphosphonates may be continued.
- Episcleritis may be treated with topical steroids or NSAIDS.
- Anterior uveitis can vary markedly in severity, and may be treated with topical or systemic steroids depending on severity. In most instances, the bisphosphonate must be discontinued for the uveitis to resolve, and they must be discontinued for cases with scleritis.

Prognosis

- Good, with resolution of symptoms in all cases, and resolution of scleritis with medical management and discontinuation of bisphosphonate therapy

REFERENCES

Fraunfelder FW, Fraunfelder FT, Jensvold B. Scleritis and other ocular side effects associated with pamidronate disodium. *Am J Ophthal.* 2003;135(2):219–222.

Moorthy RS, Valluri S, Jampol LM. Drug induced uveitis. *Surv Ophthalmol.* 1998;42(6):557–570.

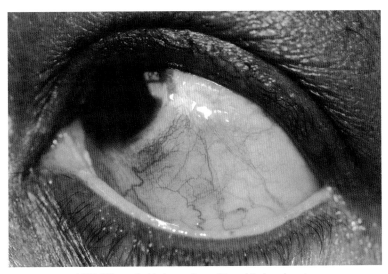

FIGURE 12-1. Mild diffuse scleritis in a patient taking a bisphosphonate.

SULFONAMIDES

Sulfonamide derivatives are a mainstay for the treatment of many gram-positive and gram-negative bacterial infections, including urinary tract infections, otitis media, bronchitis, sinusitis, and pneumonia. Visual disturbances, keratitis, conjunctivitis, and periorbital edema have been reported.

Signs and Symptoms

- Unilateral or bilateral acute iritis has been described within 24 hours of starting the medication as well as with rechallenge.

- Other autoimmune dysfunction such as erythema multiforme minor, diffuse macular vesicular rash, stomatitis, glossitis, conjunctival or scleral injection, or granulomatous hepatitis may be present concurrently. The most serious complication is Stevens-Johnson syndrome (SJS)/toxic epidermal necrolysis (TEN).

  - SJS/TEN are acute hypersensitivity reactions of the skin that are usually drug induced (Figs. 12-2 to 12-6). Most patients are young adults.

  - Patients have a flu-like prodrome of malaise, fatigue, and headache that is followed in a few days with diffuse erythematous patches that can coalesce to form blisters with full thickness epidermal necrosis. There can also be bacterial superinfection.

  - Mucosal involvement, including the conjunctiva, occurs in nearly all patients.

Treatment and Prognosis

- Discontinue agent if uveitis is severe, and treat iritis with topical steroids and cycloplegic agents as necessary.

- Patients with Stevens–Johnson syndrome may need hospitalization and care in an intensive care or burn unit. Patients may develop hypotension, renal and respiratory failure, and corneal scarring.

REFERENCE

Moorthy RS, Valluri S, Jampol LM. Drug induced uveitis. *Surv Ophthalmol.* 1998;42(6):557–570.

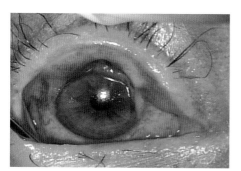

FIGURE 12-2. This patient with Stevens-Johnson syndrome has dry eye and extensive symblepharon formation. (Courtesy of Charles Bouchard, MD, Loyola University.)

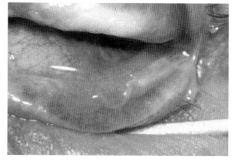

FIGURE 12-3. Another patient with Stevens-Johnson syndrome who has conjunctivitis and sloughing of the conjunctival epithelium. (Courtesy of Charles Bouchard, MD, Loyola University.)

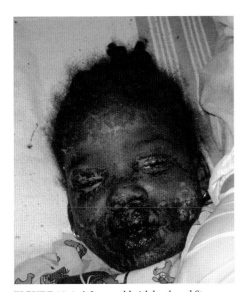

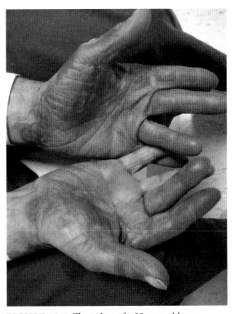

FIGURE 12-4. A 3-year-old girl developed Stevens-Johnson syndrome and suffered a desquamative eruption. Note the extensive mucositis (conjunctivitis and stomatitis) characteristic of Stevens-Johnson syndrome. Her medication was changed and she was successfully treated with intravenous immunoglobulin (IVIG). (Courtesy of Vanessa A. London, MD.)

FIGURE 12-5. The palms of a 59-year-old man diagnosed with Stevens-Johnson syndrome. Note the sharp demarcation of erythema at the edges of the palms and the classic targetoid lesions with dusky centers along his wrists. His medication was discontinued and he was treated with 60 mg prednisone for 3 days with resolution of his symptoms. (Courtesy of Vanessa A. London, MD.)

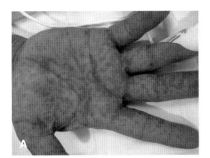

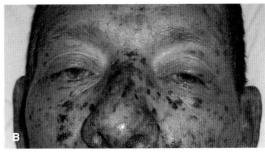

FIGURE 12-6. **A.** A 48-year-old man with AIDS presented with a diffuse morbilliform eruption that evolved into blistering with prominent palm and sole involvement. **B.** He also had conjunctivitis, stomatitis, and involvement of the glans penis. Skin biopsy confirmed a diagnosis of Stevens–Johnson syndrome. With discontinuation of trimethoprim/sulfamethoxazole, his rash and conjunctivitis eventually resolved. (Courtesy of Vanessa A. London, MD.)

METIPRANOLOL

Metipranolol is a nonselective $\beta1/\beta2$ blocker used topically in the treatment of glaucoma via suppression of aqueous humor. It is the most commonly reported beta-blocker to cause uveitis. Incidence is rare.

Signs and Symptoms

- Unilateral or bilateral granulomatous anterior uveitis with mutton-fat keratic precipitates, anterior chamber cell and flare, absence of iris nodules, with or without increased intraocular pressure.

Treatment and Prognosis

- Treat iritis with topical steroid and cycloplegic agents.

- Discontinue metipranolol and substitute another hypotensive agent for pressure control. Using another beta-blocker is usually safe.

- Symptoms usually resolve within 3 to 5 weeks.

REFERENCES

Akingbehin T, Villada JR. Metipranolol-associated granulomatous anterior uveitis. *Br J Ophthalmol.* 75(9): 519–523.

Moorthy RS, Valluri S, Jampol LM. Drug induced uveitis. *Surv Ophthalmol.* 1998;42(6):557–570.

BRIMONIDINE

Brimonidine tartrate is a highly selective α_2 adrenoreceptor agonist that lowers intraocular pressure by reducing aqueous production and increasing uveoscleral aqueous outflow. It is generally well tolerated. The most common ocular adverse events are allergic reactions severe enough to necessitate discontinuation of therapy in 7% to 15% of patients and conjunctival follicles in 8% of patients. Anterior uveitis secondary to brimonidine is rare, and develops between 11 and 15 months after starting therapy. In many cases, a previous history of allergic dermatoconjunctivitis or follicular conjunctivitis is present.

Signs and Symptoms

- Acute-onset redness, photophobia, blurred vision due to granulomatous iritis with mutton-fat keratic precipitates, with or without iris nodules or posterior synechiae, and mild anterior chamber cell and flare (Fig. 12-7).

Treatment and Prognosis

- Cessation of brimonidine
- Topical steroids and cycloplegics to treat inflammation generally leads to resolution of symptoms; permanent structural changes such as posterior synechiae may remain.

REFERENCES

Katz LJ. Brimonidine tartrate 0.2% twice-daily vs timolol 0.5% twice daily: 1-year results in glaucoma patients. Brimonidine Study Group. *Am J Ophthalmol.* 1999; 127(1):20–26.

Moorthy RS, Valluri S, Jampol LM. Drug induced uveitis. *Surv Ophthalmol.* 1998;42(6):557–570.

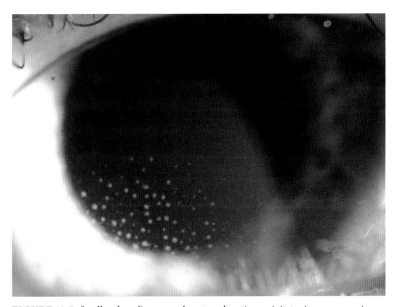

FIGURE 12-7. Small and medium granulomatous keratic precipitates in a person using topical brimonidine.

PROSTAGLANDIN ANALOGUES

Prostaglandin analogues are used in treatment of open-angle glaucoma and ocular hypertension, and act via increasing uveoscleral outflow. They are the newest class of hypotensive agents, and are often first-line agents in treating glaucoma and ocular hypertension. In one retrospective case series, anterior uveitis (iritis) was seen in 4.9% of patients treated with latanoprost within 6 months of starting the medication. This series also reported a 2.1% incidence of cystoid macular edema due to latanoprost. A previous history of cystoid macular edema, iritis, intraoperative vitreous loss, or anterior chamber intraocular lens are risk factors. Anterior uveitis has also been described with use of bimatoprost and travoprost.

Signs and Symptoms

- Eye pain and redness with a mild anterior chamber reaction

Treatment and Prognosis

- Good prognosis with complete resolution of iritis within 1 to 2 weeks of discontinuing medication

REFERENCES

Moorthy RS, Valluri S, Jampol LM. Drug induced uveitis. *Surv Ophthalmol.* 42(6):557–570.

Warwar RE, Bullock JD, Ballal D. Cystoid macular edema and anterior uveitis associated with latanoprost use. Experience and incidence in a retrospective review of 94 patients. *Ophthalmology.* 1998;105(2):263–268.

Masquerade Syndromes

PRIMARY INTRAOCULAR LYMPHOMA

H. Nida Sen and Bahram Bodaghi

Primary intraocular lymphoma (PIOL), also known as primary retinal lymphoma (PRL) or reticulum cell sarcoma, is a subset of primary CNS lymphoma (PCNSL) that involves the retina, vitreous, and optic nerve head with or without simultaneous CNS involvement. Most PIOLs are extranodal, non-Hodgkin, diffuse large B-cell lymphomas.

Epidemiology and Etiology

- More commonly seen in immuno-compromised individuals

- Incidence in the United States has tripled over the last 20 years both in immunocompromised and immunocompetent individuals.

  - 100 new cases of PIOL each year

  - The incidence of PCNSL is 4 to 5 per 1000 person-years among patients with AIDS and 0.3 per 100,000 persons-years in immunocompetent patients.

  - 25% of PCNSL patients have eye involvement at the time of presentation, whereas up to 85% of PIOL develop PCNSL.

- It typically affects an older population, usually in the fifth to sixth decades of life.

- Slight male preponderance

- Bilateral in approximately 80%, but can be very asymmetric at presentation

- Immunosuppression (secondary to AIDS or transplantation) is a risk factor. Infectious agents (Epstein-Barr virus, human herpesvirus 8, *Toxoplasma*) have been associated with PIOL. However, there have been no clear genetic or infectious markers to suggest susceptibility to PIOL.

Symptoms

- Blurry vision, floaters
- Photophobia, ocular pain (rare)

Signs (Figs. 13-1 to 13-5)

- Vitreous cells (occurring in sheets) and haze
- Multifocal, cream-colored, subretinal infiltrates

This contribution to the work was done as part of the authors' official duties as NIH employees and is a work of the United States Government.

- AC cells, keratic precipitates (KP)
- Visual acuity is far better than expected based on the amount of inflammation

Differential Diagnosis

- Sarcoidosis
- Viral retinitis (cytomegalovirus, varicella zoster virus, herpes simplex virus), acute retinal necrosis
- Toxoplasmosis
- Syphilis
- Tuberculosis
- Endophthalmitis
- Metastatic cancer

Diagnostic Evaluation

- The diagnosis is difficult, and requires malignant cells or tissue for diagnosis.
- Fluorescein angiography demonstrates diffuse retinal pigment epithelium (RPE) perturbation and late staining at the RPE level with a granular or "mottled" pattern, early blockage with late staining of retinal/subretinal lesions, optic nerve staining or leakage, and pigment epithelial detachments. Lack of cystoid macular edema (CME) and retinal vascular leakage is an interesting feature of PIOL.
- Indocyanine green angiography shows small, round hypofluorescent areas that disappear in the late phase.
- OCT: Nodular hyperreflective lesions in the RPE
- Tissue diagnosis: Cytology (large atypical lymphoma cells), flow cytometry, cytokine analysis, and molecular analyses from ocular fluids (aqueous or vitreous)
- Brain/spinal MRI and lumbar puncture (LP), (for flow cytometry and cytology) to identify CNS involvement

Treatment

- Current therapies are not curative.
- Systemic chemotherapy is the mainstay of treatment even when associated PCNSL is

not found. Adjunct local chemotherapy can be administered.

- Systemic therapy: High-dose methotrexate; cyclophosphamide, adriamycin, vincristine, and prednisone; cytarabine; radiotherapy, and rituximab have all been tried with various degrees of success.
- Local therapy: Intravitreal methotrexate (400 mcg/0.1 mL), intravitreal rituximab (1 mg/0.1 mL), and radiation can all be considered.
- Recurrence and complications tend to be higher with radiation.

Prognosis

- Prognosis is poor.
- Median progression-free survival is less than 3 years, and overall survival is approximately 5 years and appears to be unaffected by treatment type.
- Systemic spread outside of the CNS is extremely rare (<10% in autopsy specimens).
- Ocular complications can include glaucoma, cataract (both due to inflammation or radiotherapy), retinal and/or optic nerve atrophy, vitreous hemorrhage, and retinal detachment.

REFERENCES

Chan CC, Gonzalez JA. *Primary Intraocular Lymphoma.* Hackensack, NJ: World Scientific Publishing Co Pte Ltd; 2007.

Coupland SE, Damato B. Understanding intraocular lymphoma. *Clin Exp. Ophthalmol.* 2008; 36(6): 564–578.

Fardeau C, Lee CP, Merle-Béral H, et al. Retinal fluorescein, indocyanine green angiography, and optic coherence tomography in non-Hodgkin primary intraocular lymphoma. *Am J Ophthalmol.* 2009;147(5):886–894.

Grimm SA, McCannel CA, Omuro AMO, et al. Primary CNS lymphoma with intraocular involvement: International PCNSL Collaborative Group Report. *Neurology.* 2008;71:1355–1360.

Nussenblatt RB, Chan CC, Wilson WH, et al. International Central Nervous System and Ocular Lymphoma Workshop: recommendations for the future. *Ocul Immunol Inflamm.* 2006;14(3):139–144.

Sen HN, Bodaghi B, Hoang PL, et al. Primary intraocular lymphoma: diagnosis and differential diagnosis. *Ocul Immunol Inflamm.* 2009;17(3):133–141.

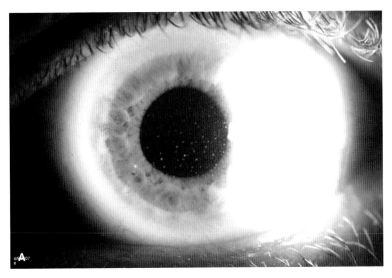

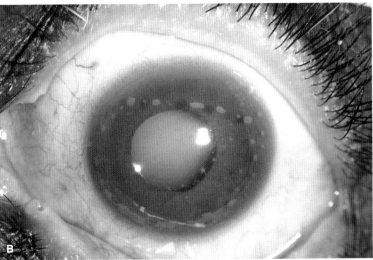

FIGURE 13-1. A. Diffuse, small- to medium-sized keratic precipitates in a patient with PIOL. **B.** There are large granulomatous-appearing pigmented KPs intermixed with stellate KPs more centrally.

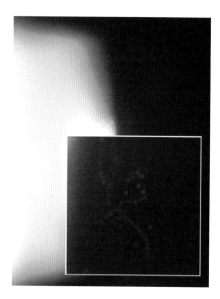

FIGURE 13-2. A 65-year-old white man developed PIOL and PCNSL. Vitreous cells in sheets are seen (inset).

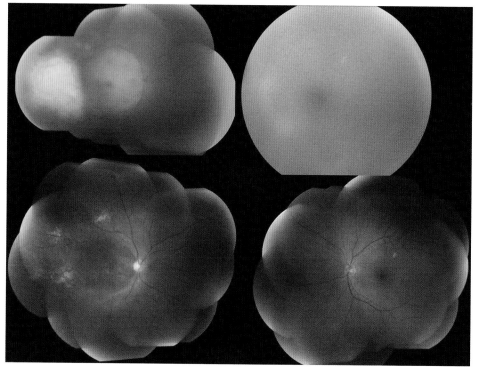

FIGURE 13-3. Top: A 67-year-old Asian man with PCNSL and PIOL had large subretinal masses in the right eye and diffuse subretinal infiltrates in the left eye with significant vitreous haze. Bottom: The same patient following treatment with resolution of tumor infiltration.

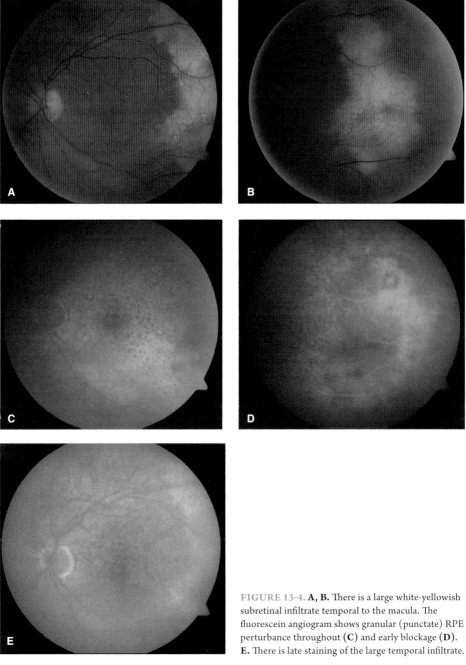

FIGURE 13-4. **A, B.** There is a large white-yellowish subretinal infiltrate temporal to the macula. The fluorescein angiogram shows granular (punctate) RPE perturbance throughout (**C**) and early blockage (**D**). **E.** There is late staining of the large temporal infiltrate.

(continued)

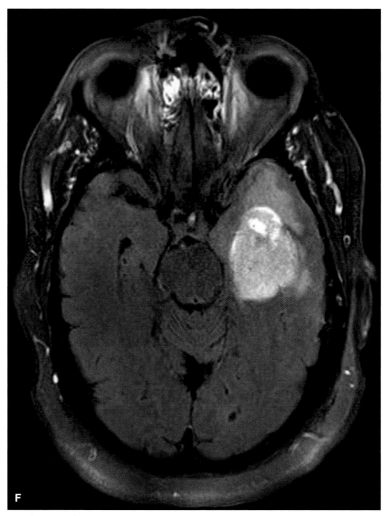

F

FIGURE 13-4. (*Continued*) **F.** MRI shows a solidly enhancing, apparently hypercellular mass in the left temporal lobe with surrounding edema. A brain biopsy was consistent with PCNSL.

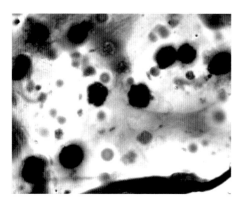

FIGURE 13-5. Vitreous cytology shows large lymphoma cells with scant cytoplasm and large convoluted nuclei.

RETINOBLASTOMA SIMULATING UVEITIS

Carol L. Shields

R etinoblastoma classically manifests as a solitary or multifocal, well-circumscribed retinal mass with dilated feeding vessels. Initially, this tumor appears as a subtle, translucent intraretinal mass. As the tumor enlarges, it assumes an exophytic, endophytic, or combined growth pattern. Exophytic retinoblastoma appears as a tumor with overlying subretinal fluid, whereas endophytic tumor appears as a mass with seeding into the vitreous cavity. A rare growth pattern is diffuse infiltrating retinoblastoma where the tumor assumes a relatively flat, ill-defined horizontal growth pattern along the retinal tissue, simulating uveitis or vitritis. Diffuse retinoblastoma seeds into the anterior segment with neoplastic pseudohypopyon and can cause intraocular hemorrhage, further confusing the findings. Often diffuse retinoblastoma is mistaken for uveitis.

Etiology and Epidemiology

- Retinoblastoma is the most common cancer of the eye in children. It is estimated that there are over 7000 cases per year worldwide with approximately 1800 in Africa, 4000 in Asia, 400 in Europe, 300 in the United States, and 600 in South America.

- The mortality rate from retinoblastoma varies depending on the continent, with 70% mortality in Africa, 40% in Asia, 20% in South America, and <5% in Europe and the United States. Diffuse retinoblastoma represents <3% of all cases.

- In the largest published report on this condition (34 cases), there were no cases of metastatic disease, as the eye was treated promptly.

Symptoms

- Painless loss of vision
- Floaters
- Red eye with conjunctival injection
- Often there are no complaints of vision loss, as young children tend to ignore visual compromise.

Signs (**Figs. 13-6 and 13-7**)

- Anterior segment
  - Iris neovascularization (50%)
  - Neoplastic pseudohypopyon (32%)
  - White tumor seeds on the corneal endothelium (24%)
  - Iris tumor nodules (18%)
  - Cornea stromal edema (9%)
  - Hyphema (9%)
- Posterior segment
  - Extensive ill-defined tumor infiltrating the retina (100%)
  - Average basal diameter of 20 mm
  - Minimal retinal thickening (100%)
  - Extensive vitreous tumor seeds (91%)
  - Visible calcification (often subtle) on ultrasonography (79%)
  - Visible calcification (often subtle) on CT (89%)
  - Vitreous hemorrhage (24%)

Differential Diagnosis

- Endophthalmitis
- Toxocariasis
- Toxoplasmosis
- Sarcoidosis
- Juvenile idiopathic arthritis
- Pars planitis

Diagnostic Evaluation

● B-scan ultrasonography: Demonstrates retinal mass with possible intralesional dystrophic calcification. One must look closely for the calcification, as it might just be a fleck of calcium and not be obvious.

● Fluorescein angiography: Demonstrates dilated feeding artery and draining vein leading to a retinal mass. The mass might be minimally thickened and subtle.

● CT: Demonstrates a thickened intraocular mass, occasionally demonstrating intralesional calcification.

● MRI: Demonstrates the intraocular mass but will not show the calcification.

● Fine-needle aspiration biopsy (FNAB): Should be reserved for cases that are diagnostically challenging. If retinoblastoma is present, tumor seeding into the orbit with risk for metastasis could occur as a result of the FNAB. This test should only be used if retinoblastoma is not high on the differential diagnosis. Usually FNAB is performed through the pars plana, but this should not be done in cases of possible retinoblastoma. Instead, the FNAB should be performed into the anterior chamber for an aqueous sample. Care should be taken not to seed tumor cells and cryotherapy should be performed at the entry site at completion of the procedure. If a vitreous specimen is needed, the pars plan route should be avoided. A preferred approach would be through the peripheral cornea, into the anterior chamber, through the peripheral iris, through the zonules (avoiding the lens), and into vitreous in an anteroposterior direction. Cryotherapy to the entry site is performed. This is a difficult procedure. Immediate cytologic preparation with preservative is important.

Treatment

● Most cases of diffuse retinoblastoma are extensive with tumor seeding into the vitreous cavity and anterior chamber, necessitating enucleation.

● Administration of intravenous or intra-arterial chemotherapy can be attempted, but the vitreous seeds might not completely respond and could show later recurrence.

● External beam radiotherapy can be employed, but a high recurrence of vitreous seeds is anticipated.

Prognosis

● Good if there is no invasion of the optic nerve, choroid, sclera, or orbit.

● Poor if there is invasion of those structures. Adjuvant systemic chemotherapy to prevent metastasis should be given in cases of invasive retinoblastoma.

REFERENCES

Shields CL, Ghassemi F, Tuncer S, et al. Clinical spectrum of diffuse infiltrating retinoblastoma in 34 consecutive eyes. *Ophthalmology.* 2008;115:2253–2258.

Shields CL, Shields JA. Retinoblastoma management: Advances in enucleation, intravenous chemoreduction, and intra-arterial chemotherapy. *Curr Opin Ophthalmol.* March 2010;21:203–212.

Shields JA, Shields CL. *Intraocular Tumors: An Atlas and Textbook.* 2nd ed. Philadelphia: Lippincott Williams & Wilkins; 2008.

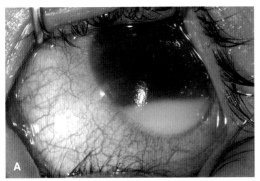
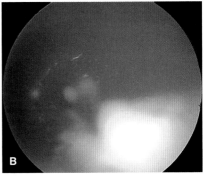

FIGURE 13-6. A young child with blurred vision and a red eye. **A.** A pseudohypopyon is noted. There are also subtle seeds along the pupillary margin at 9:00. **B.** Fundus evaluation shows diffuse vitreous tumor cells present. The vitreous cells are white and homogenous in appearance.

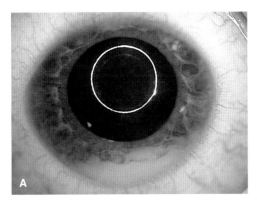
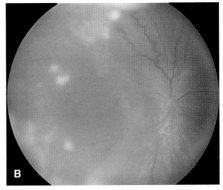

FIGURE 13-7. This child presented with a white eye and decreased vision. **A.** There is a white pseudohypopyon present. **B.** On fundus examination there are scattered vitreous seeds (opacities) that are stark white in color.

METASTATIC CANCER

Henry Wiley

Metastatic cancer can infiltrate the eyelids, conjunctiva, orbit, and most commonly to the uveal tract. It may occasionally masquerade as uveitis.

Etiology and Epidemiology

- Metastatic lesions to the eye are the most common intraocular malignancy, but many of those affected never see an ophthalmologist.
- Metastasis to the eye occurs via hematogenous dissemination.
- Breast cancer is the most common cancer to metastasize to the eye in women, while lung cancer is the most common metastasis in men. Renal, gastrointestinal tumors, prostate, and skin cancers can also metastasize to the eye.
- The uveal tract, especially the choroid, is the most frequent site of metastasis, while involvement of the vitreous, retina, or optic nerve is rare.
- Twenty-five percent of patients presenting with a choroidal metastasis to the ophthalmologist have no history of cancer.

Symptoms

- Symptoms such as blurred vision often stem from secondary effects such as exudative retinal detachment or hyphema, and many patients may have little to no symptoms.
- Patients may experience pain, most notably in cases of metastatic lung cancer.

Signs (Fig. 13-8)

- Choroidal lesions may be:
  - Solitary or multifocal: Breast cancer metastasis tends to be multifocal and bilateral, while lung cancer metastasis tends to be unilateral and unifocal.
  - Classically, they are a creamy yellow color and occasionally have overlying retinal pigment epithelial alterations.
  - They are variable in size and elevation, but usually they are less than 3 mm in thickness.
  - They may cause a secondary exudative retinal detachment.
- Iris lesions may be:
  - Solitary or multifocal
  - Variable in color, often white, yellow, or pink
  - Variable in size
  - May cause an inflammatory reaction
  - May cause hyphema or hypopyon
- Retinal, optic nerve, or vitreal lesions
  - These are uncommon.
  - Vitreous infiltration typically evolves from retinal involvement.
  - Optic disk edema may be due to metastasis to the optic nerve.

Differential Diagnosis

- Other considerations vary widely according to the presentation.
  - Iris or choroidal nevus
  - Iris or choroidal melanoma
  - Other primary uveal tumors (such as choroidal osteoma, choroidal hemangioma, etc.)
  - Retinoblastoma
  - Lymphoma or leukemia
  - Iris cyst
  - Histiocytic disorders (such as juvenile xanthogranuloma)
  - Serous or hemorrhagic ciliochoroidal detachment
  - Varix of the vortex vein
  - Benign lymphoid hyperplasia
  - Uveal effusion

This contribution to the work was done as part of the author's official duties as an NIH employees and is a work of the United States Government.

- ▦ Choroidal or iris granuloma
- ▦ Posterior scleritis
- ▦ Choroiditis

Diagnostic Evaluation

- Systemic evaluation for occult cancer is critical.
  - ▦ Eighty-five percent of patients with metastasis due to breast cancer have a known history of breast cancer. These patients may have concomitant brain metastasis.
  - ▦ If patients have no other cancer history, chest imaging (radiograph, CT, or MRI) is important.
- Standardized A-scan and B-scan ultrasonography usually shows high internal reflectivity.
- Color photographs are helpful to follow tumor response to treatment.
- Fluorescein angiography usually shows early hypofluorescence with late patchy hyperfluorescence.

Treatment

- Systemic chemotherapy is the cornerstone of treatment.
- External beam radiation or brachytherapy can be used to treat the ocular lesions if patients have significant vision loss.

Prognosis

- Many patients may have good vision for a number of years, but the long-term prognosis depends upon treatment of the underlying cancer.

REFERENCES

Shields CL, Shields JA, Gross NE, et al. Survey of 520 eyes with uveal metastases. *Ophthalmology.* 1997;104(8): 1265–1276.

Shields JA, Shields CL. Metastatic tumors to the intraocular structures. In: Shields JA, Shields CL. *Intraocular Tumors: An Atlas and Textbook,* 2nd ed. Philadelphia: Lippincott Williams & Wilkins; 2008:198–227.

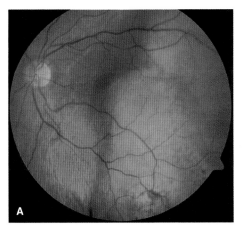 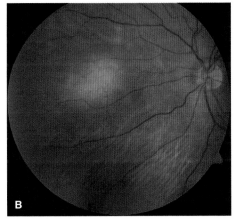

FIGURE 13-8. Choroidal metastases in the left eye of a 57-year-old woman with breast cancer. Mucinous carcinoma of the breast was diagnosed 13 years earlier and was treated with mastectomy and chemotherapy. At the time of these photographs, she also had metastases to the chest wall, skin, lymph nodes, lung, and bone. She received external beam radiation to both eyes in addition to further systemic chemotherapy. **A.** A large, elevated, yellow choroidal lesion involves the macula and temporal retina. There is pigment clumping overlying the lesion inferiorly. **B.** A much smaller, yellow choroidal lesion with subtle elevation involves the nasal retina.

RETINITIS PIGMENTOSA

Ann O. Igbre and Sunir J. Garg

R etinitis pigmentosa (RP) is a group of hereditary retinal disorders character-ized by photoreceptor degeneration. Patients with RP experience progressive visual field loss, night blindness (nyctalopia), and an abnormal electroretinogram (ERG).

Etiology and Epidemiology

- There are more than 85 different genetic types of RP, and more than 45 genes causing RP have been identified.

- RP can be inherited in any number of ways. Roughly 30% to 40% are autosomal dominant, 50% to 60% are autosomal reces-sive, and 10% are X-linked. Approximately 40% of patients with RP have no family his-tory and most of these are thought to be auto-somal recessive.

- The worldwide prevalence of RP is approximately 1 in 4000. Approximately 1 in 100 people are carriers of a gene that can cause RP.

- Most patients are legally blind by the age of 40 due to constriction of the visual field.

Symptoms

- The disease may be mild to very severe. Central visual acuity can also be normal or profoundly impaired.

- Early on, patients experience nyctalopia and trouble with dark adaptation. With time, they develop peripheral field abnormalities that can lead to tunnel vision, and occasion-ally to near total or total blindness.

- Usually divided into two large groups:

  ▪ Primary RP in which the disease pro-cess is confined to the eyes.

  ▪ Syndromic retinitis pigmentosa: Approximately 25% of patients with

RP have associated systemic disease, including:

  ▸ Usher's syndrome: RP with hearing loss and occasionally with vestibular ataxia

  ▸ Bardet-Biedl: RP associated with cognitive difficulties, obesity, hypogeni-talism, polydactyly, and kidney disease

  ▸ Bassen-Kornzweig: RP with abetalipoproteinemia

  ▸ Refsum's disease: RP with phytanic acid oxidase deficiency

Signs (Fig. 13-9)

- The classic fundus findings in RP include arteriolar narrowing, waxy pallor of the disk and variable amounts of bone spicule-like pig-ment changes in the mid and far periphery.

- In RP sine pigmento, in which bone spic-ules are absent, the peripheral retina and RPE appear atrophic.

- Posterior subcapsular cataracts can be present in up to 50% of patients.

- There is also a loss of foveal reflex and irregularity of the vitreoretinal interface.

- CME can occasionally be seen.

- Vitreous cells are also quite common and, when present in conjunction with posterior subcapsular cataracts and CME, can be mis-taken for intermediate or posterior uveitis.

Differential Diagnosis

- Congenital infections: Toxoplasmosis, Other infections, Rubella, Cytomegalovirus infection, Herpes simplex (these make up the TORCH diseases) and syphilis

- Inherited: Choroideremia, gyrate atrophy, Stargardt's disease/fundus flavimaculatus, North Carolina macular dystrophy, Bietti syn-drome, pattern dystrophies, ocular albinism, cystinosis

- Other causes: Cancer-associated retinopa-thy and intermediate uveitis can look like RP.

Previous ophthalmic artery occlusion and retinal drug toxicity should also be considered.

Diagnostic Evaluation

- ERG testing is critical to establish the diagnosis as well as to follow disease progression.

  - Pearl: ERG abnormalities often precede retinal changes and visual complaints.

- Goldmann visual field testing is necessary to assess the degree of visual field impairment.

- Color vision testing can be helpful. Patients with RP often have deficiency in blue cone function (tritanopia).

- Optical coherence tomography can be useful for assessing CME, for measuring retinal thickness, and for evaluating atrophy of the outer retina.

Treatment

- Patients with RP should have regular ophthalmic evaluations every 1 to 2 years with Goldmann visual field testing and ERG evaluation to monitor progression.

- Low-vision aids can also be helpful in patients with subnormal visual fields and reduced night vision.

- Vitamin A palmitate (15,000 IU/day) has been shown to slow the progression of RP by about 20% per year. High doses of vitamin A may be hepatotoxic, so liver function tests should be performed at baseline and every 6 months thereafter. Women should not become pregnant while taking vitamin A.

Patients who have smoked in the past 7 years should not be given supplemental vitamin A.

- Supplemental vitamin E appears to have a deleterious effect and should be avoided.

- Diets high in omega-3 fatty acids (specifically docosahexaenoic acid) may also slow disease progression.

- Supplemental lutein 12 mg daily may also be of benefit.

- Patients with CME may respond to topical or oral carbonic anhydrase inhibitors.

Prognosis

- RP is a slowly progressive disease in which many patients do well for decades. Complete blindness is uncommon and prognosis should be individualized for each patient based on their clinical findings.

REFERENCES

Berson EL, Rosner B, Sandberg MA, et al. Clinical trial of lutein in patients with retinitis pigmentosa receiving vitamin A. *Arch Ophthalmol.* 2010;128(4):403–411.

Berson EL, Rosner B, Sandberg MA, et al. A randomized trial of vitamin A and vitamin E supplementation for retinitis pigmentosa. *Arch Ophthalmol.* 1993; 111:761–772.

Berson EL, Rosner B, Sandberg MA, et al. Further evaluation of docosahexaenoic acid in patients with retinitis pigmentosa receiving vitamin A treatment: subgroup analyses. *Arch Ophthalmol.* 2004;122:1306–1314.

Genead MA, Fishman GA. Efficacy of sustained topical dorzolamide therapy for cystic macular lesions in patients with retinitis pigmentosa and usher syndrome. *Arch Ophthalmol.* 2010;128(9):1146–1150.

Hartong DT, Berson EL, Dryja TP. Retinitis pigmentosa. *Lancet.* 2006;368(9549):1795–1809.

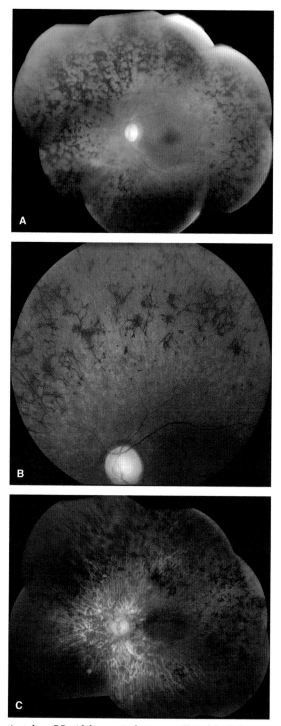

FIGURE 13-9. These patients have RP with bone spicules, waxy pallor of the disk, and attenuated retinal vessels.

OCULAR ISCHEMIC SYNDROME

Ann O. Igbre and Sunir J. Garg

Ocular ischemic syndrome (OIS), also known as venous stasis retinopathy, is due to chronic ocular hypoperfusion and includes a number of clinical findings. Due to variable presentation, it can be a diagnostic challenge. It can cause chronic intraocular inflammation and can occasionally be misdiagnosed as ocular inflammatory disease.

Etiology and Epidemiology

- OIS is almost always a result of severe underlying carotid occlusive disease and less commonly due to other causes of reduced blood flow to the eye or orbit, such as systemic vasculitis. Reduced vascular perfusion results in ocular hypoxia/ischemia, which can also lead to retinal and/or anterior segment neovascularization.

- OIS is associated with a significant risk of both cardiovascular and cerebrovascular mortality. It usually occurs in men with a mean age of 65 years. It is bilateral in 20% of cases.

Symptoms

- Progressive vision loss occurs over several weeks to several months, but may be sudden.

- At presentation, one-third of patients have vision of 20/40 or better and one-third have vision of count fingers or worse.

- Patients often complain of transient visual loss and visual field loss.

- An achy orbital pain due to ocular ischemia or to anterior segment neovascularization.

- Prolonged visual recovery following exposure to bright light.

Signs (Figs. 13-10 and 13-11)

- Anterior segment
  - Dilated conjunctival and episcleral vessels
  - Corneal edema
  - Fixed pupil
  - Anterior chamber cells
  - Advanced cataract
  - Neovascularization of the iris/angle
  - Neovascular glaucoma (but the IOP may only be in the mid-20s)
  - Patients may also have a low intraocular pressure due to ciliary body hypotony.

- Posterior segment
  - Narrowed retinal arteries
  - Dilated but not tortuous retinal veins
  - Midperipheral dot-and-blot retinal hemorrhages
  - Microaneurysms
  - Cotton-wool spots
  - Neovascularization of the disk and/or retina
  - Anterior ischemic optic neuropathy

Differential Diagnosis

- Central retinal vein occlusion
- Giant cell arteritis
- Diabetic retinopathy
- Anterior uveitis
- Hyperviscosity syndromes

Diagnostic Evaluation

- Systemic workup includes carotid artery Doppler testing and angiography (conventional and/or magnetic resonance angiography [MRA] or CT angiography).

- Fluorescein angiography usually demonstrates delayed choroidal filling (normal is less than 5 seconds) and a prolonged arterio-venous transit time. Staining of the retinal vessels also commonly occurs. Fifteen percent of patients have macular edema.

- Digital ophthalmodynamometry (pushing on the eye with the examiner's finger) may demonstrate artery pulsations with minimal pressure. This occurs because the perfusion pressure into the eye is reduced in OIS.

- Pearl: ERG often shows a diminished amplitude of the a- and b-waves as a result of outer and inner layer retinal ischemia.

Treatment

- The aim of management is to prevent further ocular damage as well as to prevent and/or treat systemic co-morbidities.

- Carotid artery stenting and endarterectomy may reduce the risk of a stroke, and may help improve the vision in patients with mild to moderate vision loss.

- Full-scatter panretinal photocoagulation is used to treat eyes with rubeosis, but it may cause regression of visible neovascularization in only one-third of patients. Intravitreal bevacizumab may also be considered for short-term control.

- Ocular hypertension/glaucoma can often be medically managed.

- A referral to a neurovascular specialist is also recommended.

- Patients should also be evaluated and treated for systemic vascular disease such as cardiac ischemia, cerebrovascular ischemia, peripheral vascular ischemia, dyslipidemia, and hypertension.

Prognosis

- As most patients with OIS also have ischemic cardiovascular disease, the 5-year mortality rate is approximately 40% and the majority of the deaths occur secondary to complications of cardiovascular disease.

- Many patients have progressive vision loss. When rubeosis is present, greater than 90% of those eyes are legally blind within a year after diagnosis.

REFERENCES

Brown GC, Magargal LE. The ocular ischemic syndrome. Clinical fluorescein angiographic and carotid angiographic features. *Int Ophthalmol.* 1988;11(4):239–251.

Hazin R, Daoud YJ, Khan F. Ocular ischemic syndrome: recent trends in medical management. *Curr Opin Ophthalmol.* 2009;20(6):430–433.

Malhotra R, Gregory-Evans K. Management of ocular ischaemic syndrome. *Br J Ophthalmol.* 2000; 84(12):1428–1431.

Mendrinos E, Machinis TG, Pournaras CJ. Ocular ischemic syndrome. *Surv Ophthalmol.* 2010;55(1):2–34.

Sivalingam A, Brown GC, Magargal LE, et al. The ocular ischemic syndrome. II. Mortality and systemic morbidity. *Int Ophthalmol.* 1989;13(3):187–191.

Sivalingam A, Brown GC, Magargal LE. The ocular ischemic syndrome. III. Visual prognosis and the effect of treatment. *Int Ophthalmol.* 1991;15(1):15–20.

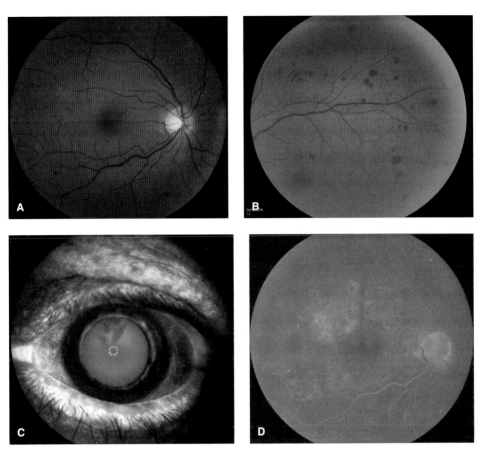

FIGURE 13-10. A 67-year-old man presented with a several-month history of blurry vision and ocular discomfort. **A** and **B.** Fundus exam revealed round retinal hemorrhages typical of OIS. **C.** Anterior segment fluorescein angiography reveals anterior segment neovascularization. **D.** Fluorescein angiography reveals nonspecific leakage.

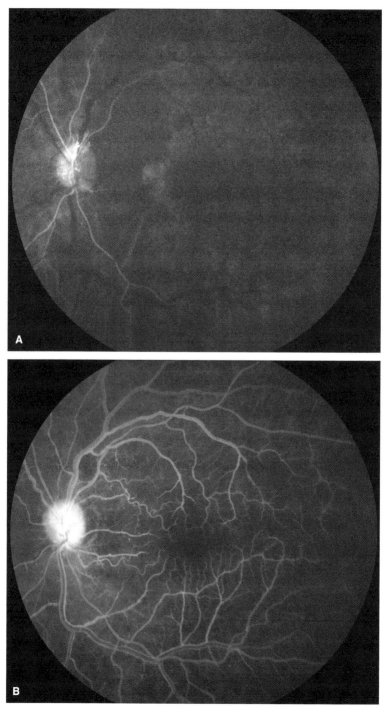

FIGURE 13-11. **A.** Fluorescein angiography at 22 seconds reveals delayed arm to retina time. **B.** At 35 seconds, the venous phase is still not complete. This is typical of OIS.

CANCER-ASSOCIATED RETINOPATHY SYNDROME

John F. Payne and Sunil K. Srivastava

The autoimmune retinopathies, including cancer-associated retinopathy (CAR) and melanoma-associated retinopathy (MAR), are uncommon paraneoplastic processes in which formation of antiretinal antibodies lead to retinal degeneration and vision loss.

Epidemiology and Etiology

- There is no gender predisposition and affected patients are typically older.
- Often patients have a family history of other autoimmune diseases.
- These paraneoplastic autoimmune retinopathies are caused by antibodies produced in response to antigens expressed by the tumor. These antibodies may then cross-react with similar retinal antigens.
- The most commonly identified antigen in CAR is recoverin (a 23-kDa calcium binding protein found in rods and cones). Other autoantibodies associated with CAR include α-enolase, transducin-β, carbonic anhydrase, arrestin, heat-shock protein (HSP) 70, and TULP1.
- Malignancies most often associated with CAR include small cell lung cancer (most common), non–small cell lung cancer, ovarian carcinoma, endometrial carcinoma, uterine carcinoma, breast carcinoma, and prostate carcinoma. Patients with CAR often have vision changes that occur before they have been diagnosed with underlying cancer.
- MAR is thought to be caused by antibodies to the retinal bipolar cells.
- The autoantibodies ultimately lead to apoptosis of the photoreceptors and to retinal degeneration.

Symptoms

- CAR syndrome
  - Patients have bilateral subacute, progressive, vision loss occurring over weeks to months.
  - The eyes may be asymmetrically involved.
  - Patients often note shimmering or flickering lights.
  - Decreased visual acuity, color vision abnormalities, glare, and photosensitivity may also occur. Paracentral scotomas may also occur.
  - Impaired dark-adaptation or night blindness occurs due to damage to the rods.
  - Visual symptoms may precede signs of systemic malignancy by 3 to 12 months.
- MAR syndrome
  - Patients describe acquired night blindness.
  - Similar to patients with CAR, they have photopsias.
  - Although many patients retain good visual acuity and color vision, some patients develop bilateral nonprogressive central scotomas with vision loss.
  - Patients may develop vitiligo (depigmentation) of the skin and uveal tract.
  - In general, most affected patients have a known diagnosis of cutaneous malignant melanoma at the time the ocular symptoms develop.

Signs (Figs. 13-12 and 13-13)

- Early in the disease course, the funduscopic examination may be normal.
- With disease progression, the fundus exam may show arteriole attenuation, mottling of

the retinal pigment epithelium, and optic disk pallor.

- Patients can have CME.
- Anterior chamber and vitreous cells may be seen.

Differential Diagnosis

- Nonneoplastic autoimmune retinopathy
- Retinitis pigmentosa
- Birdshot retinopathy
- Acute zonal occult outer retinopathy
- Multiple evanescent white dot syndrome
- Toxic or ischemic optic neuropathy
- Punctate inner choroiditis
- Intraocular lymphoma or metastasis
- Intermediate uveitis

Diagnostic Evaluation

- CAR syndrome

  ▪ ERG will show a negative waveform with decreased and delayed amplitudes for both rods and cones.

  ▪ Visual field testing may show a ring, central, or paracentral scotoma.

  ▪ Optical coherence tomography (OCT) often shows diffuse retinal atrophy.

  ▪ Western-blot analysis, immunohisto-chemistry, or enzyme-linked immuno-sorbent assay are used to detect antiretinal antibodies. False-negatives are not infrequent, and thus a negative titer does not exclude the diagnosis.

    ▸ Antirecoverin antibodies are most strongly associated with CAR. Antiarrestin antibodies and anti-α-enolase antibodies are helpful in supporting the diagnosis of CAR.

    ▸ Western blot testing can demonstrate multiple antiretinal antibodies.

- In patients with suspected CAR, a thorough systemic workup to look for an underlying malignancy should be performed.

- MAR syndrome

  ▪ ERG typically shows a markedly decreased scotopic b-wave with a normal a-wave. However, the ERG can show reduced a- and b-waves in both scotopic and photopic conditions.

  ▪ Antibodies against retinal bipolar cells may be found using Western-blot analysis, but often are not found.

Treatment

- Immunosuppression may be useful in stabilizing the visual function in some CAR patients. This should be done in consultation with an oncologist, as treatment may have a negative effect on the patient's own tumor immunosurveillance.

- Treatment of primary malignancy has not been shown to improve visual outcomes.

Prognosis

- The visual prognosis tends to be poor.

- The duration of treatment response has been limited by high mortality rates from the underlying malignancies.

REFERENCES

Ferreyra HA, Jayasundera T, Khan NW, et al. Management of autoimmune retinopathies with immunosuppression. *Arch Ophthalmol.* 2009;127(4):390–397.

Keltner JL, Thirkill CE, Yip PT. Clinical and immunologic characteristics of melanoma-associated retinopathy syndrome: eleven new cases and a review of 51 previously published cases. *J Neuro-ophthalmol.* 2001;21(3):173–187.

Khan N, Huang JJ, Foster CS. Cancer associated retinopathy (CAR): an autoimmune-mediated paraneoplastic syndrome. *Semin Ophthalmol.* 2006;21:135–141.

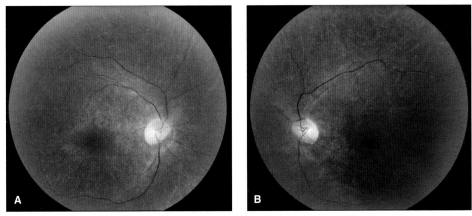

FIGURE 13-12. Color photographs showing attenuated arterioles and mottling of the retinal pigment epithelium in the central macula.

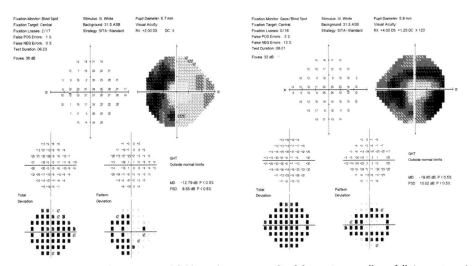

FIGURE 13-13. Humphrey 24-2 visual field test showing generalized depression as well as a full ring scotoma in the right eye and a partial ring scotoma in the left eye.

Treatment of Uveitis

LOCAL THERAPY

Sam S. Dahr

Local therapy of uveitis consists of topical drops, periocular injections, and intravitreal modalities, including injections and implants.

TOPICAL THERAPY

PREDNISOLONE AND DIFLUPREDNATE

- Prednisolone acetate 1% ophthalmic suspension is a commonly used steroid eye drop marketed under the brand names Pred-Forte, Econopred, and Omnipred. Numerous generic formulations are also available.

- Difluprednate ophthalmic emulsion 0.05% (Durezol) is a newer alternative that is currently FDA approved for the treatment of inflammation and pain associated with ocular surgery and is being evaluated for the treatment of uveitis.

- It is thought to be at least as effective as prednisolone acetate 1%, and some evidence suggests that it is approximately twice as effective.

- Unlike prednisolone acetate, which is a suspension, difluprednate does not require shaking, and due to its higher potency, it may allow for a less frequent dosing regimen.

Indication and Dosing

- Topical drops should be used to treat anterior uveitis. It may also be used to treat the *anterior component* of uveitis that also affects the intermediate or posterior compartments. Drops *should not* be used as monotherapy for intermediate uveitis, posterior uveitis, or panuveitis.

- The drops should be dosed according to disease activity and can be used as frequently as every half hour while awake.

- Brand name Pred-Forte is felt to be more effective than generic prednisolone acetate 1%.

- The goal is to eliminate the anterior chamber cell activity whenever possible.

- A common regimen is to taper by 1 drop per week, but tapering should not occur until the eye is inflammation free (if able to be achieved within a reasonable period of time).

Complications and Side Effects

- The main side effects of topical steroids are an elevated intraocular pressure and cataract formation. This risk may be higher with difluprednate.

- Secondary infections, such as reactivated herpetic keratitis, bacterial keratitis, or fungal keratitis are also possible side effects.

- Patients should not use contact lenses while using topical steroid therapy.

CYCLOPLEGICS AND MYDRIATICS

- Cycloplegics and mydriatics such as tropicamide, cyclopentolate, scopolamine, homatropine, and atropine dilate the pupil and can prevent the development of posterior synechiae and may ameliorate pain associated with ciliary body inflammation and spasm.

Indication and Dosing

- It can be used for all cases with significant anterior chamber inflammation or eye pain suggestive of ciliary body spasm.

- Usually shorter acting agents such as tropicamide provide a few hours of dilation followed by subsequent pupillary constriction. Three times a day dosing allows several cycles of dilation and constriction during a 24-hour period; by keeping the pupil moving, posterior synechiae development is reduced.

- Eyes with darker irides or higher levels of inflammation may require stronger/longer acting agents such as scopolamine, homatropine, or atropine, both to facilitate the dilation/constriction cycle and to relieve ciliary pain.

- Some pupillary motility should be encouraged. If the pupil is immobile while dilated, posterior synechiae can still form.

Complications and Side Effects

- These medications are anticholinergics; therefore they may induce dryness of the mouth, facial flushing, headache, and rarely vasomotor or cardiorespiratory disturbances. Patients at risk of such complications may be advised to perform nasolacrimal occlusion for 1 minute after drop instillation.

PERIOCULAR THERAPY

TRIAMCINOLONE

- Triamcinolone acetonide is an injected long-acting steroid suspension, obtained under the brand names Kenalog or Kenalog-40.

- Kenalog has been used for periocular injections in an off-label fashion for decades.

Indication and Dosing

- It is useful for all types of intraocular inflammation: Anterior, intermediate, posterior, and panuveitis, as well as uveitic macular edema.

- Transconjunctival, transdermal, anterior sub-Tenon's, and posterior sub-Tenon's (Nozik style) injection techniques may be used.

- Typically 40 mg (usually in 1 mL) is given, although 20 mg/0.5 mL may be used for an anterior sub-Tenon's injection.

Complications and Side Effects

- The most feared complication is inadvertent ocular penetration.

- Patients may develop ptosis, even after a single injection.

- Septal atrophy with protuberance of the lower eyelid may also occur.

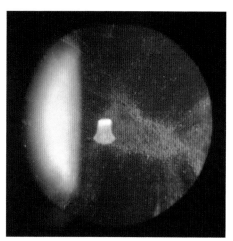

FIGURE 14-1. This patient developed a posterior subcapsular cataract due to both her uveitis and periocular steroid injections. (Courtesy of Julia Monsonego, CRA.)

- Increased intraocular pressure and cataract may occur months or even years later, so patients need to have regular intraocular pressure measurements (**Fig. 14-1**).

- A triamcinolone injection may increase the risk of secondary infections and contact lens use should be discouraged.

- Chorioretinal scars suggestive of previous *Toxoplasma* infection and a positive *Toxoplasma* serum IgG titer are a strong relative contraindication to steroid injection.

INTRAVITREAL THERAPY

TRIAMCINOLONE

- Triamcinolone acetonide is an injectable long-acting steroid suspension.

- Trivaris (Allergan) and Triesence (Alcon) are preservative-free and are FDA-labeled for intraocular use in uveitis and ocular inflammatory conditions.

- Preservative-free triamcinolone can be obtained from some compounding pharmacies.

Indication and Dosing

- It can be used in cases of intermediate, posterior, and panuveitis, as well as in cases of uveitic cystoid macular edema, in cases in which systemic therapy is insufficient and/or contraindicated.

- The traditional dose is 4 mg. However, a lower dose of 1 to 2 mg may be considered, particularly for uveitic macular edema. One mg may also be associated with a lower rate of side effects.

Side Effects

- Patients may develop:
  - True infectious endophthalmitis
  - A paradoxical noninfectious inflammatory response to the drug ("sterile endophthalmitis")
  - A "pseudoendophthalmitis" due to triamcinolone particles settling in the anterior chamber and appearing as a hypopyon

- Increased intraocular pressure and cataract may occur months or years later.

- As with sub-Tenon's steroid injection, when possible, periocular steroid injection should be avoided in eyes with a previous *Toxoplasma* infection and a positive *Toxoplasma* serum IgG titer.

RANIBIZUMAB AND BEVACIZUMAB

- Ranibizumab (Lucentis) and bevacizumab (Avastin) are genetically engineered monoclonal antibodies that bind to and inhibit the biologic activity of human vascular endothelial growth factor (VEGF). Ranibizumab is FDA approved for intraocular injection to treat wet macular degeneration and macular edema associated with retinal vein occlusion. Bevacizumab is FDA approved for IV use for various forms of cancer; the intraocular use of bevacizumab is off label, but its use is well established both in the ophthalmic literature and in clinical practice.

Indication and Dosing

● Anti-VEGF therapy may be used in conjunction with steroid therapy (usually sub-Tenon's or intravitreal triamcinolone) for inflammatory choroidal neovascularization associated with white dot syndromes, sarcoidosis, and other forms of uveitis. It is also useful for peripheral retinal and anterior segment neovascularization.

● While anti-VEGF therapy may be considered for patients with uveitic macular edema unresponsive to steroid and steroid-sparing therapy, any effect tends to be mild and transient, with a need for repeated injections over time. Therefore, anti-VEGF treatment should not be considered first-line therapy for uveitic macular edema.

● The typical dosing is a 0.05-mL injection of either ranibizumab 0.5 mg or bevacizumab 1.25 mg.

Complications and Side Effects

● The standard potential complications of an intravitreal injection apply.

● Rarely, anywhere from days to weeks after an injection, patients may develop a mild inflammatory response with anterior chamber and vitreous cells but without significant vitreous haze.

FLUOCINOLONE IMPLANT (RETISERT)

● The fluocinolone acetonide intravitreal implant is a long-acting implant marketed under the name Retisert. It is inserted through a pars plana incision performed in the operating room (Fig 14-2).

Indication and Dosing

● The FDA label states that the fluocinolone implant is indicated for the treatment of chronic noninfectious uveitis affecting the posterior segment of the eye. In terms of the SUN classification, the implant can be used

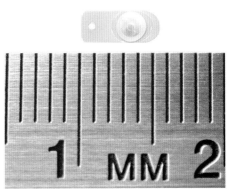

FIGURE 14-2. The Retisert implant. The Retisert implant is surgically placed through the pars plana. The anchoring suture is passed through the hole in the anchoring strut. The drug is released over 30 months. The implant can be left in place, and if needed, a second implant can be place elsewhere in the eye. (Courtesy of Bausch and Lomb.)

to treat significant intermediate, posterior, or panuveitis.

● The fluocinolone implant may be especially useful for unilateral disease or for patients who are intolerant of systemic immunomodulatory therapy. In patients previously on systemic steroid-sparing therapy, the fluocinolone implant does not necessarily eliminate a patient's need for such therapy, but may allow dose reductions during the life of the implant.

● The 0.59-mg implant releases fluocinolone acetonide for approximately 30 months. Another implant can be placed without need for removal of the previous implant.

Side Effects

● The fluocinolone implant shares all the potential complications of a vitreoretinal procedure, including endophthalmitis and hemorrhage.

● In the phase 3 trials, 60% of patients needed intraocular pressure lowering therapy, and at 2 years 32% of patients needed glaucoma filtering surgery. Greater than 90% of phakic eyes needed cataract surgery by 2 years postimplantation.

- Electing to perform fluocinolone implant surgery essentially commits a uveitic eye to at least two surgeries: the implant surgery itself and subsequent cataract surgery. Patients may also need glaucoma surgery and/or implant replacement; thus, over a few-year period, an eye may undergo several surgeries; due to the efficacy of the implant, these subsequent surgeries have a good success rate.

DEXAMETHASONE IMPLANT (OZURDEX)

- The dexamethasone implant (Ozurdex) is a solid polymer drug delivery system containing 0.7 mg of micronized dexamethasone.

- The rod-shaped implant is injected in an office procedure into the vitreous through the pars plana utilizing a 22-gauge single-use injector/applicator. The implant is preservative free and will completely biodegrade over time.

Indication and Dosing

- The dexamethasone (Ozurdex) implant is currently FDA approved for the treatment of noninfectious uveitis affecting the posterior segment of the eye.

- The recent phase 3 trials suggest the peak effect of the drug is achieved around days 60 to 90, and the drug may last up to 6 months in the vitreous.

Side Effects

- The dexamethasone (Ozurdex) implant shares all the potential complications of an intravitreal injection. Elevated intraocular pressure and cataract may occur. The rate of these complications may be less than with intravitreal triamcinolone but longer term studies are needed to assess this.

- Chorioretinal scars suggestive of previous *Toxoplasma* infection and a positive *Toxoplasma* serum IgG titer should be considered a strong relative contraindication to intraocular steroid injection.

METHOTREXATE

- Methotrexate in a preservative-free formulation of 25 mg/mL exists for IV and intrathecal use. This formulation can be injected intravitreally in an off-label fashion.

Indication and Dosing

- Significant literature exists on the use of intraocular methotrexate for lymphoid malignancies of the eye, in particular primary intraocular lymphoma (PIOL). Secondary lymphoid malignancies involving the eye can also be treated with intravitreal methotrexate.

- Intravitreal methotrexate can also be used to treat noninfectious uveitis.

- A single intraocular dose typically ranges from 200 mcg in 0.05 or 0.1 mL to 400 mcg in 0.1 mL. Recent practice tends more toward the 400 mcg dose, for both malignancy and noninfectious uveitis.

- For lymphoma, some practitioners utilize an "induction" phase of 400 mcg twice weekly for a month, followed by "consolidation" of 400 mcg once weekly for 1 to 2 months, followed by "maintenance" of 400 mcg once monthly for 6 to 12 months. A less rigorous initial injection regimen consisting of a weekly injection for a month followed by a monthly injection for a period of time titrated to the clinical exam (e.g., absence of significant cells or infiltrates) can also work well and may minimize surface epitheliopathy (see below).

Side Effects

- The standard potential complications of an intravitreal injection apply.

- The major complication is surface epitheliopathy affecting the cornea, conjunctiva, or both. Patients may develop significant epitheliopathy after only a few injections, and the effect is cumulative. Typically the epitheliopathy will resolve once injections cease, but recovery time is usually proportional to the cumulative number of injections.

RITUXIMAB (RITUXAN)

- Rituximab (Rituxan) is a genetically engineered chimeric murine/human monoclonal antibody against the CD20 antigen and is FDA approved for the systemic treatment of non-Hodgkin's lymphoma, chronic lymphocytic leukemia, and rheumatoid arthritis. Any intraocular use of rituximab is off label.

Indication and Dosing

- A small number of patients with PIOL treated with intravitreal rituximab have been reported in the literature. Indications for intraocular rituximab therapy in the setting of PIOL may include: combination therapy with intravitreal methotrexate in treatment-naïve patients, rescue therapy in patients with recurrence after intravitreal methotrexate or who show resistance to intravitreal methotrexate, or patients who cannot tolerate intravitreal methotrexate secondary to epitheliopathy.
- A suggested dose is 1 mg/0.1 mL. A suggested initial regimen for PIOL is a once-a-week injection for 4 weeks followed by clinical assessment.

Side Effects

- The standard potential complications of an intravitreal injection apply.
- An immunologic reaction to the murine components of the humanized antibody may develop after repeated intraocular rituximab injections and would need to be distinguished from lymphoma-related inflammation.

GANCICLOVIR

- Ganciclovir is a synthetic nucleoside analogue that inhibits replication of herpes viruses. Two forms of ganciclovir local therapy may be utilized:

  - Ganciclovir for intravenous infusion (Cytovene) may be injected into the vitreous in an off-label manner.
  - The ganciclovir implant (Vitrasert) may be surgically implanted into the pars plana.

Indication and Dosing

- Ganciclovir may be injected intravitreally to treat CMV retinitis and other necrotizing herpetic retinopathies such as acute retinal necrosis (ARN) and progressive outer retinal necrosis (PORN).
- The ganciclovir implant is FDA-labeled for the treatment of CMV retinitis in patients with AIDS. The ganciclovir implant may be used in an off-label fashion to treat other necrotizing herpetic retinopathies such as ARN and PORN.
- Ganciclovir is typically injected as 2 mg/0.05 mL.
- Ganciclovir injections may be given in tandem with foscarnet intravitreal injections. The injections may be given two to three times a week in an "induction" phase of 2 weeks followed by a "maintenance" phase of injections one to two times a week as indicated.
- Alternatively, foscarnet injections may be given to supplement the ganciclovir implant.
- The injection dosages may be reduced by half in silicone oil-filled eyes.
- Each ganciclovir implant contains 4.5 mg of ganciclovir, which is released over 5 to 8 months.

Side Effects

- The standard potential complications of an intravitreal injection apply.
- The ganciclovir implant shares all the potential complications of a vitreoretinal procedure.

FOSCARNET

- Foscarnet is a pyrophosphate analog that selectively inhibits virus-specific DNA polymerases, inhibiting the replication of herpes viruses.

Indication and Dosing

- Foscarnet may be injected intravitreally in an off-label fashion to treat CMV retinitis and other necrotizing herpetic retinopathies such as ARN and PORN.

- Intravitreal foscarnet may be used as monotherapy, in combination with systemic antiviral therapy, or in combination with additional local therapy such as ganciclovir injections or the ganciclovir implant.

- Doses of 1.2 mg and 2.4 mg have been utilized, with a trend toward the higher dose.

- The injection may be given two to three times a week in an "induction" phase of 2 weeks followed by a "maintenance" phase of injections one to two times a week as indicated.

Side Effects

- The standard potential complications of an intravitreal injection apply.

CLINDAMYCIN

- Clindamycin is FDA approved for IV and IM use against severe bacterial infections. Case reports and small case series, however, have suggested some efficacy against the *Toxoplasma* parasite.

Indication and Dosing

- Clindamycin may be injected intravitreally in an off-label fashion to treat *Toxoplasma* retinochoroiditis. The injection may be used in combination with systemic therapy or as monotherapy in patients who do not tolerate systemic therapy.

- For ophthalmic use, usually a single dose of 1 mg/0.1 mL is given. The dose may be repeated, however, if needed.

Side Effects

- The standard potential complications of an intravitreal injection apply.

REFERENCES

Callanan DG, Jaffe GJ, Martin DF, et al. Treatment of posterior uveitis with a fluocinolone acetonide implant: three-year clinical trial results. *Arch Ophthalmol.* 2008; 126(9):1191–1201.

Chan CC, Wallace DJ. Intraocular lymphoma: update on diagnosis and management. *Cancer Control.* 2004; 11285–11295.

Itty S, Pulido JS. Rituximab for intraocular lymphoma. *Retina.* 2009;29129–29132.

Lasave AF, Diaz-Llopis M, Muccioli C, et al. Intravitreal clindamycin and dexamethasone for zone 1 toxoplasmic retinochoroiditis at twenty-four months. *Ophthalmology.* 2010;1171831–1171838.

Lowder C, Belfort R, Lightman S, et al. Dexamethasone intravitreal implant for noninfectious intermediate or posterior uveitis. *Arch Ophthalmol.* epub Jan 2011.

Martin DF, Parks DJ, Mellow SD, et al. Treatment of cytomegalovirus retinitis with an intraocular sustained-release ganciclovir implant. A randomized controlled clinical trial. *Arch Ophthalmol.* 1994;1121531–1121539.

SYSTEMIC THERAPY

Theresa Larson and H. Nida Sen

STEROIDS

- Systemic corticosteroids are the mainstay of therapy for uveitis and are effective treatments for both severe anterior uveitis not responsive to topical medication and to vision-threatening posterior uveitis.

- Steroids are typically started at 1 mg/kg/day for up to a month or until the disease is under control, at which point the steroids should be tapered. The prednisone should be tapered gradually, with periodic visits during the tapering process to assess for recurrent inflammation.

- For acute flares of vision-threatening inflammatory diseases such as Behçet's retinitis, treatment with high-dose pulse IV methylprednisolone is indicated.

- Corticosteroids come in different potencies and duration of action. The most commonly used steroids for the treatment of uveitis are prednisone and methylprednisolone (**Table 14-1**). However, systemic corticosteroid use is often limited due to the potentially severe side effects of cushingoid effects, mood changes, diabetes, hypertension, osteoporosis, and fluid retention. In children, steroids suppress the adrenal system and can cause growth retardation.

- Ocular side effects include cataract and glaucoma.

- Patients should be maintained on no more than 10 mg of prednisone daily for long-term disease control. If more than 10 mg of prednisone is needed to achieve quiescence, other steroid-sparing agents should be considered.

IMMUNOSUPPRESSIVE AGENTS

- Often immunosuppressive agents are referred to as corticosteroid-sparing agents or in the rheumatologic literature as disease-modifying antirheumatic drugs. They are indicated when inflammation is not controlled with high doses of prednisone (>60 mg/day), or prednisone doses cannot be tapered below 10 mg, or if side effects from prednisone require discontinuation.

- Several classes of drugs are currently in use in uveitis and are listed below. See **Table 14-2** for their mechanism of action and dosing.

TABLE 14-1. Corticosteroids

Corticosteroid Type	Relative Potency	Duration of Action
Cortisone	0.2	8–12 hours
Hydrocortisone	0.25	8–12 hours
Prednisone*	1	12–36 hours
Prednisolone	1	12–36 hours
Methylprednisolone	1.25	12–36 hours
Triamcinolone	1.25	12–36 hours
Dexamethasone	6.7	36–72 hours
Betamethasone	7.0	36–72 hours

*Prednisone is the most commonly used oral steroid for uveitis in the United States. The potency scale is approximate. For example, 10 mg of prednisone would provide similar efficacy to 40 mg of hydrocortisone.

This contribution to the work was done as part of the authors' official duties as NIH employees and is a work of the United States Government.

TABLE 14-2. Systemic Treatment for Uveitis

Drug	Class	Mechanism of Action	Dosing	Laboratory Monitoring
Prednisone	Glucocorticoid	Multiple mechanisms	1 mg/kg/day	BP, blood glucose
Azathioprine	Antimetabolite	A purine nucleoside analog that interferes with DNA and RNA synthesis	2–2.5 mg/kg/day or 150 mg/day	CMP & CBC
Methotrexate	Antimetabolite	Inhibits dihydrate folate reductase	7.5–25 mg per week given with folic acid	CMP & CBC
Mycophenolate mofetil	Antimetabolite	Inhibits inosine monophosphate dehydrogenase	500–1500 mg b.i.d.	CMP & CBC
Cyclosporine	T cell inhibitor	Calcineurin inhibitor	3–5 mg/kg/day in divided doses	CMP including creatinine
Tacrolimus	T cell inhibitor	Calcineurin inhibitor	0.05 mg/kg/day	CMP including creatinine
Sirolimus	T cell inhibitor	Inhibits mTOR pathway	Loading dose of 6 mg followed by 2 mg/day	Lipid panel
Cyclophosphamide	Alkylating agent	DNA cross-linking	1–3 mg/kg	CBC with differential
Chlorambucil	Alkylating agent	DNA cross-linking	Long term: 0.1–0.2 mg/kg; short term: 2 mg/day for 1 week followed by 2 mg/wk	CBC with differential
Infliximab	Biologic	Anti-TNFα	3–10-mg/kg infusions at 0, 2, 6, 8 weeks and then every 4 to 8 weeks	Hepatitis B & C; latent tuberculosis; CMP & CBC
Adalimumab	Biologic	Anti-TNFα	40-mg subcutaneous injection every 1–2 weeks	Hepatitis B & C; latent tuberculosis; CMP & CBC
Etanercept	Biologic	Anti-TNFα	25-mg subcutaneous injection 1–2 times weekly	Hepatitis B & C; latent tuberculosis; CMP & CBC
Daclizumab	Biologic	Blocks IL-2 receptor (CD25)	1–2 mg/kg every 2–4 weeks	CMP & CBC
Interferon α2a	Biologic	Anti-immunomodulatory effects	3–9 million units once daily to three times a week	CMP & CBC
Rituximab	Biologic	Anti-CD20	1000 mg given twice at 2-week intervals	CMP & CBC

ANTIMETABOLITES

- Antimetabolites refers to a class of drugs which inhibit nucleic acid synthesis and thus inhibit cell proliferation. Drugs commonly used in the treatment of uveitis in this class include methotrexate, azathioprine (Imuran), and mycophenolate mofetil (CellCept).

- The most common side effects of this class include hepatotoxicity, thrombocytopenia and suppression of the white blood cell count, all of which require regular monitoring of liver function tests and complete blood counts.

T-CELL INHIBITORS

- T-cell inhibitors include the commonly used calcineurin inhibitors, cyclosporine and tacrolimus (FK506), as well as rapamycin (Sirolimus), which work through the mammalian target of rapamycin (mTOR) pathway.

- All of these drugs suppress T-cell proliferation.

- Both cyclosporine and tacrolimus need regular laboratory monitoring for possible nephrotoxicity. Cyclosporine often causes hypertension as well. Rapamycin may cause pneumonitis, elevated cholesterol, and diarrhea.

ALKYLATING AGENTS

- Alkylating agents include cyclophosphamide and chlorambucil and work by crosslinking DNA, thus inhibiting DNA transcription and replication.

- They are associated with more severe side effects including thrombocytopenia, leucopenia, increased infection, malignancy, teratogenicity, and sterility. In younger patients, banking sperm and oocytes should

be considered. Cyclophosphamide may also cause hemorrhagic cystitis and subsequent secondary bladder cancer. As a result, use of this class is deferred for severe, sight-threatening uveitis not responsive to other immunosuppressive treatment.

BIOLOGICS

- Biologics represent the newest class of drugs used for the treatment of autoimmune disease. They are designed to modulate the immune response and currently include antibodies and cytokine-based factors.

- Infliximab, adalimumab, and etanercept are all tumor necrosis factor-α inhibitors (TNF-α); daclizumab is a monoclonal antibody to CD25 (the alpha subunit of the IL-2 receptor of T-cells); rituximab is a monoclonal antibody to CD20 on B-cells; and interferon-α (INF-α2a) is a cytokine released in viral infections. Of the TNF-α inhibitors, infliximab and adalimumab are the most efficacious in uveitic diseases.

- Daclizumab is currently limited in supply, rituximab use is not well established, and INF-α2a works best in Behçet's disease.

REFERENCES

Galor A, Perez VL, Hammel JP, et al. Differential effectiveness of etanercept and infliximab in the treatment of ocular inflammation. *Ophthalmology.* 2006; 113:2317–2323.

Jabs DA, Rosenbaum JT. Guidelines for the use of immunosuppressive drugs in patients with ocular inflammatory disorders: recommendations of an expert panel. *Am J Ophthalmol.* 2001;131:492–513.

Jap A, Chee SP. Immunosuppressive therapy for ocular diseases. *Curr Opin Ophthalmol.* 2008;19:535–540.

Kempen JH, Gangaputra S, Daniel E, et al. Long-term risk of malignancy among patients treated with immunosuppressive agents for ocular inflammation: a critical assessment of the evidence. *Am J Ophthalmol.* 2008; 146:802–812.

Index

NOTE: Locators followed by 'f' and 't' refer to figures and tables respectively.

A

Acetaminophen, 179
Acetylsalicylic acid, 170
ACR. *see* American College of
      Rheumatology (ACR)
Active choroiditis, 198f
Active perivasculitis, 101
Acute idiopathic blind spot enlargement
      syndrome (ADIBSES), 132
Acute macular neuroretinopathy
      (AMN), 153, 155–156
Acute-onset postoperative
      endophthalmitis, 238–240,
      240f
  diagnosis, 239
  etiology and epidemiology, 238–239
  prognosis, 240
  symptoms and signs, 239
  treatment, 239–240
Acute posterior multifocal placoid
      pigment epitheliopathy
      (APMPPE), 124–127
  acute multifocal ischemic
      choroidopathy, 124
  diagnosis, 125
  epidemiology and etiology, 124
  ocular histoplasmosis syndrome, 125
  PIC, 125
  prognosis, 125
  RPE, 124
  signs and symptoms, 124–125
  treatment, 125
  VKH disease, 125
Acute retinal necrosis (ARN), 163, 255
  diagnosis, 261
  epidemiology and etiology, 261
  ganciclovir, 305
  prognosis, 262
  signs, 261
  symptoms, 261
  syndrome, 163–168
    blurred vision and floaters, 167f
    clinical characteristics of, 170t
    diagnosis, 164
    epidemiology and etiology, 163
    granulomatous anterior uveitis,
      167f
    nonviral necrotizing retinopathies,
      165t
    peripheral retinal necrosis, 167f
    prognosis, 166
    retinal detachment, 168f
    signs, 164
    treatment, 164–166, 166t

  treatment, 261–262
  VZV, 163
Acute retinal pigment epitheliitis,
      159–162, 161–162
  diagnosis, 159
  etiology and epidemiology, 159
  prognosis, 160
  signs, 159
  symptoms, 159
  treatment, 159
Acute zonal occult outer retinopathy
      (AZOOR), 132
  blind spot and photopsias, 154f
  diagnosis, 153
  epidemiology and etiology, 153
  prognosis, 154
  signs, 153
  symptoms, 153
  treatment, 154
Adalimumab, 48, 309
Adaptive immunity, 1
ADIBSES. *see* Acute idiopathic blind
      spot enlargement syndrome
      (ADIBSES)
AIDS-related eye disease
  acute retinal necrosis,
      261–262
  CMV retinitis, 255–259
  fungal retinitis, 265–266
  HIV retinopathy, 253–254
  IRU, 260
  KS, 268–269
  PC choroiditis, 267
  PORN, 263–264
Albendazole, 221
Alkylating agents, 309
American College of Rheumatology
      (ACR), 122
American Uveitis Society (AUS), 59,
      76, 261
Amikacin, 239, 240, 242, 243, 244,
      246
AMN. *see* Acute macular
      neuroretinopathy (AMN)
Amphotericin B, 250
ANA. *see* Antinuclear antibodies
      (ANA)
ANCA. *see* Antineutrophil cytoplasmic
      antibody (ANCA)
Angiotensin converting enzyme (ACE),
      37
Ankylosing spondylitis, 36
  right ankle arthritis, 38f
Anterior uveitis

FUS, 43–45
  diagnosis, 44
  epidemiology, 43
  etiology and pathogenesis, 43
  prognosis, 44
  signs, 43–44
  symptoms, 43
  treatment, 44
HLA B27, 35–40
  etiology and epidemiology, 35
  seronegative
      spondyloarthropathies,
      36–37
  signs, 36
  symptoms, 35
JIA, 46–50
  diagnosis, 47
  epidemiology and etiology, 46
    risk factors in children, 46t
    schedule for screening in
      Children, 46t
  prognosis, 48–49
  signs, 46–47
  symptoms, 46
  treatment, 47–48
    anti-TNF-α therapy, 48
    DMARD, 47
    periocular steroid injections,
      48
    topical corticosteroids, 47
PSS, 41–42
  ancillary tests, 41
  diagnosis, 41
  epidemiology, 41
  etiology, 41
  prognosis, 42
  signs, 41
  symptoms, 41
  treatment, 42
  white keratic precipitates, 41,
      42f
TINU, 51–52
  diagnosis, 51
  etiology and epidemiology,
      51
  prognosis, 52
  signs, 51
  symptoms, 51
  treatment, 52
Antibodies, 3–4
Anti-citrullinated cyclic protein (CCP),
      15
Antihistamines, 230
Antimetabolites, 309

Antineutrophil cytoplasmic antibody
    (ANCA), 82
Antinuclear antibodies (ANA), 82
Antinuclear antibodies (ANA +), 46
Antiphospholipid syndrome
    choroidal infarction, 95
    deep vein thrombosis, 95
    diagnosis, 97
    etiology and epidemiology, 95
    pathophysiology of, 96f
    prognosis, 98
    recurrent fetal loss, 95
    signs, 95–97
    symptoms, 95
    systemic manifestations of, 96t
    treatment, 97–98
        algorithm for management, 100f
Anti-SS-A and B antibodies, 82
Anti–vascular endothelial growth
        factor (VEGF) therapy,
        129, 303
APMPPE. *see* Acute posterior
        multifocal placoid
        pigment epitheliopathy
        (APMPPE)
ARN. *see* Acute retinal necrosis (ARN)
Aspirin, 109
Atovaquone, 205
AUS. *see* American Uveitis Society
        (AUS)
Auxiliary cells, 3
Avastin. *see* Ranibizumab and
        bevacizumab
Azathioprine, 32, 48, 61, 76, 105, 115,
        120, 123, 129, 136
AZOOR. *see* Acute zonal occult outer
        retinopathy (AZOOR)

B

Band keratopathy, 37, 48, 59
    in child, 49f
BARN. *see* Bilateral acute retinal
        necrosis (BARN)
Bartonella henselae, 212
Basophils and mast cells, 3
B Cells (Bursa), 3–4
BD. *see* Behçet's disease (BD)
Behçet's disease (BD), 51
    diagnosis, 85–86
    diagnostic criteria for, 87t
    epidemiology and etiology, 85
    oral ulcer, 90f
    prognosis, 86
    retinal vasculitis
        ischemia and, 88f
        macular retinitis and, 88f
        retinal hemorrhages, 90f
        sclerotic vessels with, 89f
    signs and symptoms, 85
    treatment, 86

Bilateral acute retinal necrosis (BARN),
        163
Bilateral microphthalmos, 175f
Bilateral posterior capsular cataract,
        175f
Birdshot chorioretinopathy
    CME, 152f
    diagnosis, 149, 150
    epidemiology and etiology, 149
    prognosis, 150–151
    signs and symptoms, 149
    treatment, 150
Bisphosphonates, 273
Blood urea nitrogen (BUN) levels,
        51
Bone marrow transplantation and CMV
        retinitis, 257f
Borrelia afzelii, 188
Borrelia burgdorferi, 188
Bowel disease, inflammatory, 60
Brimonidine, 277
Bullous central serous
        chorioretinopathy, 76

C

Calcineurin inhibitors, 309
Cancer-associated retinopathy
        syndrome, 297–299
Candidemia and vitreous snowballs,
        248f
Candle-wax drippings, 68, 69f
c-antineutrophil cytoplasmic antibody
        (c-ANCA), 105
Caspofungin, 250
Cataract, 175f
    phacoantigenic
        corneal edema, 55f
        diagnosis, 54
        etiology and epidemiology, 53
        intraocular lens implantation,
            55f
        prognosis, 54
        signs and symptoms, 53
        treatment, 54
    surgery, 56–58
Cat-scratch disease (CSD)
    diagnosis, 212–213, 213
    etiology and epidemiology, 212
    optic disk edema and chorioretinitis,
        215f
    Parinaud's oculoglandular syndrome,
        216f
    prognosis, 213
    signs and symptoms, 212
    stellate neuroretinitis, 214f
    treatment, 213
Ceftazidime, 239
Ceftriaxone, 244
Cervical lymphadenopathy, 108
Chemokines, 5

Chikungunya, 179–180
Chlorambucil, 32
Chloroquine, 179
Chorioretinitis pattern, 252f
Choroidal infarction, 95
Choroidal neovascularization (CNV),
        128
Choroidal tubercle, 197f
Choroidal tumors, 19
Chronic vitritis, 255
Cidofovir, 256, 272
Ciliochoroidal effusion, 104
Clindamycin, 205, 306
CME. *see* Cystoid macular edema
        (CME)
CMV retinitis. *see* Cytomegalovirus
        (CMV) retinitis
CNV. *see* Choroidal neovascularization
        (CNV)
Complement system, 5
Congenital rubella syndrome
        (CRS)
    bilateral microphthalmos, 175f
    bilateral posterior capsular cataract,
        175f
    cataract, 175f
    cornea clouding, 174f
    corneal scarring and buphthalmos,
        175f
    diagnosis, 172–173, 173
    etiology and epidemiology, 172
    leukocoria due to cataract, 174f
    prognosis, 173
    signs and symptoms, 172
    treatment, 173
Conjunctivitis, 104
Cornea
    clouding, 174f
    degeneration, 32
    edema, 53, 55f
    melt, 32
    scarring and buphthalmos, 175f
Coronary artery aneurysms, 108
Corticosteroids, 67, 114–115, 120, 129,
        136, 170, 179, 307t
    cycloplegic and topical, 183
    sparing immunosuppressive agents,
        73
CRS. *see* Congenital rubella syndrome
        (CRS)
CSD. *see* Cat-scratch disease (CSD)
Cutaneous calcification, 121f
Cyclophosphamide, 105, 129, 309
Cycloplegics and mydriatics, 301
Cyclosporine, 48, 76, 150, 309
Cyclosporine A, 32, 129
Cystoid macular edema (CME), 37,
        48, 56, 59, 63f, 101, 135,
        209, 255
Cytokines and cytokine receptors, 5

Cytomegalovirus (CMV) retinitis, 163, 258–259
  bone marrow transplantation and, 257f
  cidofovir, 272
  diagnosis, 255
  epidemiology and etiology, 255
  prognosis, 256
  signs and symptoms, 255
  treatment, 255–256
Cytovene. *see* Ganciclovir

D

Daclizumab, 150, 308, 309
Dacryocystitis and dacryoadenitis, 181
DEC. *see* Diethylcarbamazine citrate (DEC)
Deep vein thrombosis, 95
Delayed-onset (chronic) postoperative endophthalmitis, 242f
  diagnosis, 241
  etiology and epidemiology, 241
  prognosis, 242
  symptoms and signs, 241
  treatment, 241–242
Dendritic keratitis, 24, 25f
Dermatomyositis and polymyositis
  cutaneous calcification, 121f
  diagnosis, 119
  etiology and epidemiology, 119
  Gottron rash, 119
  heliotrope rash and edema, 121f
  prognosis, 120
  scarring and pigmentation, 120f
  signs and symptoms, 119
  telangiectasis of upper eyelid skin, 121f
  treatment, 120
Dexamethasone, 239, 242, 244
  implant, 304
Diethylcarbamazine citrate (DEC), 230
Diffuse unilateral subacute necrosis (DUSN), 153
Diffuse unilateral subacute neuroretinitis, 222f, 223f
  diagnosis, 220–221, 221
  etiology and epidemiology, 220
  prognosis, 221
  symptoms and signs, 220
  treatment, 221
Disciform stromal keratitis, 24, 25f
Disease-modifying antirheumatic drugs (DMARD), 47, 82
DMARD. *see* Disease-modifying antirheumatic drugs (DMARD)
Doxycycline, 189, 213, 226
Drug-induced nephritis, 51

DUSN. *see* Diffuse unilateral subacute necrosis (DUSN)

E

Eales' disease
  active perivasculitis, 101
  cystoid macular edema, 101
  diagnosis, 101
  etiology and epidemiology, 101
  prognosis, 102
  retinal detachment, 101
  retinal ischemia, 101
  signs and symptoms, 101
  treatment, 101–102
ELISA testing, 189, 209, 213
Endogenous endophthalmitis
  candidemia and vitreous snowballs, 248f
  diagnosis, 245–246
  etiology and epidemiology, 245
  infected foot wound, 247f
  intense vitreous inflammation, 248f
  multifocal posterior, 247f
  prognosis, 246
  symptoms and signs, 245
  treatment, 246
Endogenous fungal endophthalmitis
  Aspergillus fumigatus -associated, 251f
  Candida albicans-associated chorioretinitis, 251f
  chorioretinitis pattern, 252f
  diagnosis, 250
  epidemiology, 249
  etiology and pathogenesis, 249
  prognosis, 250
  subretinal hemorrhage, 252f
  symptoms and signs, 249
  treatment, 250
  vitreous abscesses, 251f
Endophthalmitis
  postoperative
    acute-onset, 238–240
    delayed-onset (chronic), 241–242
    endogenous, 245–248
    endogenous fungal, 249–252
    filtering bleb-associated, 243–244
Endophthalmitis Vitrectomy Study (EVS), 230, 241
Eosinophils, 3
Epiretinal membrane (ERM), 135
Episcleritis, 92, 104
  bisphosphonates, 273
  diagnosis, 13–14
  etiology and epidemiology, 13
  prognosis, 14
  signs, 13, 14f
  symptoms, 13
  treatment, 14

ERM. *see* Epiretinal membrane (ERM)
Erythema, 108
Erythromycin, 189
Etanercept, 48, 309
Ethambutol, 195
EVS. *see* Endophthalmitis Vitrectomy Study (EVS)

F

Familial exudative vitreoretinopathy (FEVR), 209
Fascicular keratitis, 21
FEVR. *see* Familial exudative vitreoretinopathy (FEVR)
Filtering bleb-associated endophthalmitis
  diagnosis, 243
  etiology and epidemiology, 243
  symptoms and signs, 243
  treatment, 243–244
Floaters, 43
Fluorescent treponema antibody-absorption (FTAAbs), 182
Fomivirsen, 256
Foscarnet, 256, 306
Frosted branch angiitis, 255
Fuchs' heterochromic iridocyclitis. *see* Fuchs' uveitis syndrome (FUS)
Fuchs' uveitis syndrome (FUS), 43–45
Fungal retinitis, 265–266
FUS. *see* Fuchs' uveitis syndrome (FUS)

G

Ganciclovir, 170, 256, 305
Glaucoma, 48, 53, 61
Glomerulonephritis, 104
Gottron rash, 119
Granulomatous uveitis, 27f
  anterior, 194

H

HAART. *see* Highly active antiretroviral therapy (HAART)
Hansen's disease, 200
Hansen uveitis. *see* Leprosy
Heliotrope rash and edema, 121f
Hemorrhagic cystitis, 105
Herpes zoster ophthalmicus, 26
  lipid and fibrotic keratopathy, 27f
Herpetic keratouveitis
  herpes simplex virus
    dendritic keratitis, 24, 25f
    diagnosis, 24
    disciform stromal keratitis, 24, 25f

etiology and epidemiology, 24
oral acyclovir, 25
prognosis, 25
signs, 24
symptoms, 24
tarsorrhaphy, 25
treatment, 24–25
varicella zoster virus
cycloplegic agents, 27
diagnosis, 26
etiology and epidemiology, 26
granulomatous uveitis, 27f
Hutchinson's sign, 26
Heterochromia, 41, 43, 45f
Highly active antiretroviral therapy
(HAART), 170, 253
Hilar lymphadenopathy, 196f
HIV retinopathy
epidemiology and etiology, 253
prognosis, 253
signs, 253
symptoms, 253
treatment, 253
see also ELISA testing
HLA B27, 35–40
Human leukocyte antigen (HLA), 4,
5, 46, 128
Hutchinson's teeth, 182
Hypersensitivity reactions, 5–6
Hyphema, 44, 56, 58f, 285, 288
Hypotony, 37

I

IBD. see Inflammatory bowel disease
(IBD)
Ibuprofen, 109
ICGA. see Indocyanine green
angiography (ICGA)
Immune recovery uveitis (IRU), 260
Immune response
adaptive immunity, 1
building blocks of
cytokines and cytokine receptors, 5
leukocytes, 2–3
lymphocytes, 3–4
MHC molecules, 2, 3
complement system, 5
hypersensitivity reactions, 5–6
immunity and eye, 6
innate immunity, 1
Immunity and eye, 6
Immunoglobulins. see Antibodies
Immunomodulatory therapy (IMT),
136
Immunosuppressive agents, 307
IMT. see Immunomodulatory therapy
(IMT)
Inactive uveitis, 11
Indocyanine green angiography
(ICGA), 125

Infectious endophthalmitis, 56, 57
Inflammatory bowel disease (IBD), 36
Infliximab, 111
Innate immunity, 1
Interferons, 5
Interferon-α (INF-α2a), 309
Interleukins, 5
Intermediate uveitis
diagnosis, 60
lymphoma, 60, 64f
epidemiology and etiology, 59
evaluation, 60
prognosis, 61
signs, 59
RetCam photos, 62f
snowballs and snowbank, 62f, 63f
symptoms, 59
treatment, 60–61
International Uveitis Study Group
(IUSG) criteria, 7
Intraocular lenses (IOL), 173
implantation, 55f
Intraocular pressure (IOP), 41
Intraocular tuberculosis
active choroiditis, 198f
choroidal tubercle, 197f
diagnosis, 194–195
epidemiology and etiology, 194
hilar lymphadenopathy, 196f
intermediate uveitis with CME, 196f
Koeppe nodules and posterior
synechiae, 195f
prognosis, 195
retinal vasculitis choroiditis, 199f
signs and symptoms, 194
treatment, 195
Intravenous gamma globulin, 109
Intravitreal amphotericin B, 242, 250,
265
Intravitreal triamcinolone acetonide, 61
IOL. see Intraocular lenses (IOL)
IOP. see Intraocular pressure (IOP)
Iridocyclitis, 26
Iris synechiae, 37
Iritis, 91, 224, 278
IRU. see Immune recovery uveitis (IRU)
Ischemic optic neuropathy, 171
Ivermectin, 225, 230

J

Jarisch-Herxheimer reaction, 183
JIA. see Juvenile idiopathic arthritis (JIA)
Juvenile idiopathic arthritis (JIA),
46–50

K

Kaposi's sarcoma (KS), 268–269
Kawasaki's disease
diagnosis, 108–109

etiology and epidemiology,
108
prognosis, 109
signs, 108
symptoms, 108
treatment, 109
Kenalog. see Triamcinolone
Keratic precipitates (KP), 43, 45f, 47,
53, 55f, 56, 204
Keratitis, 82
Keratoconjunctivitis sicca, 81, 91, 92,
95, 114
Keratoderma blennorrhagicum,
36
Koeppe nodules, 44
and posterior synechiae, 195f
KP. see Keratic precipitates (KP)
KS. see Kaposi's sarcoma (KS)

L

Lamellar or penetrating keratoplasty,
33
Large granular lymphocytes, 4
Laser flare photometry (LFP), 47
Lens-induced uveitis
corneal injury, 58f
diagnosis, 56–57
etiology and epidemiology, 56
hyphema, 56, 58f
iris transillumination defects, 58f
prognosis, 57
signs, 56
symptoms, 56
treatment, 57
Leprosy, 203
conjunctival lepromas, 202f
diagnosis, 200
diffuse scleritis, 202f
etiology and epidemiology, 200
Madarosis, 201f
pinna deformity, 201f
prognosis, 201
signs, 200
symptoms, 200
tissue loss in lepromatous, 202f
treatment, 200–201
tropic ulcers and finger deformation,
202f
Leptospirosis
diagnosis, 191
etiology and epidemiology, 191
leptospiral uveitis, 192f
prognosis, 192
signs, 191
symptoms, 191
treatment, 192
Leukocytes, 2–3
Lipid and fibrotic keratopathy,
27f
Loa loa filariasis, 229

Loiasis, 231f
  diagnosis, 229
  etiology and epidemiology, 229
  signs and symptoms, 229
  treatment, 230
Low-grade endophthalmitis, 54
Lucentis. *see* Ranibizumab and
      bevacizumab
Lyme disease, 76
  diagnosis, 188, 189
  etiology and epidemiology, 188
  intermediate uveitis, 189f
  prognosis, 189
  retinal venules, 189f
  signs, 188
  symptoms, 188
  treatment, 189
Lyme titers, 60
Lymphocytes, 3–4

M

MAC. *see* Mycobacterium avium
      complex (MAC)
Macrophages, 3
Maculopapular rash, 224
Maculopathy, 47
Major histocompatibility complex
      (MHC) molecules, 5
Mammalian target of rapamycin
      (mTOR) pathway, 309
Mango fly, 229
Mantoux skin test, 194
Marginal keratitis, 32
Masquerade syndromes, 19
  cancer-associated retinopathy
        syndrome, 297–299
  metastatic cancer, 288–289
  OIS, 293–296
  PIOL, 279–284
  retinitis pigmentosa, 290–292
  retinoblastoma, 285–287
MAT. *see* Microscopic agglutination test
      (MAT)
Metastatic cancer, 288–289
Methotrexate, 47, 61, 105, 136, 304
Metipranolol, 276
MEWDS. *see* Multiple evanescent white
      dot syndrome (MEWDS)
MFCP. *see* Multifocal choroiditis
      and panuveitis syndrome
      (MFCP)
Microscopic agglutination test (MAT),
      191
Mononuclear phagocytes, 3
Mooren's ulcer
  clinical spectrum of, 29f
  diagnosis, 28
  epidemiology and etiology, 28
  infectious keratitis, 28
  ocular rosacea, 28

peripheral ulcerative keratopathy,
        28
  prognosis, 29
  signs, 28
  symptoms, 28
  Terrien's marginal degeneration, 28
  treatment, 28–29
Mucous plaque keratopathy, 26
Multibacillary leprosy, 201
Multifocal choroiditis and panuveitis
        syndrome (MFCP),
        135–140
  birdshot retinochoroidopathy, 135
  CME, 135
  diagnosis, 135–136, 136
  epidemiology and etiology, 135
  multiple choroidal lesions, 135
  multiple creamy lesions, 137f–138f
  ocular histoplasmosis, 135
  prognosis, 136–137
  punctate inner choroidopathy, 135
  signs, 135
  with subfoveal CNV, 139f
  with subretinal fibrosis, 140f
  symptoms, 135
  treatment, 136
  vitreous haze, 135
Multiple evanescent white dot
        syndrome (MEWDS),
        132–133
  diagnosis, 132
  epidemiology and etiology, 132
  prognosis, 133
  signs, 132
  symptoms, 132
  treatment, 132–133
Multiple sclerosis (MS), 60
Mycobacterium avium complex
      (MAC), 270
Mycobacterium leprae, 200
Mycobacterium tuberculosis, 194
Mycophenolate mofetil, 48, 61, 76, 120,
      129, 136

N

Natural killer (NK) cell, 4
Necrotizing retinopathies, 163
Necrotizing scleritis, 104
Neovascularization and vitreous
      hemorrhage, 261
Niclosamide, 232–233
Nodular scleritis, 82

O

Ocular cysticercosis
  diagnosis, 232
  etiology and epidemiology, 232
  intracranial cysticercosis, 234f
  prognosis, 233

scolex, 234f
  subretinal cysticercosis, 233f
  symptoms and signs, 232
  treatment, 232–233
Ocular histoplasmosis syndrome
      (OHS), 125, 135, 145–146
  diagnosis, 145
  "histo spots," 145
  prognosis, 146
  signs and symptoms, 145
  treatment, 145
Ocular ischemic syndrome (OIS),
      293–296
Ocular lymphoma, 76, 85
Ocular toxocariasis
  diagnosis, 209
  epidemiology and etiology, 208
  prognosis, 209
  retinal detachment and hyperechoic
        subretinal granuloma, 210f
  signs, 208–209
  subretinal granuloma with central
        scar formation, 211f
  symptoms, 208
  treatment, 209
  vitritis and, 210f
Ocular toxoplasmosis
  congenital, 207f
  diagnosis, 204–205
  etiology and epidemiology, 204
  Kyrieleis plaques, 207f
  prognosis, 205–206
  recurrence of, 206f
  retinochoroiditis with vasculitis,
        206f
  signs, 204
  symptoms, 204
  treatment, 205
OHS. *see* Ocular histoplasmosis
      syndrome (OHS)
OIS. *see* Ocular ischemic syndrome
      (OIS)
Oncho-C27 antigen, 225
Onchocerciasis, 228f
  atrophic inguinal skin, 227f
  diagnosis, 225
  etiology and epidemiology, 224
  keratitis, 226f
  "leopard-spot" pattern of skin
        depigmentation, 227f
Opsonization, 5
Optical coherence tomography (OCT),
      47, 60
Optic disk edema and chorioretinitis,
      215f
Optic neuritis, 19
Oral acyclovir, 25, 179
Oral amoxicillin, 189
Oral cefixime, 218
Oral corticosteroids, 230

Oral dapsone, 235
Oral fluconazole and voriconazole, 250
Oral prednisone, 101
Orbital inflammation/pseudotumor, 91
Ozurdex. *see* Dexamethasone, implant

P

PAN. *see* Polyarteritis nodosa (PAN)
Parinaud's oculoglandular syndrome, 216f
Pars plana vitrectomy (PPV), 101, 238
Pars planitis, 60
   snowballs and snowbank of, 62
Paucibacillary leprosy, 200–201
PCNSL. *see* Primary CNS lymphoma (PCNSL)
Pellucid marginal degeneration, 32
Penicillin allergy, 189
Penicillin G sodium, 182
Periarteritis nodosa, 122
Peripheral ulcerative keratitis (PUK), 104
   corneal melt, 32, 34f
   diagnosis, 32
   etiology, 31
   Mooren's ulcer and, 31
   pathophysiology, 31
   prognosis, 33
   signs, 32
   symptoms, 31
   treatment, 32–33
Peripheral vascular sheathing, 59
Persistent hyperplastic primary vitreous (PHPV), 209
Phacolytic uveitis, 53–55
   see also Cataract
Phagocytes, 2–3, 2f
Pharyngeal edema, 108
Phlyctenular keratoconjunctivitis, 21–22
Phlyctenulosis, 21, 22f, 32
PHPV. *see* Persistent hyperplastic primary vitreous (PHPV)
Phthisis bulbi, 54
PIC. *see* Punctuate inner choroidopathy (PIC)
PIOL. *see* Primary intraocular lymphoma (PIOL)
Plaque psoriasis, 40f
Plasmapheresis, 123
Platelets, 3
Pneumocystis carinii (PC) choroiditis, 267
Polyarteritis nodosa (PAN)
   diagnosis, 122–123
   etiology and epidemiology, 122
   prognosis, 123
   scleritis with scleromalacia, 123f
   sclerokeratitis, 123f

signs, 122
symptoms, 122
treatment, 123
Polymorphonuclear neutrophils (PMN), 2–3
PORN. *see* Progressive outer retinal necrosis (PORN)
Posner-schlossman syndrome (PSS), 41–42
Posterior scleritis, 76
Posterior synechiae, 56
Posterior uveitis and collagen vascular diseases, 65–123
PPV. *see* Pars plana vitrectomy (PPV)
Praziquantel, 232–233
Pred-Forte. *see* Prednisolone and difluprednate
Prednisolone and difluprednate, 300–301
Prednisone, 76, 82, 111, 114, 129
Primary CNS lymphoma (PCNSL), 279
Primary intraocular lymphoma (PIOL), 304
   diagnosis, 280
   epidemiology and etiology, 279
   prognosis, 280
   signs, 279–280
   symptoms, 279
   treatment, 280
Primary retinal lymphoma (PRL), 279
PRL. *see* Primary retinal lymphoma (PRL)
Prognosis, 226
Progressive outer retinal necrosis (PORN), 163, 169–171, 255, 264
   clinical characteristics of, 170t
   diagnosis, 169, 263
   epidemiology and etiology, 169, 263
   medical treatment of, 169–170, 263
   prognosis, 170–171, 263
   retinal necrosis, 171f
   retina thickness, 171f
   signs, 169, 263
   symptoms, 169, 263
   treatment, 169–170, 170t, 263
   VZV-associated, 171f
Prophylactic argon laser retinopexy, 170
Propionibacterium acnes, 56
Proptosis, 104
Prostaglandin analogues, 278
Pseudo-subconjunctival hemorrhage, 269f
Psoriatic arthritis, 36–37
PUK. *see* Peripheral ulcerative keratitis (PUK)
Punctate keratitis, 226f

Punctuate inner choroidopathy (PIC), 125, 141–144
   diagnosis, 141–142
   epidemiology and etiology, 141
   inactive scars band secondary CNV, 143f
   prognosis, 142
   signs, 141
   subfoveal CNV, 143f
   symptoms, 141
   treatment, 142
   unilateral, 144f
Purified protein derivative (PPD) test, 6, 60

Q

Quantiferon-TB gold test (QFT-G), 60, 194

R

Ranibizumab and bevacizumab, 302–303
Rapamycin, 309
Rapid plasmin reagin (RPR), 182
Reactive arthritis syndrome, 36
Recurrent glaucomatocyclitic crisis syndrome, 41
Reiter's syndrome. *see* Reactive arthritis syndrome
Relapsing polychondritis
   auricular edema, 112f, 113f
   diagnosis, 110
   epiglott itis, 110
   etiology and epidemiology, 110
   laryngotracheal- bronchial stricture, 110
   nasal inflammation, 110
   prognosis, 111
   "saddle-nose" deformity, 113f
   signs, 110
   symptoms, 110
   treatment, 111
   voice hoarseness, 110
Renal biopsy, 51
Retinal detachments, 101, 256
Retinal hemorrhage, 91
Retinal ischemia, 101
Retinal S-antigen, 149
Retinal vascular occlusions, 104
Retinal vasculitis, 91, 92
   choroiditis, 199f
Retinal venous occlusive disease, 91
Retinitis, 183
   pigmentosa, 290–292
Retinoblastoma, 285–287
Retisert. *see* Fluocinolone acetonide implant
Rhegmatogenous retinal detachment, 19, 61

Rhegmatogenous retinal detachments (RRD), 255
Rheumatoid arthritis (RA), 51
   ocular complications of
      diagnosis, 81, 82
      diffuse anterior scleritis, 81
      diffuse scleritis, 83f
      epidemiology and etiology, 81
      episcleritis, 81
      keratoconjunctivitis sicca, 81
      nodular scleritis, 83f
      peripheral ulcerative keratitis, 81, 83f
      prognosis, 82
      signs, 81
      symptoms, 81
      treatment, 82
      uveal prolapse, 83f
      vasculitis of skin, 84f
Rheumatoid factor (RF), 82
Rhinosporidosis
   conjunctival polyp, 236f
   conjunctival rhinosporidiosis, 236f
   diagnosis, 235
   etiology and epidemiology, 235
   prognosis, 235
   scleral ectasia, 237f
   signs and symptoms, 235
   treatment, 235
   uveal prolapse, 237f
Rifabutin, 270–271
Rituximab, 105, 120, 305, 309
Rosacea keratitis, 32
RPR. see Rapid plasmin reagin (RPR)
RRD. see Rhegmatogenous retinal detachments (RRD)
Rubella, 172–175

S

Salt and pepper retinopathy, 172
Sarcoidosis, 6, 37, 41, 47, 51, 60, 65–67, 76
Sarcoidosis-associated uveitis
   Blau syndrome and juvenile idiopathic arthritis in children, 66
   candle-wax drippings, 68f, 69f
   choroidal granulomas, 66
   diagnosis, 66–67
   diagnostic criteria for ocular, 67t
   epidemiology and etiology, 65–66
   Heerfordt's syndrome, 66
   lacrimal gland enlargement, 66
   multifocal choroiditis, 66
   multiple skin nodules, 70f
   mutton fat keratic precipitates, 66, 69f
   optic neuritis, 66
   primary intraocular lymphoma, 66
   prognosis, 67
   signs, 66

snowballs, snowbanking, 66, 70f
subconjunctival granulomas, 66
sympathetic ophthalmia, 66
symptoms, 66
syphilis, 66
tent-shaped peripheral anterior synechiae, 66
treatment, 67
tuberculosis, 66
vitreous cells and haze, 66
Vogt-Koyanagi-Harada (VKH) syndrome, 66
Scleritis, 82, 104
   anterior, 91
      diagnosis, 15–16
      etiology and epidemiology, 15
      necrotizing scleritis, 18f
      nodular scleritis and peripheral ulcerative keratitis, 18f
      prognosis, 16
      rheumatoid arthritis and, 18f
      signs, 15
      symptoms, 15
      systemic disease associations, 16t
      treatment, 16
   clinical subtypes and prevalence, 15t
   phlectenulosis
      diagnosis, 21
      etiology and epidemiology, 21
      prognosis, 21–23
      signs, 21
      symptoms, 21
      treatment, 21
   posterior, 20f
      diagnosis, 19
      etiology and epidemiology, 19
      fluorescein angiogram, 19, 20f
      prognosis, 19
      signs, 19
      symptoms, 19
      treatment, 19
      T-sign on B-scan ultrasound, 19, 20f
Scleroderma
   classic features of, 115f
   diagnosis, 114
   "en coup de sabre," 114
   etiology and epidemiology, 114
   facial skin creases and tight skin, loss of, 116f
   ischemic digital ulcer, 118f
   mild scleritis and nasal corneal ulcer, 117f
   prognosis, 115
   sclerodactyly, 117f
   signs, 114
   symptoms, 114
   telangiectasis of eyelids, 114
   treatment, 114–115
Scopolamine, 27

Sector iris stromal atrophy, 26
Septicemic phase, 191
Seronegative spondyloarthritis, 39f
Serous retinal detachment, 91
Serpiginous chorioretinopathy, 128–131
   choroiditis, 130f, 131f
   diagnosis, 129
   diferential diagnosis, 128–129
   epidemiology and etiology, 128
   prognosis, 129
   signs, 128
   symptoms, 128
   treatment, 129
Serpiginous choroiditis, 128, 194
Sjögren syndrome, 51
SJS. see Stevens-Johnson syndrome (SJS)
Spiramycin, 205
Standardization of Uveitis Nomenclature (SUN), 7
Stellate keratic precipitates, 27f
Stellate neuroretinitis, 214f
Steroids, 307
   sparing agents, 123
   sparing immunomodulatory agents, 150
Steroid-sparing systemic immunosuppression, 61
Stevens-Johnson syndrome (SJS), 274, 274f, 275f
Subretinal fibrosis, 135
Sulfadiazine, 205
Sulfonamides, 274–275
Sympathetic ophthalmia, 6, 54, 92
   bullous serous retinal detachment, 74f
   cerebrospinal fluid pleocytosis, 72
   choroidal neovascularization, 72
   chronic retinal detachment and choroidal thickening, 73f
   Dalen-Fuchs nodules, 72, 74f
   diagnosis, 72
   etiology and epidemiology, 72
   intraocular lymphoma, 72
   iris thickening and synechiae, 72
   optic atrophy, 72
   phthisis, 72
   phthisis bulbi, 73f
   prognosis, 73
   sarcoidosis, 72
   signs, 72
   symptoms, 72
   syphilis, 72
   treatment, 73
   tuberculosis, 72
   VKH, 72
Syphilis, 76
   acute syphilitic posterior placoid chorioretinitis, 185f
   angular stomatitis, 186f
   bilateral decreased vision, 186f–187f
   diagnosis, 182

etiology and epidemiology, 181
interstitial keratitis, 183f
prognosis, 183
"salt and pepper" chorioretinitis, 184f
signs, 181–182
symptoms, 181
treatment, 182–183
uveitis associated, 184f
Systemic lupus erythematosus
anterior scleritis, 91, 93f
arthritis, 91
diagnosis, 92
discoid rash, 91
etiology and epidemiology, 91
keratoconjunctivitis sicca, 91
Malar rash, 91, 93f
oral ulcers, 91
prognosis, 92
serositis, 91
signs, 91
symptoms, 91
treatment, 92
Systemic lupus erythematosus (SLE), 51

T

Taciolimus, 120
Tacrolimus (FK506), 76, 309
TASS. *see* Toxic anterior segment
syndrome (TASS)
TB-SLC. *see* Tuberculous serpiginous-
like choroiditis (TB-SLC)
T-cell inhibitors, 309
T-cell receptors (TCR), 4
T cells (Thymus), 4
Telangiectasis of upper eyelid skin, 121f
TEN. *see* Toxic epidermal necrolysis
(TEN)
Terrien's marginal ulceration, 32
TINU. *see* Tubulointerstitial nephritis and
uveitis syndrome (TINU)
Toxic anterior segment syndrome
(TASS), 239
Toxic epidermal necrolysis (TEN), 274
Toxocara canis, 208
Toxocariasis titers, 60
Toxoplasma gondii, 204
Toxoplasma retinochoroiditis, 169
Toxoplasmosis, 255
Trachomatous pannus, 32
Transforming growth factor beta
(TGF-β), 6
Treponema pallidum, 181, 182
Triamcinolone, 82, 301–302
Triesence, 302
Trimethoprim-sulfamethoxazole, 205
Trivaris, 302
Tropheryma whipplei, 217
Tuberculin skin test, 194
Tuberculous serpiginous-like
choroiditis (TB-SLC), 128

Tubulointerstitial nephritis and uveitis
syndrome (TINU), 51–52
Tumor necrosis factors, 5

U

Unilateral acute idiopathic maculopathy
diagnosis, 157
etiology and epidemiology, 157
prognosis, 158
signs and symptoms, 157
treatment, 157
Urinalysis, 51
Uveal effusion, 91
Uveal effusion syndrome, 19
Uveal metastasis, 76
Uveitis
anatomic classification of, 12
differential diagnosis of , 8t–9t
National Eye Institute grading
scheme, 10t
SUN classification, 7
SUN working group, 8t, 10t
Vitreous haze grading, 11f
drug-induced
bisphosphonates, 273
brimonidine, 277
cidofovir, 272
metipranolol, 276
prostaglandin analogues, 278
rifabutin, 270–271
sulfonamides, 274–275
infectious posterior
acute retinal necrosis syndrome,
163–168
chikungunya, 179–180
congenital rubella syndrome,
172–175
CSD, 212–216
DUSN, 220–223
intraocular tuberculosis, 194–199
leprosy, 200–203
leptospirosis, 191–193
loiasis, 229–231
Lyme disease, 188–190
ocular cysticercosis, 232–234
ocular toxocariasis, 208–211
ocular toxoplasmosis, 204–207
onchocerciasis, 224–228
progressive outer retinal necrosis,
169–171
rhinosporidosis, 235–237
syphilis, 181–187
west nile virus, 176–178
Whipple's disease, 217–219
Uveitis, treatment of
intravitreal therapy
clindamycin, 306
dexamethasone implant, 304
fluocinolone implant, 303
foscarnet, 306

ganciclovir, 305
methotrexate, 304–305
ranibizumab and bevacizumab,
302–303
retisert implant, 303f
rituximab, 305
triamcinolone, 301
periocular therapy
triamcinolone, 302
systemic therapy, 308t
alkylating agents, 309
antimetabolites, 309
biologics, 309
immunosuppressive agents, 307
steroids, 307
T-cell inhibitors, 309
topical therapy
cycloplegics and mydriatics, 301
prednisolone and difluprednate,
300–301
Uveitis-glaucomahyphema (UGH)
syndrome, 56

V

Valgancyclovir, 256
Vancomycin, 239–240, 242, 243, 244, 246
Varicella zoster virus (VZV), 163
Vascular endothelial growth factor
(VEGF), 302
Vasculitis, 122
Vaso-occlusive retinopathy, 91
VDRL. *see* Venereal Disease Research
Laboratory (VDRL)
VEGF. *see* Vascular endothelial growth
factor (VEGF)
Venereal Disease Research Laboratory
(VDRL), 182
Venous stasis retinopathy, 293
Vernal keratoconjunctivitis, 32
Visceral larva migrans (VLM), 208
Vitiliginous chorioretinitis. *see* Birdshot
chorioretinopathy
Vitreous abscesses, 251f
Vitritis, 56
VLM. *see* Visceral larva migrans (VLM)
Vogt-Koyanagi-Harada syndrome,
19, 91
AUS criteria for diagnosis of, 80t
choroidal melanocytes, loss of, 80f
diagnosis, 76
epidemiology and etiology, 76
prognosis, 77
serous retinal detachment, 79f, 80f
and choroiditis, 79f
signs, 76
skin depigmentation, 78f
subretinal fibrosis, 80f
treatment, 76
Voriconazole, 242, 250
VZV. *see* Varicella zoster virus (VZV)

W

Wegener's granulomatosis, 6, 32
  CT scan of sinuses, 106f
  diagnosis, 104–105, 105
  etiology and epidemiology, 104
  gingivitis in gums, 107f
  inferior and posterior globe
      displacement, 106f
  peripheral choroidal mass,
      106f
  prognosis, 105
  scleritis, 106f
  signs, 104
  symptoms, 104
  treatment, 105
Wegener syndrome, 51
Weil's syndrome, 191

West Nile virus
  atrophic chorioretinal lesions, 177f
  diagnosis, 176–177
  etiology and epidemiology, 176
  inactive chorioretinal lesions, 178f
  prognosis, 177
  signs, 176
  symptoms, 176
  treatment, 177
Whipple's disease
  chronic posterior uveitis, 219f
  diagnosis, 217–218, 218
  epidemiology, 217
  etiology, 217
  periodic acid-Schiff positive
      macrophage inclusions, 219f
  prognosis, 218

  signs and symptoms, 217
  treatment, 218
White Dot syndromes
  acute retinal pigment epitheliitis,
      159–162
  AMN, 155–156
  APMPPE, 124–127
  AZOOR, 153–154
  birdshot chorioretinopathy, 149–152
  MEWDS, 132–133
  MFCP, 135–140
  OHS, 145–146
  PIC, 141–144
  serpiginous chorioretinopathy,
      128–131
  unilateral acute idiopathic
      maculopathy, 157–158